SIDE-EFFECTS OF ANTI-INFLAMMATORY DRUGS

SIDE-EFFECTS OF ANTI-INFLAMMATORY DRUGS

PART ONE
CLINICAL AND EPIDEMIOLOGICAL ASPECTS

EDITED BY

K. D. Rainsford
Department of Pharmacology
University of Cambridge, and
Strangeways Research
Laboratory, Cambridge UK

G. P. Velo
Institute of Pharmacology
University of Verona, Verona
Italy

Proceedings of the 2nd International Meeting on the Side-effects of Anti-inflammatory Analgesic Drugs held at Cambridge, England, 31st July - 2nd August, 1985

MTP PRESS LIMITED
a member of the KLUWER ACADEMIC PUBLISHERS GROUP
LANCASTER / BOSTON / THE HAGUE / DORDRECHT

Published in the UK and Europe by
MTP Press Limited
Falcon House
Lancaster, England

British Library Cataloguing in Publication Data

International Meeting on the Side-Effects of
Anti-Inflammatory Drugs (2nd :
1985 : Cambridge)
Side-effects of anti-inflammatory drugs :
proceedings of the 2nd International Meeting
on the Side-effects of Anti-Inflammatory
Analgesic Drugs, held at Cambridge, 31st
July - 2nd August 1985.
Vol. 1 : Clinical and epidemiological aspects
1. Anti-inflammatory agents--side-effects
I. Title II. Rainsford, K.D. III. Velo, G.P
615'.7042 RM405

ISBN 978-94-010-9774-1 ISBN 978-94-010-9772-7 (eBook)
DOI 10.1007/978-94-010-9772-7

Published in the USA by
MTP Press
A division of Kluwer Academic Publishers
101 Philip Drive
Norwell, MA 02061, USA

Library of Congress Cataloging-in-Publication Data

International Meeting on the Side-effects of
Anti-inflammatory Analgesic Drugs (2nd :
1985 : Cambridge, Cambridgeshire)
Side-effects of anti-inflammatory drugs.

Contents: v. 1. Clinical and epidemiological
aspects -- v. 2. Studies in major organ systems.
Includes bibliographies and index.
1. Anti-inflammatory agents--Side-effects--
Congresses. I. Rainsford, K.D., 1941- .
II. Velo, G.P. (Giampaolo) II. Title.
[DNLM: 1. Analgesics, Anti-inflammatory--adverse
effects--congresses. 2. Anti-Inflammatory Agents--
adverse effects--congresses. W3 IN7612 2nd 1985s /
QV 247 I612 1985s]

RM405.I58 1985 615'.77 86-27805
ISBN 978-94-010-9774-1

Frome and London

Part 1 Table of Contents

PART 1 TABLE OF CONTENTS

Part 2 Table of Contents

SECTION III GASTROINTESTINAL TRACT (EXPERIMENTAL ASPECTS)

PART 2 TABLE OF CONTENTS

PART 2 TABLE OF CONTENTS

Preface

These two volumes contain the proceedings of a 3 day international meeting held at the University of Cambidge and Queens' College Cambridge from 31st July to 2nd August 1985 on the Side-Effects of Anti-Inflammatory Analgesic Drugs. The first meeting was held in Verona, (Italy) in 1982 and the organisers felt that, with a number of recent developments including the withdrawal of a number of new anti-inflammatory drugs, and concern being expressed in the lay and specialist medical press and other media about the safety of these drugs, that it was appropriate to have a second such meeting.

The meeting was attended by some 300 delegates and the discussion focussed most intently on the recent issues, e.g. the value of adverse drug reaction reporting of the non-steroidal anti-inflammatory (NSAI) drugs, certain side-effects associated with particular NSAI drugs, the predictive value of animal models etc.

Organising a meeting de novo without outside help would not have been possible without the immensely valuable help given enthusiastically by people and financial assistance given most generously by those pharmaceutical companies listed below. These financial contributions were given despite current economic difficulties and moves to restrict the proportion of profits towards educational activities. Also, the topics relating to the side-effects of drugs are not exactly those which would naturally attract commercial interest, yet the open donations shown by those listed companies and participation by scientists from industry in the meeting are in fact a reflection of the genuine interest and concern being shown by industry in the current problems from drug usage and in development of procedures and education in preventing the untoward side effects from the anti-inflammatory drugs.

We would like to record the help given by those people who gave much time and energy in the preparation, advice and running of the meeting, among these being: Mrs Veronica Rainsford, Mrs Janet Eastwell, Mrs Vanessa Woodward, Mr George Archer, Mr David Bennett, Dr Brian Callingham, (all of University of Cambridge), Mr Joe Kerridge and staff at A. H. Robins Co. Ltd.,

Horsham, U.K. (for assistance with advertising and printing), members of the technical and secretarial staff of the Department of Pharmacology, University of Cambridge, and Mr Lee Bollam and staff of Queens' College Cambridge. We thank Professor A. W. Cuthbert FRS, for allowing the use of facilities in the Department of Pharmacology, University of Cambridge, and for his generous encouragement of this meeting. We also thank members of the Scientific Advisory Committee comprising:

Dr W Dawson, Lilly Research Centre Ltd., Windlesham.
Dr B L Hazleman, Addenbrooke's Hospital, Cambridge.
Professor D V Parke, University of Surrey, Guildford
Professor M J H Smith, King's College Hospital School of Medicine and Dentistry, London
Dr J C P Weber, Medicines Division, Department of Health & Social Security, London

as well as the section chairmen for their help and valuable advice.

Our thanks go to the contributors to these volumes who provided much valued efforts and were patient in the unforeseen delays which occurred as a result of the decision to change publishers. This decision was necessary because there would have been a further years delay if we had progressed with the original publisher. We do, however, thank Dr Peter Clarke, Mr Martin Lister and their staff at MTP for all their efforts in trying to ensure rapid publication subsequent upon the above decision.

The papers in this book have been organized into approximately the same order as they were presented at the conference. For the sake of completeness we have included summaries of the brief reports of some poster presentations in the relevant sections. The discussion was recorded and later transcribed from tape and in some four cases the comments were unclear or otherwise unsatisfactory for publication. Much effort has gone into accurate presentation of the valuable comments and questions which were recorded, but in some cases it has not been possible to attribute comments (hence these are simply recorded as "Anonymous") or in the case of that following the Experimental Gastroenterology section were not recorded because of technical difficulties. In the main, however, most of the discussion has been successfully recorded and carefully edited for the sake of accuracy and cogency. We hope the reader will glean at least some of the liveliness of the discussion that formed an essential part of the success which was apparent of this meeting.

We wish to thank the following companies for their generous financial support towards the cost of the meeting:

A.H. Robins Co. Ltd. (U.K.)
Wyeth Laboratories Inc. (U.S.A.)
Pfizer International Inc. (U.S.A.)
Ciba-Geigy Ltd. (U.K.)
Hoechst A.G. (F.R.G.)
Merrell-Dow Pharmaceuticals Ltd. (U.K.)
Schering A.G. (F.R.G.)
Lederle Laboratories (U.K.)

Lepetit S.p.A. (Italy)
Rorer Italiana S.p.A (Italy)
F. Hoffman-La Roche & Co. (Switzerland)
Squibb S.p.A. (Italy)
Glaxo Holdings p.l.c. (U.K.)
Glaxo S.p.A. (Italy)
A. Natterman & Cie G.m.b.H. (F.R.G.)
Merck Sharp & Dohme Ltd. (U.K.)
Stuart Pharmaceutical-I.C.I.Americas (U.S.A.)
Lilly Research Centre Ltd. (U.K.)
Cilag S.p.A. (Italy)
De Angeli (Italy)
Upjohn Ltd. (U.K.)
E. Merck (U.K.)
American Cynamid (U.S.A.)
Roche Products Ltd. (U.K.)
Syntex Pharmaceuticals (U.K.)

The Editors

List of Contributors

S Adami
Istituto di Semeiotica e Nefrologia
Medica dell'Università di Verona
Verona
Italy

BF Allam
Department of Biochemistry
Stobhill General Hospital
Glasgow G21 3UW
UK

E Arosio
Istituto di Farmacologia
Clinica Medica
University of Verona
Verona
Italy

PH Bach
Robens Institute of Industrial and Environmental Health and Safety
University of Surrey
Guildford
Surrey GU2 5XH
UK

PA Bacon
Department of Rheumatology
University of Birmingham
Birmingham
UK

P Ballanti
Dipartimento di Biopatologia Umana
dell'Università "La Sapienza" di Rome
Rome
Italy

EF Barker
Anti-Inflammatory Drug Group
Department of Health and Human Services
Public Health Service
Rockville, MD 20857
USA

A Baumgartner
Gastrointestinal Unit
Inselspital
University of Berne
Berne
Switzerland

H Beck
Department of Pharmacological and Toxicological Research
Heumann-Pharma
D-8500 Nürnberg
Federal Republic of Germany

R Behrens
Department of Gastroenterology
Addenbrooke's Hospital
Hills Road
Cambridge CB2 2QD
UK

N Bellamy
University of Western Ontario
London, Ontario
N6A 3K7
Canada

G Benoni
Istituto de Farmacologia
University of Verona
Verona
Italy

A Bennett
Department of Surgery
King's College School of Medicine and Dentistry
The Rayne Institute
123 Coldharbour Lane
London SE5 9NU
UK

U Bergman
Department of Clinical Pharmacology
Karolinska Institutet
Huddinge Hospital
Huddinge
Sweden

E Bonnucci
Dipartimento di Biopatologia Umana
dell'Università "La Sapienza" di Roma
Rome
Italy

J Bourgouin
McMaster University
Hamilton
Ontario
L85 4L8
Canada

EJS Boyd
Department of Therapeutics
University of Dundee
KGW Ninewells Hospital
Dundee DD1 9SY
UK

C Bracq
Blood Bank
Hôpital Henri Mondor
Université Paris-Val de Maine
Creteil
France

J Braun
Institute for Nephrology
University of Erlangen-Nürnberg
D-8500 Nürnberg
Federal Republic of Germany

PM Brooks
Department of Medicine
University of Sydney
Sydney
New South Wales
Australia

K Brune
Dept of Pharmacology and Toxicology
University of Erlangen-Nürnberg
D-8520 Erlangen
Federal Republic of Germany

A Buchanan
McMaster University
Hamilton
Ontario
L85 4L8
Canada

G Caille
McMaster University
Hamilton
Ontario
L85 4L8
Canada

J Caldwell
Department of Pharmacology
St Mary's Hospital Medical School
London W2 1PG
UK

J Calvin
Department of Clinical Pathology
M.R.C., Dunn Clinical Nutrition Centre,
Trumpington Street
Cambridge CB2 2QD
UK

MG Capuzzo
Istituto di Farmacologia
Clinica Medica
University of Verona
Verona
Italy

GJ Carroll
Department of Rheumatic Diseases
Royal Perth Hospital
Perth, W.A.
Australia

J Ceuppens
Division of Rheumatology
Department of Medicine
University of Leuven
B-3041 Pellenberg
Belgium

G Ciabattoni
Department of Pharmacology
Catholic University School of Medicine
00168 Rome
Italy

GA Cinotti
Division of Nephrology
Department of Medicine
University of Rome
La Sapienza
00100 Rome
Italy

D StJ Collier
Department of Surgery
Addenbrooke's Hospital
Hills Road
Cambridge
UK

PO Collins
Department of Surgery
King's College School of Medicine and Dentistry
The Rayne Institute
123 Coldharbour Lane
London SE5 9NU
UK

G Cove
Istituto di Farmacologia
Clinica Medica
University of Verona
Verona
Italy

NL Cox
Royal Hants County Hospital
Winchester
Hants
UK

K Crowshaw
Director of Scientific Relations
Ono Pharmaceutical Comapny
London Office
St. Alphage House
2 Fore Street
London EC2Y 5DA
UK

L Cuzzolin
Institute of Pharmacology
University of Verona
Verona
Italy

PF D'Arcy
Department of Pharmacy
The Queens University of Belfast
Medical Biology Centre
Lisburn Road
Belfast BT9 7BL
UK

J Debeugher
Department of Rheumatology and Physical Medicine
Hôpital Universitaire St Pierre
322 rue Haute
B-1000 Bruxelles
Belgium

L De Clerck
Division of Rheumatology
Department of Internal Medicine
University of Leuven
B-3041 Pallenberg
Belgium

C Della Rocca
Dipartimento di Biopatologia Umana
dell'Università "La Sapienza" di Roma
Rome
Italy

LIST OF CONTRIBUTORS

P Del Soldato
Pierrel S.p.A.
via Bisceglie 96
Milan
Italy

CW Denko
Case Western Reserve
University and Fairview
General Hospital
Cleveland OH 44111
USA

J Dequeker
Division of Rheumatology
Department of Internal
Medicine
University of Leuven
B-3041 Pellenberg
Belgium

M Deveraux
Department of Rheumatology
Addenbrooke's Hospital
Hills Road
Cambridge CB2 2QD
UK

SM Doherty
Hull Royal Infirmary
Humberside
UK

KW Dreyling
Department of Experimental
Clinical Medicine
Ruhr-University of Bochum
D-4630 Bochum
Federal Republic of Germany

BP Ekholm
Riker Laboratories
St Paul
Minnesota
USA

E Ekman
Department of Drugs
National Board of Health
and Welfare
Uppsala
Sweden

H Engler
Department of
Pharmacological &
Toxicological Research
Heumann Pharma
D-8500 Nürnberg
Federal Republic of Germany

E Ezer
Pharmacological Research
Centre
Chemical Works of Gideon
Richter Ltd
Budapest H-1475
Hungary

JP Famaey
Department of Rheumatology
and Physical Medicine
Hôpital Universitaire St.
Pierre
322 rue Haute
B-1000 Bruxelles
Belgium

M Farr
Department of Rheumatology
University of Birmingham
Edgbaston
Birmingham
UK

MS Feldman
Robens Institute of
Industrial and
Environmental Health and
Safety
University of Surrey
Guildford
Surrey GU2 5XH
UK

KH Fok
Department of
Gastroenterology
Whittington Hospital
Highgate Hill
London N19
UK

J Fontaine
Laboratory of Pharmacology
Hôpital Universitaire St
Pierre
322 rue Haute
B-1000 Bruxelles
Belgium

D Foschi
Institute of Biomedical
Science
University of Milan
Milan
Italy

L Frost
Department of Surgery
University of Lund
Malmö General Hospital
Malmö
Sweden

B Fuller
Academic Department of
Surgery
Royal Free Hospital
London
UK

A Garner
Bioscience Department
ICI Pharmaceutical Division
Alderley Park
Macclesfield
Cheshire SK10 4TG
UK

J Gauthier
McMaster University
Hamilton
Ontario
L85 4L8
Canada

M Geldmacher von Mallinckrodt
Institute for Legal
Medicine of the University
of Erlangen-Nürnberg
D-8520 Erlangen
Federal Republic of Germany

PJM George
Department of
Gastroenterology
Whittington Hospital
Highgate Hill
London N19
UK

U Gessler
Institute of Nephrology
University of Erlangen-
Nürnberg
D-8500 Nürnberg
Federal Republic of Germany

SC Gilman
Department of Experimental
Therapeutics
Wyeth Laboratories, Inc
PO Box 8299
Philadelphia, PA 19101
USA

M Giordano
Medical Clinic
1st Faculty of Medicine
University of Naples
Naples
Italy

AJ Gordon
Pfizer International Inc.
235 East 42 Street
New York
USA

S Gotzkowsky
Clinical Research Center
New Orleans
Louisiana
USA

C Green
Division of Comparative
Medicine
Clinical Research Centre
Northwick Park Hospital
Harrow
Middlesex
UK

G Guarrera
Istituto di Semeiotica e
Nefrologia Medica
dell'Università di Verona
Verona
Italy

HA Guess
Merck Sharp and Dohme
Research Laboratories
West Point, PA 19486
USA

J-C Guillaume
Department of Dermatology
Hôpital Henri Mondor
Université Paris-Val de
Maine
Creteil
France

K Gyires
Semmelweis University of
Medicine
Department of Pharmacology
Budapest 1445
Nagyvarad ter 4
Hungary

U Haglund
Dept of Surgery
General Hospital
S-214 01 Mälmo
Sweden

F Halter
Gastrointestinal Unit
Inselspital
University of Berne
Berne
Switzerland

RC Hamdy
Department of Clinical
Gerontology
St John's Hospital
London SW11
UK

BL Hazleman
Rheumatology Department
Addenbrooke's Hospital
Hills Road
Cambridge CB2 2QD
UK

G Healing
Division of Comparative
Medicine
Clinical Research Centre
Northwick Park Hospital
Harrow
Middlesex

ML Heide
Riker Laboratories
St Paul
Minnesota
USA

D Helston
Department of Health
Regina
Saskatchewan
S4S 6X6
Canada

M Hemmerlein
Carl Korth Institute for
Cardiovascular Research
Division of Clinical
Pharmacology
D-8520 Erlangen
Federal Republic of Germany

H Hopf
Institute for Legal
Medicine of the University
Erlangen-Nürnberg
D-8520 Erlangen
Federal Republic of Germany

U Hoppe
Department of Pharmacology
Ruhr University of Bochum
D-4630 Bochum
Federal Republic of Germany

JRS Hoult
Department of Pharmacology
King's College
Strand
London WC2R 2LS
UK

H Howard Lock
McMaster University
Hamilton
Ontario
L85 4L8
Canada

HM Høyeraal
Pediatric Division
Oslo Sanitetsforening
Rheumatism Hospital
Oslo
Norway

AM Huther
Pharmacological Research
A Natterman & Cie, GmbH
PO Box 350120
D-5000 Cologne 30
Federal Republic of Germany

AJ Hutt
Department of Pharmacy
Brighton Polytechnic
Moulsecoomb
Brighton
West Sussex
UK

B Imbimbo
Istituto di Semeiotica e
Nefrologia
Medica dell'Università di
Verona
Verona
Italy

RGD Improta
Medical Clinic
1st Faculty of Medicine
University of Naples
Naples
Italy

WHW Inman
Drug Surveillance Research
Unit
University of Southampton
North Croft House
Botley
Southampton SO3 2BX
UK

G Janning
Department of Nephrology
Georg-August-Universität
D-3400 Göttingen
Federal Republic of Germany

LIST OF CONTRIBUTORS

H Jick
Boston Collaborative Drug Surveillance Program
Boston University Medical Center
Boston
Massachusetts
USA

ME Jones
Human Morphology
Flinders University of South Australia
Adelaide, S.A.
Australia

RA Jones
Research Division
The North East Wales Institute
Deeside
Clwyd CH5 4BR
UK

E Käss
Oslo Sanitetsforening
Rheumatism Hospital
Oslo
Norway

WF Kean
Rheumatic Disease Unit
McMaster University
Hamilton
Ontario
L85 4L8
Canada

A Kleine
Department of Experimental Clinical Medicine
Ruhr University of Bochum
D-4630 Bochum
Federal Republic of Germany

J Knoll
Semmelweis University of Medicine
Department of Pharmacology
Budapest 1445
Nagyvarad ter 4
Hungary

HR Koelz
Gastrointestinal Unit
Inselspital
University of Berne
Berne
Switzerland

SJ Konturek
Institute of Physiology
31-531 Krakow ul
Grzegorzecka 16
Poland

R Koob
Carl Korth Institute for Cardiovascular Research
Division of Clinical Pharmacology
D-8520 Erlangen
Federal Republic of Germany

W Kozuschek
Department of Surgery
Clinic Langendreer
Ruhr-University of Bochum
D-4630 Bochum
Federal Republic of Germany

I Krakau
Carl Korth Institute for Cardiovascular Research
Division of Pharmacology
D-8520 Erlangen
Federal Republic of Germany

DC Kvam
Riker Laboratories
St Paul
MN
USA

TK Kvien
Department of Rheumatology
Diakonhjemmet Hospital
PO Box 23 Vinderen
N-0319 Oslo 3
Norway

N Kwiecien
Institute of Physiology
Academy of Medicine
31-531 Krakow, ul,
Grzegorzecka 16
Poland

PP Lamy
Department of Epidemiology and Preventive Medicine
University of Maryland at Baltimore
Baltimore, MD 21201
USA

E Lang
Carl Korth Institute for Cardiovascular Research
Division of Clinical Pharmacology
D-8520 Erlangen
Federal Republic of Germany

MJS Langman
University Department of Therapeutics
Queens Medical Centre
Nottingham NG7 2UH
UK

A Lechi
Istituto di Farmacologia
Clinica Medica
University of Verona
Verona
Italy

J Leggate
Department of Biochemistry
Stobhill General Hospital
Glasgow G21 3UW
UK

M Levy
Clinical Pharmacology Unit
Department of Medicine A
Hadassah University Hospital
Jerusalem
Israel

AJ Lewis
Department of Experimental Therapeutics
Wyeth Laboratories, Inc.
PO Box 8299
Philadelphia, PA 19101
USA

S Leyck
Pharmacological Research
A Nattermann & Cie, GmbH
PO Box 350120
D-5000 Cologne 30
Federal Republic of Germany

V LoCascio
Istituto di Semeiotica e Nefrologia Medica
dell'Università "La Sapienza" di Verona
Verona
Italy

CJL Lock
McMaster University
Hamilton
Ontario
L85 4L8
Canada

J Lunec
Department of Biochemistry
Selly Oak Hospital
Birmingham B29 6JD
UK

F Luyten
Department of Rheumatology
Ghent University Hospital
Ghent
Belgium

E Lydick
Merck Sharp & Dohme
Research Laboratories
West Point
PA 19486
USA

WH Lyle
Courtaulds plc
Medical Department
18 Hanover Square
London
UK

B McConkey
Dudley Road Hospital
Birmingham B18 7QH
UK

JC McElnay
Department of Pharmacy
The Queen's University of
Belfast
Medical Biology Centre
Lisburn Road
Belfast BT9 7BL
UK

PE McGill
Rheumatic Diseases Unit
Stobhill General Hospital
Glasgow G21 3UW
UK

FG McMahon
Clinical Research Center
New Orleans
Louisiana
USA

E McNiven
McMaster University
Hamilton
Ontario
L85 4L8
Canada

PJ Meffin
Department of Clinical
Pharmacology
Flinders University of
South Australia
Adelaide, S.A.
Australia

S Migliaresi
Medical Clinic
1st Faculty of Medicine
University of Naples
Naples
Italy

H Mielants
Department of Rheumatology
University Hospital
Ghent
Belgium

K Miller
Immunotoxicology Department
The British Industrial
Biological Research
Association
Woodmansterne Road
Carshalton
Surrey
UK

P Minuz
Istituto di Farmacologia
University of Verona
Verona
Italy

J Morley
Preclinical Research
Sandoz Ltd
CH-4002 Basle
Switzerland

B Murnane
Department of Clinical
Gerontology
St. John's Hospital
London SW11
UK

M Myrhed
Department of Drugs
National Board of Health
and Welfare
Uppsala
Sweden

S Navaratnam
Research Division
The North East Wales
Institute
Deeside
Clwyd, CH5 4BR
UK

G Neale
Department of
Gastroenterology
Addenbrooke's Hospital
Hills Road
Cambridge CB2 2QQ
UK

S Nicklin
Immunotoxicology Department
The British Industrial
Biological Research
Association
Woodmansterne Road
Carshalton
Surrey
UK

Y Noguchi
Research and Development
Division
Taito-Pfizer
Nagoya
Japan

B Nürnberg
Department of Pharmacology
and Toxicology
University of Erlangen-
Nürnberg
D-8520 Erlangen
Federal Republic of Germany

WM O'Brien
Division of Rheumatology
Department of Internal
Medicine
University of Virginia
Hospital
Charlottesville
Virginia
USA

J Oleksy
Institute of Physiology
Academy of Medicine
31-531 Krakow, ul
Grzegorzecka 16
Poland

CP Page
Preclinical Research
Sandoz Ltd
CH-4002 Basle
Switzerland

JA Paine
Department of Surgery
Addenbrooke's Hospital
Hills Road
Cambridge CB2 2QD
UK

AL Parke
Division of Rheumatic
Diseases
University of Connecticut
Health Center
Farmington
Connecticut
USA

LIST OF CONTRIBUTORS

DV Parke
Department of Biochemistry
University of Surrey
Guildford
Surrey GU2 5XH
UK

MJ Parnham
Pharmacological Research
A Nattermann & Cie, GmbH
PO Box 350120
D-5000 Cologne 30
Federal Republic of Germany

BJ Parsons
Research Division
The North East Wales
Institute
Deeside
Clwyd CH5 4BR
UK

C Patrono
Department of Pharmacology
Catholic University School
of Medicine
00168 Rome
Italy

S Perry
Poisons Unit
New Cross Hospital
London SE14
UK

BM Peskar
Department of Experimental
Clinical Medicine
Ruhr-University of Bochum
D-4630 Bochum
Federal Republic of Germany

GO Phillips
Research Division
The North East Wales
Institute
Deeside
Clwyd CH5 4BR
UK

U Picillo
Medical Clinic
1st Faculty of Medicine
University of Naples
Naples
Italy

A Pierucci
Division of Nephrology
Department of Medicine
University of Rome
La Sapienza
00100 Rome
Italy

YJ Purdi
Department of Clinical
Pharmacology
Flinders University of
South Australia
Adelaide, S.A.
Australia

T Radecki
Institute of Physiology
Academy of Medicine
31-531 Krakow, ul
Grzegorzecka 16
Poland

MG Raimondi
Institute of Pharmacology
University of Verona
Verona
Italy

KD Rainsford
Dept of Pharmacology
University of Cambridge
Hills Road
Cambridge CB2 2QD
UK

NSB Rawson
Drug Surveillance Research
Unit
University of Southampton
North Croft House
Botley
Southampton SO3 2BX
UK

J Revuz
Department of Dermatology
Hôpital Henri Mondor
Université Paris-Val de
Maine
Creteil
France

J Rischke
McMaster University
Hamilton
Ontario
L85 4L8
Canada

J-C Roujeau
Department of Dermatology
Hôpital Henri Mondor
Universite Paris-Val de
Maine
Cretail
France

PH Rowe
Guy's Hospital
London Bridge
London SE1
UK

JR Ryan
Clinical Research Centre
New Orleans
Louisiana
USA

R Sachs
Pfizer Pharmaceuticals
235 East 42 Street
New York
USA

B C Sallustio
Department of Clinical
Pharmacology
Flinders University of
South Australia
Adelaide, S.A.
Australia

B Sandstad
University of Oslo
Oslo
Norway

F Scheler
Department of Nephrology
Georg-August-Universität
D-3400 Göttingen
Federal Republic of Germany

M Schmidz Schulmann
Abteilung Pneumologie
Robert-Koch Clinic
University of Freiberg
Freiberg-im-Breisgau
Federal Republic of Germany

DGI Scott
Department of Rheumatology
Univerisity of Birmingham
Birmingham
UK

I Scott
Medical Laboratory
Scientific Officer
Department of Biochemistry
Stobhill General Hospital
Glasgow G21 3UW
UK

TY Shen
Chemistry Department
University of Virginia
Charlottesville, VA
USA

BM Simonetti
Division of Nephrology
Department of Medicine
University of Rome
La Sapienza
00100 Rome
Italy

RD Situnayake
Dudley Road Hospital
Birmingham B18 7QH
UK

F Sörgel
Carl Korth-Institute for
Cardiovascular Research
Division of Clinical
Pharmacology
D-8520 Erlangen
Federal Republic of Germany

G Stappaerts
Department of Rheumatology
University Hospital
Ghent
Belgium

LM Strand
Department of Health
Regina
Saskatchewan
S4S 6X6
Canada

P Streete
Poisons Unit
New Cross Hospital
London SE14
UK

K Szaz
Department of Nuclear
Medicine
M.R.C., Dunn Clinical
Nutrition Centre
Trumpington Road
Cambridge
UK

A Szczeklik
Professor of Medicine
Department of Medicine
Copernicus Academy of
Medicine
Skawinska 8
31-006 Krakow
Poland

I Szelenyi
Department of Biological
Research
Heumann AG
D-8500 Nürnberg
Federal Republic of Germany

D Tartatotti
Istituto di Semeiotica e
Nefrologia
Medica dell'Università di
Verona
Verona
Italy

IA Tavares
Department of Surgery
King's College School of
Medicine and Dentistry
The Rayne Institute
123 Coldharbour Lane
London SE5 9NU
UK

J Tillman
Senior Biochemist
Department of Biochemistry
Stobhill General Hospital
Glasgow G21 3UW
UK

G Tirri
Associate Professor of
Medicine and Chief of the
Rheumatology Unit
Medical Clinic
1st Faculty of Medicine
University of Naples
Naples
Italy

R Tocchio
McMaster University
Hamilton
Ontario
L85 4L8
Canada

R Touraine
Department of Dermatology
Hôpital Henri Mondor
Université Paris-Val de
Maine
Creteil
France

L Varga
Gastrointestinal Unit
Inselspital
University of Berne
Berne
Switzerland

R Vargas
Clinical Research Center
New Orleans
Louisiana
USA

GP Velo
Istituto di Farmacologia
Clinica Medica
University of Verona
Verona
Italy

G Verbruggen
Department of Rheumatology
Ghent University Hospital
Ghent
Belgium

H Vergin
Department of Biological
Research
Heumann AG
D-8500 Nürnberg
Federal Republic of Germany

EM Veys
Dept of Rheumatology
Ghent University Hospital
Ghent
Belgium

FR Vicary
Department of
Gastroenterology
Whittington Hospital
Highgate Hill
London N19
UK

GN Volans
Poisons Unit
New Cross Hospital
London SE14
UK

FS Walker
AH Robins Company Ltd
Horsham
Surrey
UK

JCP Weber
Association of the British
Pharmaceutical Industry
Whitehall
London
UK

MH Weber
Department of Nephrology
Georg-August-Universität
D-3400 Göttingen
Federal Republic of Germany

LIST OF CONTRIBUTORS

R West
Department of Health
Regina
Saskatchewan
S4S 6X6
Canada

MW Whitehouse
Adelaide Rheumatology
Research Group
c/o Department of Pathology
University of Adelaide
Adelaide, S.A.
Australia 5001

BE Wiholm
Dept of Clinical
Pharmacology
Karolinska Institute
Huddinge University
Hospital
Huddinge
Sweden

BE Wilson
Department of Drugs
National Board of Health
and Welfare
Uppsala
Sweden

EH Wiseman
Central Research Division
Pfizer Inc.
Groton, CT 06340
USA

K Wolski
Merck Sharp & Dohme
Research Laboratories
West Point, PA 19486
USA

KG Wormsley
Department of Therapeutics
University of Dundee
Ninewells Hospital
Dundee DD1 9SY
UK

E Zielonka
Institute of Physiology
31-531 Krakow, ul
Grzegorzecka 16
Poland

SECTION I

CLINICAL AND EPIDEMIOLOGICAL ASPECTS

1
Introduction and historical aspects of the side-effects of anti-inflammatory analgesic drugs

KD Rainsford
Department of Pharmacology
University of Cambridge
Hills Road, Cambridge CB2 2QD, UK

CONTENTS

I. INTRODUCTION

During this decade much concern has been expressed both in the lay and specialist medical press and the media about the increasing incidence and severity of the side-effects which occur with the various groups of anti-inflammatory, anti-arthritic and analgesic drugs. The interest shown previously in the first conference of this series held in Verona (Italy) in 1982[1] and now in the present

Side-effects of Anti-inflammatory Drugs. Rainsford, KD and Velo, GP (eds)
Part 1: Clinical and Epidemiological Aspects. (Lancaster: MTP Press)

international conference on this topic is in fact a reflection of this concern. Our purpose should be (i) to establish the real basis for occurrence of such side-effects from epidemiological and clinical aspects and (ii) to establish the real incidence and factors responsible for the occurrence of such side-effects through to detailed biochemical, cellular and physio-pathological studies in experimental models and isolated cell systems in laboratory animals and, where appropriate, in man. While political influences and demands are ever pervasive and even persuasive it is imperative that where possible these should be differentiated from the scientific issues which we are concerned with at this meeting.

To place the overall problems and issues about the side-effects of anti-inflammatory-analgesic and anti-arthritic drugs it is important to consider some of the historical associations of the appearance of such side-effects. Some of the more recent problems which have developed with particular drugs or groups of drugs can then be viewed with some perspective. In this introduction consideration will also be given to what issues are currently of concern and might be so in the future, and will indicate those aspects of importance which will be considered by the contributors to this meeting.

II. HISTORICAL ASPECTS

A. The salicylates

Before the introduction of aspirin in 1899, therapy with the salicylates involved the use of various plant extracts containing salicylates in various chemical forms (chiefly as salicin, saligenin and salicylic acid) or, from the mid-19th century, when the purified forms of salicylic acid (either as the acid or more frequently as the sodium salt) and salicin (the glucose conjugate of salicyl alcohol) became available[2]. It was when the highly purified forms were synthesized or obtained from plant extracts during the mid-later 19th century that particular concern was expressed about their toxicity[2].

Probably the first report of a salicylate-associated adverse drug reaction (ADR) was by Longmore in 1797[3]. Fourteen men of the Royal Artillery at Quebec drank a herbal tea containing Gaultheria, and suffered symptoms of poisoning by oil of Wintergreen (methyl salicylate) which is present in this herb[3]. The symptoms they incurred comprised vertigo, vomiting and diarrhoea, respiratory distress and coma, and while severe there was no fatal outcome[3].

There were also reports in the USA as early as 1834 of a number of fatalities due to the oil prepared from Gaultheria[4].

1. Salicylic acid and salicin

In Britain during the period of the mid-1870s onwards there was much debate in the medical press about the toxicity in the gastrointestinal (GI) tract of the purified forms of the salicylates when these had become available in that country[5-9]. In 1874-80 Dr TJ Maclagan of Dundee, who appears to have been responsible for instigating interest in this period in salicylate therapy, also published several reports about the toxic symptoms from salicylic acid and salicin[6-8]. These comments were reinforced by Drs Stricker, Myers, Senator, Wolffberg and other British and German physicians who were obviously very concerned about the potential hazards of these drugs[1,4,5-9]. The points to note here are that:

(a) an appreciable number of reports of toxicity associated with salicylates appeared shortly after their introduction in pure forms;
(b) the correct dosage to achieve therapeutic benefit and at the same time minimize toxic side-effects was very much on a trial-and-error basis and a matter of considerable debate (e.g. see ref. 5); and
(c) the real therapeutic benefits and costs of the salicylates were rather debatable[5-7].

These very problems concern us today, especially as applied to those drugs introduced in more recent years.

The matter of dosage was of particular concern, for some patients were given or prescribed up to 30 grains (2 grams) of salicin and 7-15 grains (0.5-1 gram) of salicylic acid hourly for the treatment of fever either in rheumatism or infectious diseases such as typhoid (which was then rampant in Europe). It is therefore not surprising, with hourly intake of such large doses of these salicylates, that potentially toxic levels of salicylate could be achieved relatively quickly.

Maclagan[7] noted in 1874 that salicylic acid "benefited the rheumatism, but caused at the same time, so much irritation of the throat and stomach that I abandoned it in favour of salicin, and did not try it again until after the publication of Stricker's observations" (in 1876). Maclagan took issue with Stricker's comments concerning the relative efficacy and actions of salicin compared with salicylic acid and challenged Stricker's notion that salicylic acid was produced from salicin, and as well the safety of these drugs[7]. He pointed out that salicylic acid or its sodium salt could cause "considerable and even alarming depression" which today is not surprising in view of the high dosages (up to 20 grains or approx. 1.3 grams) he employed. He mentioned in 1876-9 that this drug was as efficacious as the alkaloid (salicin) but was more irritating to the alimentary canal[6-8]. A Dr Wolffberg is also mentioned at the time (by Myers[5]) as having found "haemorrhagic erosions in the mucous membrane of the stomach and intestines in several persons who had died after taking the acid made up into wafers; and in the large intestine of a dog, which had an enema containing 2 grams suspended in 50 g of water, there were numerous haemorrhagic ulcerations".

A young Swiss physician, Dr Carl Buss, must take much credit for recording at about the same time observations of the toxic effects of the salicylates, including those on himself[10]. He should also be credited with having reported the first detailed experiments of the effects of salicylates on the gastrointestinal tract of rabbits, in which he demonstrated the pronounced local irritant effects of the drug compared with the absence of gastric irritancy when the drug was give parenterally. He also was the first to establish that the local irritant effects of salicylic acid in the stomach could be ameliorated by co-administration of sodium bicarbonate[10].

2. Aspirin

As is well known, aspirin was developed to obviate the GI side-effects of salicylic acid and its sodium salt (see refs 2 and 4 for historical account), and in early reports at the beginning of this century after it was introduced suggested that aspirin was less likely to cause GI disturbances than sodium salicylate or salicylic acid. It was not long before a spate of reports appeared showing that aspirin could cause GI haemorrhage, ulcerations and other associated side-effects[2,4,11]. Dr Roch of Geneva in 1911 appears to have been the first to challenge the idea that aspirin could be more tolerable than sodium salicylate from his observations on 10 patients who had proven gastrointestinal intolerance to aspirin but who could tolerate salicylate. Very soon studies in animals[2] and the pioneering gastroscopic studies of Douthwaite, Hurst and Lintott[12,13] soon established that aspirin was indeed irritant to the stomach. The high incidence of aspirin-induced GI haemorrhage which was observed during the famous 'flu epidemic of 1918-19[14], attested to the frequent occurrence of this side-effect in the community.

In addition to the GI toxicity of aspirin a considerable number of reports appeared, some as early as 1903, on a range of other toxic effects of this drug[15-17]. Amongst these were included case reports on a number of hypersensitivity reactions manifest in the form of urticaria or angioedema[18-22]. It has been said by many authorities that any application for new product licence of a drug with the GI profile of aspirin would probably be refused today. Doubtless few have appreciated the nature and severity of some of the hypersensitivity reactions in these early reports, and likewise these would arouse concern today.

The fact is, however, that we have learned to "live" with aspirin, and it is through this understanding of the benefits and the ways by which we can minimize the occurrence of the range of side-effects from this drug and its congeners. As we have seen in the past with aspirin, we can see in recent years the pattern of the early awareness of side-effects following the introduction of a new drug, and Dr Peter Weber showed this in statistical terms at the previous meeting in this series, i.e. where there is a peak at 2 years of ADR (adverse drug reaction) reports[1].

The problems of considering the side-effects in relation to beneficial effects of drugs, as well as in the whole problem of ADR reporting, will be considered by many authors in these proceedings. Clearly this is an old problem, as we have seen it follows the introduction of aspirin. As with the early problems that beset those using the salicylates this must be seen in the problems of optimizing the dosage of the drug to achieve therapeutic effects and at the same time minimize side-effects.

B. Phenylbutazone and indomethacin

The above-mentioned problems of safe and effective dosage have also entered into the historical consideration of occurrence of side-effects with both these drugs; the forerunners to the modern non-steroidal anti-inflammatory drugs (NSAIDs) we have today. While Professor Levy has here highlighted the inadequacies in assessing the incidence of pyrazolone-associated agranulocytosis, this side-effect, as well as other blood dyscrasias, has been shown to occur with phenylbutazone and oxyphenbutazone since their introduction in 1952 and 1959 respectively[23]. There has been an increasing amount of evidence over the past few years suggesting that these side-effects are related to the tendency of both these butazones to accumulate in the body; a consequence of their long plasma half-life as well as their complex metabolism[24]. Recognition of the tendency of these butazones to cause serious blood dyscrasias has led to considerable debate[25,26] (some of it with an appreciable emotive content) concerning their continued use, with resultant restriction in the availability of both butazones in some countries.

As history has a habit of repeating itself, so we now see increasing concern that those drugs with long plasma half-lives (e.g. benoxaprofen, piroxicam) may exhibit higher incidence of serious side-effects, especially in the elderly arthritic patient whose renal and liver metabolic functions and plasma albumin levels are subnormal. These aspects will be considered here by Professors Lamy, Parke and O'Brien, and Dr Whitehouse, as well as being alluded to by a number of other authors.

Indomethacin led to a particularly worrying situation following its introduction from the frequent occurrence of upper GI ulceration and haemorrhage with the tablet formulation of this drug[27,28]. The change of formulation to the now familiar capsules of this drug caused a reduction, but certainly did not eliminate the occurrence of this side-effect. More recently the osmotic slow release formulation of this drug Osmosin (GITS formulation) was associated with a few cases of intestinal perforation[29], (see also paper by Dr Shen, Chapter 18). Some data considered in these proceedings by Professors Inman and Langman challenges the statistical incidence of lower intestinal tract injury associated with Osmosin, but still the few cases that have occurred have been a concern necessitating withdrawal of this drug formulation. Studies considered in these proceedings by Professor Brune and by the author emphasize problems of delivering or recirculating NSAIDs with the lower small and large intestine where this region of the GI tract may well be more sensitive to injury than in the stomach.

C. Problems with formulations

Problems associated with formulating NSAIDs as tablets have occurred quite frequently. A well-known, but still little appreciated, problem is the enhanced upper GI injury induced by aspirin in various tablet formulations (even as the much-favoured enteric-coated tablet), compared with suspensions or solutions as sodium or other salts[2]. Some further aspects of this matter of drug formulation as applied to other NSAIDs are considered here by Whitehouse and Rainsford.

Skin rashes associated with alclofenac were more frequent with the tablet form (10.3%) compared with capsule (2.1%) formulations of this drug[30]. Likewise tableting and possibly some manufacturing problems probably contributed to the occurrence of skin side-effects, Stevens-Johnson syndrome and GI toxicity of Clozic; in many respects an unfortunate situation in view of the apparent novel "anti-rheumatic" actions of this drug.

D. The proliferation of NSAIDs

The period in the 1960s-1970s has seen the development and introduction of a vast array of non-steroidal anti-inflammatory drugs (NSAIDs) many of which are acids. This is a recognition in itself of (a) the real need for more effective and safer pain-relieving and anti-inflammatory therapy than traditionally provided by aspirin and its congeners, indomethacin and phenylbutazone, and (b) the commercial gains which could obviously be obtained from the development of such therapies. Table 1 shows a list of drugs which have been or are currently well advanced in development for clinical use, and while not completely exhaustive (some minor developments having been omitted), it is apparent that about 100 drugs or drug variants (i.e. formulations) have appeared for full-scale clinical trials and/or extensive use.

Table 1 Non-steroidal anti-inflammatory drugs currently available or in advanced stages in clinical trials

Generic (INN) name	Trade mark names	Manufacturer(s)
Acemetacin (indomethacin glycolate)	Rantudil	Bayer Troponwerke: Kowa
Acetyl salicylic acid/aspirin	Aspirin, Ecotrin	Various (Trademark for Aspirin held by Bayer in certain European countries)
*Alclofenac		Continental Pharma: Berk
Alminoprofen	Minalfen, Minalfene	Bouchara

Drug withdrawn* or restricted[*] in use because of untoward side-effects

Table 1 continued

Generic (INN) name	Trade mark names	Manufacturer(s)
[*]Amfenac sodium		AH Robins: Meiji Seika
Amorfazone		Morishita
Antrafenine	Stakane	Synthelabo
Azapropazone	Rheumox	Siegfried: AH Robins: Robapharm
Benorylate (paracetamol-ester of aspirin)	Benoral	Winthrop
*Benoxaprofen	Opren: Coxigon	Lilly: Shionogi
Benzydamine hydrochloride	Benalgin: Benzyrin: Dorinamin: Epiroten: Imotryl: Indolin: Ririlim Salyzoron: Tamas: Tantum	Angelini: Palazzo: Fawns McAllan
BPPC		Syntex
Bufexamic acid	Droxarol: Droxaryl Feximac: Flogocid: Parfenac	Continental Pharma: American Cyanamid
Butyl fenamate	Fenazole, Combec	Hokuriku
Carprofen	Imadyl: Rimadyl	Roche
Choline salicylate	Actosal: Arret: Arthropan: Atrobione: Mundisal	Various
*Cincophen	Atophan: Quinophen Phenoquin (+various)	ICN
Cinmetacin	Cindomet	Chiesi: Lorens: Sanitas: Sam Jin

Drug withdrawn* or restricted[*] in use because of untoward side-effects

Table 1 continued

Generic (INN) name	Trade mark names	Manufacturer(s)
Clidanac	Indanal: Britai	Bristol Meyers: Takeda
Cloximate		Solvay/Duphar
CS-600		Sankyo
Diclofenac	Voltaren: Voltarol	Ciba-Geigy
Difenpyramide	Difenax	Zambeletti
Diflunisal	Dolisal: Dolobid Unisal	Merck
Disalcid (diplosal)	Salsalate	Riker
Epirizole	Mebron: Experizole	Dauchi Seiyaku
Eterylate	Daital	Alter
Etodolac	Lodine: Romadar	American Home Products: Maggioni: Med Import
Etofenamate		Bayer
Fenamole Fenbufen	Bufenid: Cinopal Lederfen: Nabanol Stimsen	American Cyanamid
*Fenclofenac	Flenac: Gidalon	Reckitt & Colman: Boehringer Mannheim: Morton Norwich
Fenclorac		Roter
*Fenclozic acid	Myalex	ICI
Fendosal	Alnovin	Hoechst: Roussel Uclaf
Fenoprofen	Nalfon	Lilly
Fenflumizole		CDC Life Sciences

Drug withdrawn* or restricted[*] in use because of untoward side-effects

Table 1 continued

Generic (INN) name	Trade mark names	Manufacturer(s)
Fentiazic	Atilan: Donorest Flogene: Norvedan Regilon	American Home Products: LPB: Niphon Chemiphar: Gist Brocades
Feprazone	Danfenona: Methrazone: Zepelan: Zepelin	Boehringer-Ingelheim: Teijin
Flufenamic acid	Archless: Arlef: Fullsafe: Paraflu Parlef: Restogen: Surika: Tecramine	Parke Davis - Warner Lambert
*Flufenisal		Merck
Flunixin	Banamine	Schering-Plough
Flunoxaprofen		Ravizza
Flurbiprofen	Ansaid: Cebutid Froben	Boots: Smith-Kline: Upjohn
Fluquazone		Sandoz
Fosfosal		Uriach
Furobufen		American Home Products
Furofenac		Alfa Farmaceutici
Glutametacin	Indicin; Indoglucin: Teorema: Teoremec	SIR
*Ibufenac	Dytransin	Boots
Ibuprofen	Brufen	Boots: Upjohn American Home Products

Drug withdrawn* or restricted[*] in use because of untoward side-effects

Table 1 continued

Generic (INN) name	Trade mark names	Manufacturer(s)
Ibuprofen guaicol-ester		Lab Angelini
Ibuproxam	Ibudros	Ferrer: Manetti & Roberts
*ICI 55,897 clobuzarit	Clozic	ICI
[*]Indoprofen	Endyne: Flozin: Flosint: Flozin	Montedison: Adria: Farmitalia Carlo Erba
Indomethacin	Amuno: Artrinovo: Artrivia: Conforted: Indomethine: Inacid: Indocid: Indocin: Indomed: Infrocin: Inteban SP: Mezolin Osmosin: Oraflex	Merck
Ionazolac calcium		Byk Gulden
Isofezolac		Pharmuka
Isonixin	Nixyn	Hermes
*Isoxepac	Moxicam	Hoechst: Roussel Uclaf: Daiichi Seiyaku
*Isoxicam	Moxicam	Warner Lambert/ Parke Davis
Ketoprofen	Alrheumat: Alrheumun: Orudis Prafenid	Rhone Poulenc/ May & Baker American Home Products
Lofemizole		Farmitas
Loxoprofen sodium	Loxonin	Sankyo
Magnesium salicyate	Trilisate	

Drug withdrawn* or restricted[*] in use because of untoward side-effects

Table 1 continued

Generic (INN) name	Trade mark names	Manufacturer(s)
Meclofenamate sodium	Arquel: Meclofen	Warner Lambert/ Parke Davis
Mefenamic acid	Coslan: Lyzalgo: Parkemed: Poustan: Poustel: Poustel: Poustyl: Poutal: Tauston: Vialidon	Warner Lambert/ Parke Davis
*Meseclazone		Carter Wallace
Methyl salicylate	Various	Various
Miroprofen		Yoshimoto
Nabumitone		Beecham: Ferrosan
Naproxen sodium	Anaprox: Flanax: Flanex: Naproxen: Naprozyn-S: Synflex	Syntex
Nictindole		Sanofi
Niflumic acid	Actol: Forenol: Landruma: Nifluril	UPSA
Oxametacin (indoxamic acid)	Flogar: Restid	ABC: UBC
Oxaprozin	Duraprox	American Home Products: Talsho
Oxepinac		Daiichi
[*]Oxyphenbutazone	Tanderil	Ciba-Geigy
Parsalmide	Parsal	Sanofi
Perisoxal citrate	Isoxal	Shionogi
[*]Phenylbutazone	Butazolindine: Butacote: Butazolidin	Ciba-Geigy

Drug withdrawn* or restricted[*] in use because of untoward side-effects

Table 1 continued

Generic (INN) name	Trade mark names	Manufacturer(s)
Pirprofen	Rengasil	Ciba-Geigy
Pirproxen	Numide	Hosbon
Piroxicam	Feldene	Pfizer; Toyama: Chiesi
Pranoprofen	Niflan	Yoshimoti
Proglumetacin maleate	Afloxan: Protaxil: Proxil	Rorer: Rotta Products
Proquazone	Biarison: Biarson	Sandoz
Sfericase	Ponase	Meiji Seika
Sodium salicylate	Various	Various
*Sudoxicam		Pfizer
Sulindac	Arthrocine: Clinoril Imberal: Sulindac Udolac	Merck: Banyu
Sulphinpyrazone	Anturan	Ciba-Geigy
Superoxide dismutase	Orgetein	Diagnostic Data: Astra: Bristol-Myers: Toyo Jozo: Zambeletti
Suprofen	Sutoprofen: Maldocil	Janssen: Johnson & Johnson: Cilag
Talniflumate	Somalgen	Bago: Norpro
Tenoxicam		Roche
Tiabinac		
Thiazolinobutazone	Deflogix	Almirall: UCB

Drug withdrawn* or restricted[*] in use because of untoward side-effects

Table 1 continued

Generic (INN) name	Trade mark names	Manufacturer(s)
Tiaprofenic acid	Artiflam: Surgam	Roussel-Uclaf: Eisai
*Tiflamizole		Du Pont
Timegadine		Leo Denmark
Tioxaprofen	Thioxaprofene	E. Merck
Tolfenamic acid	Clotam	Tobisha: Medica: GEA
Tolmetin sodium	Midocil: Tolectin: Tolecgin	McNiel Johnson & Johnson
Trimethazone		
Zidometacin		Pierrel: Forest
*Zomepirac	Zomax	Johnson & Johnson

Drug withdrawn* or restricted[*] in use because of untoward side-effects

What is very sobering is that even after the most thorough pre-clinical and toxicological testing it is apparent that some 17 of these have been withdrawn or restricted since their introduction because of untoward side-effects, thus representing roughly a 17% failure rate. This has been both tragic for the patient (in some cases fatal) and at the same time immensely costly for the drug industry. Inspection of Figures 1-4 will show that such drug failures have encompassed nearly all major structural classes (i.e. chemically speaking). Furthermore, it can be seen from these summary diagrams that many of these side-effects have occurred under clinical situations which are probably unique to man, and to some albeit as yet largely unspecified conditions in the arthritic patient. As seen in later chapters a whole variety of situations or conditions may play a significant part in creating the conditions for the development of a particular side-effect attributed to a drug (e.g. age, sex, disease or drug interactions).

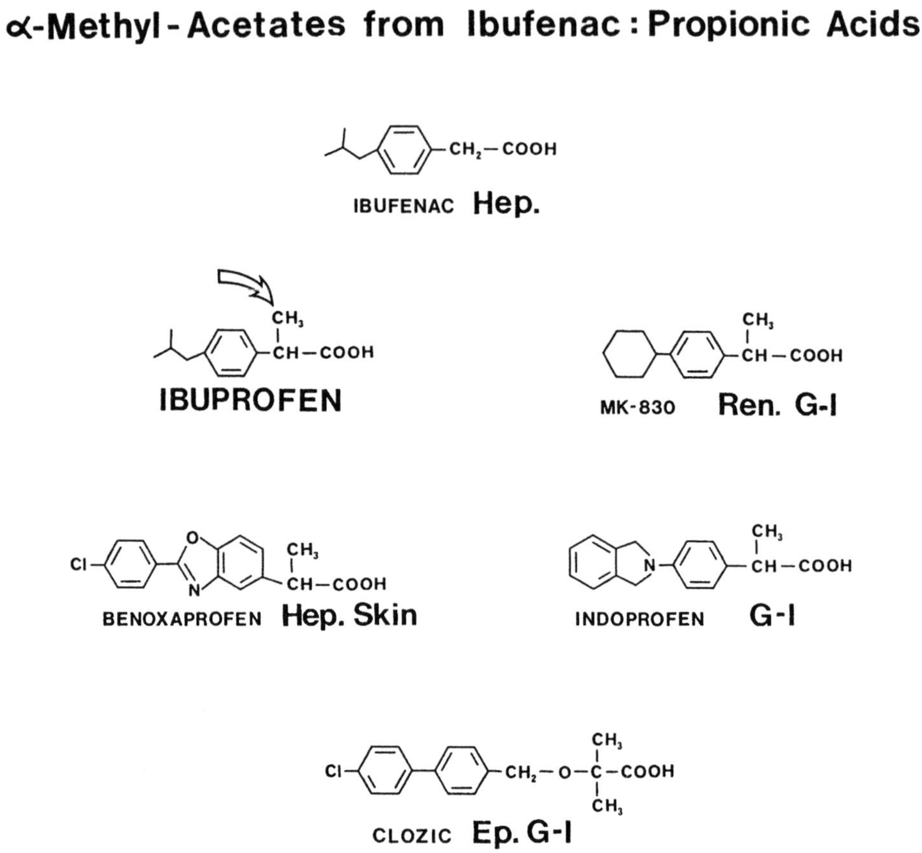

Figure 1 Side-effects of NSAIDs by structural class: the case of α-methylacetates, or propionates, derived originally from the phenyl acetate moiety typified here by ibufenac. Note that the simple insertion of a methyl group at the α-carbon of ibufenac was successful in eliminating the hepatotoxicity (abbreviated Hep) of ibufenac. **Abbreviations** for toxicities of other propionates: Ren. = renal toxicity; GI = gastrointestinal toxicity; Ep. = epithelial toxicity; Skin = skin toxicity.

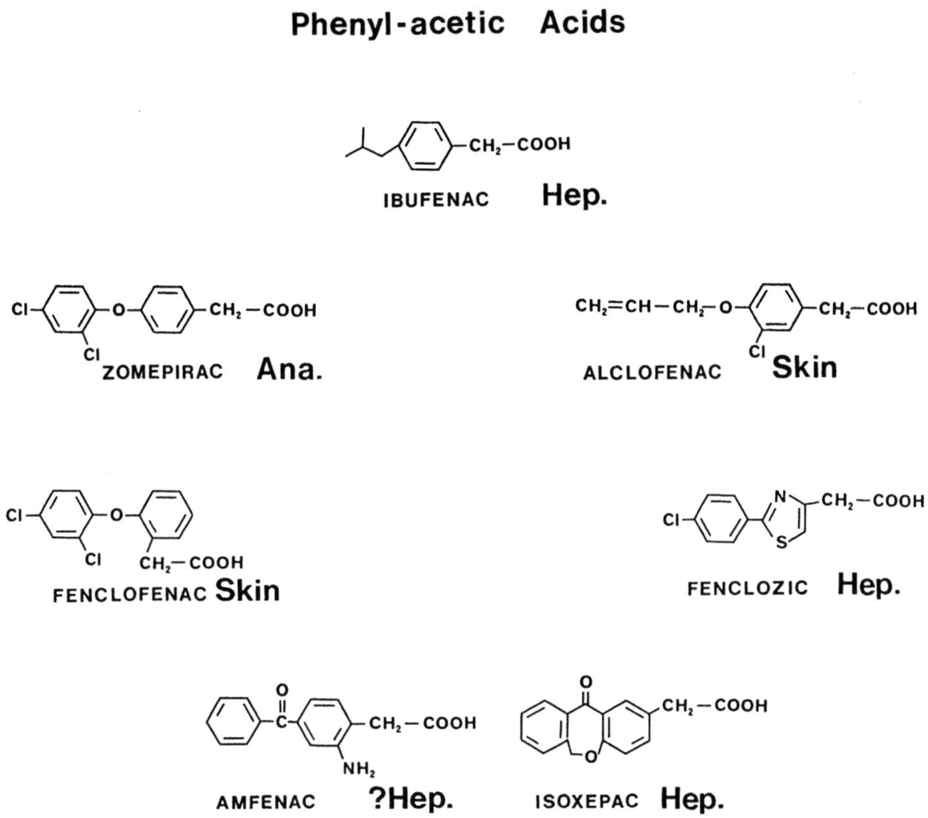

Figure 2 Side-effects of NSAIDs by structural class: phenyl acetates. The development of side-effects is independent of chemical structure. Abbreviations for particular side-effects as in Figure 1, and in addition: Ana = anaphylactoid reactions. There is a query over hepatotoxicity of amfenac and this is still under investigation.

Benzoic Acids

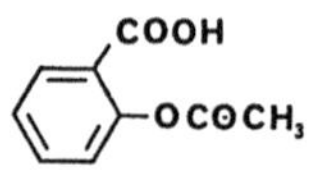

ASPIRIN

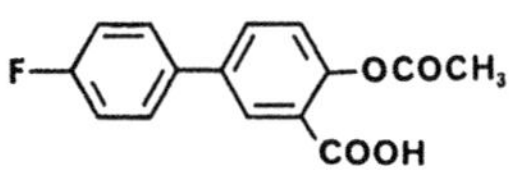

FLUFENISAL **Ren.**

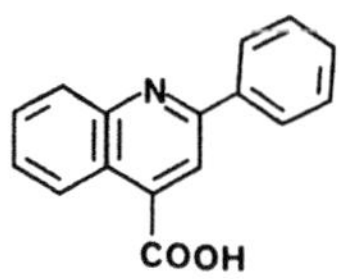

CINCOPHEN **Hep.**

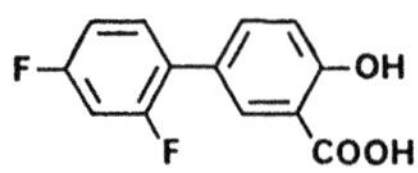

DIFLUNISAL

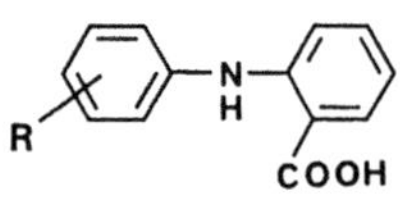

N-ANTHRANILIC ACIDS

R = 3-CF_3 , Flufenamic Acid
2,3-Me_2, Mefenamic Acid
3-Me,2,6-Cl_2, Meclofenamic Acid

Figure 3 Side-effects of NSAIDs by structural class: benzoic acids. Hepatotoxicity from cincophen and renal toxicity from flufenisal resulted in withdrawal of these drugs. However, small structural variations of flufenisal resulted in successful development of diflunisal, a drug with relatively low nephrotoxicity. Likewise other benzoic acids, actually anthranilic acids, have proven relatively safe and effective agents.

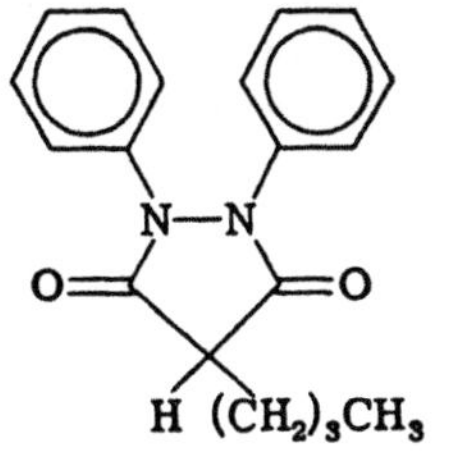

Phenylbutazone

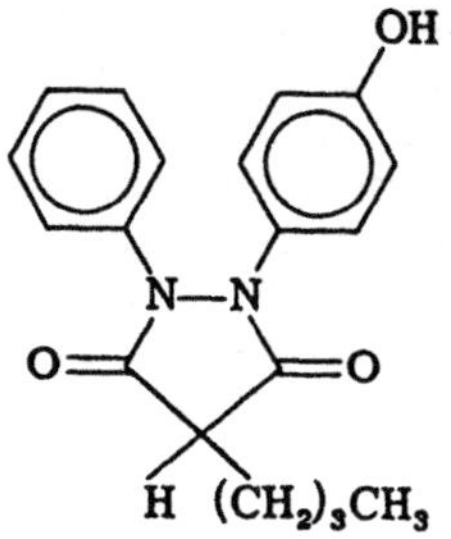

Oxyphenbutazone

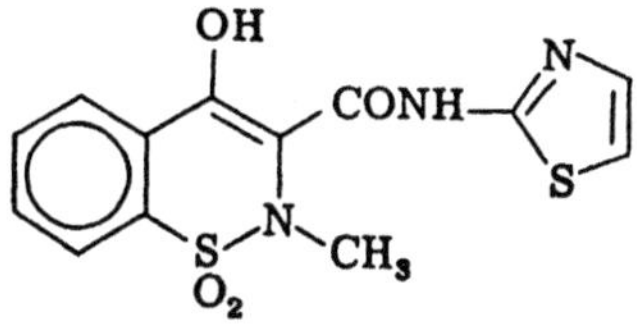

Sudoxicam

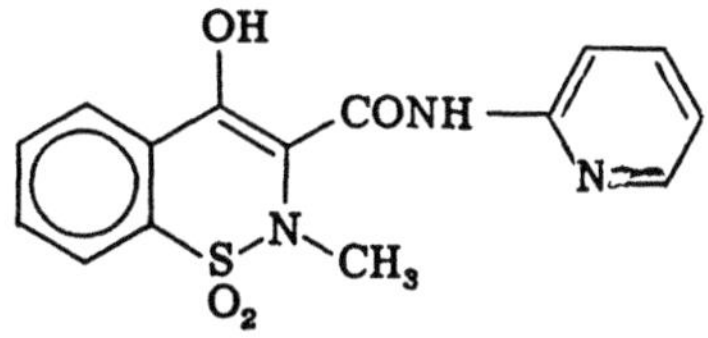

Piroxicam

Figure 4 Side-effects by structural class: non-carboxylic acids enolic acids/oxicams. Butazones: phenylbutazone and oxyphenylbutazone have been shown to induce blood dyscrasias, albeit at somewhat variable frequency (see Chapter 7 in this volume). However, other enolic acids clearly do not have this propensity (e.g. azapropazone - see Chapter 45 in Part 2 of this volume), feprazone, etc. Oxicams: the GI and possibly other toxicity of sudoxicam did not present in such a way as to limit successful development and use of piroxicam, or indeed other oxicams, e.g. tenoxicam.

Initial developments along the lines of anti-inflammatory/analgesic compounds during the 1960s were essentially based on somewhat empirical grounds, and can be summarized as:

1. Modifications of the salicylate molecular structure. A recent review of these historical developments can be found in ref. 2. These modifications also involved the development of the fenamates whose essential structure derived from benzoic acid to the anthranilic acid structure of the fenamates.
2. Progression from benzoates (i.e. from salicylates, fenamates), by increase in C-atoms between the aryl and carboxylic acid moieties[32].

carboxylic acid moieties[32].
3. Developments of non-carboxylate enolic acids (including oxicams) deriving essentially on phenylbutazone[32,34].
4. Modifications of the indole acetic acids (see ref. 33 and chapter by Dr Shen in these proceedings).
5. Development of non-acidic NSAIDs (e.g. proquazone) and NSAI pro-drugs (e.g. meseclazone, butyl-fenamate, etofenamate, fenbufen, sulindac)[34].
6. Development of dermal preparations[34].

In these developments the objectives have been to:

(a) promote anti-inflammatory activity, and
(b) reduce gastric and other toxicity

The latter objective has been a particular aim of the non-acidic and/or pro-drug types, and a reduction in GI irritancy/ulcerogenity appears to have been partially successful[2,35].

Following the initial empirical approach of the early 1960s, the pioneering observations of Smith and Willis[36], and Vane and his colleagues[37,38] on the role of prostaglandins (PGs) in the inflammatory process, led to an immediate thrust during the 1970s to develop potent synthesis inhibitors in the belief that these would achieve the objectives in (a) and (b) above. The situation was summarized by JR Vane in 1979, who stated in the context of the development of propionic acids that:

> It could be that the second generation of anti-inflammatory compounds, [could be] based on the propionic acids, because they have less gastrointestinal side-effects than the earlier ones are in fact demonstrating some of this specificity [i.e. towards selective inhibition of prostaglandin synthesis in different tissues][39].

The concept that there could be selective inhibition of PG synthesis in different tissues such that potent inhibition of PGs could be achieved at inflammatory sites but with much lower inhibition of cytoprotective PGs in the GI tract and kidney (whose reduction could be seen to be detrimental to the functions of these systems) was a powerful impetus towards the development of several propionates and other classes of drugs (e.g. see refs 40-42). That such selective actions could be a reality for all the propionates is indeed doubtful and may, as Dr Caldwell has suggested in these proceedings (Chapter 17) depend entirely on the rates of conversion of inactive R(-) to active S(+) forms of this group of drugs. For at least one such drug, tiaprofenac acid, there may be a small margin of selectivity in inhibiting PGs in some tissues in vitro[40] but there is no doubt that it is a potent inhibitor of PG production in the gastric mucosa (of man) in vivo[43]. Also, the proposed selective PG effect of the non-acidic experimental drug BW755c on gastric PG production[42] has now been shown to be inconsistent, with inhibition being evident at high concentrations such as would be expected in the stomach[44,45]. Such selective effects may, however, be evident with other classes of NSAIDs (and obviously is critically dependent upon the pharmacokinetics of the drugs)[46,47].

It is now clear that inhibition of PG production may be more evident in the stomach with some drugs, and this may or may not be related to their propensity to develop GI damage (refs 46,47, see Rainsford these proceedings Chapter 1, Part 2), and also there may be other biochemical and cellular actions of NSAIDs even with the propionic acids, which accounts for their anti-inflammatory actions[48]. Thus the whole basis for the actions of drugs, especially the phenylpropionates and phenylacetates, may in fact be more complex than envisaged when their search was initiated on the basis of inhibiting (either selectively or non-selectively) PG production.

III. DEVELOPMENTS IN THE 1980s

This decade will be renown no doubt for the dramatic withdrawals of some possibly very promising NSAIDs reflecting very special problems relating to the use and possibly basic properties of these drugs. Among the major problems have been:

1. The development of jaundice, renal failure, and other severe toxic reactions, especially in some elderly patients, and exceptionally high incidence of onycholysis and photosensitivity skin reactions in patients of all age groups on benoxaprofen (Opren, Coxigon)[49-55]. The possibility also exists from studies in mice that this drug might be carcinogenic[55].
2. The reports of GI haemorrhage and ulceration from the osmotic slow-release (GITS) formulation of indomethacin, Osmosin[29,56], a high incidence of deaths and side-effects including those from GI side-effects with indoprofen (Flosint[57-59], and GI ulceration and haemorrhage from piroxicam (Feldene) (refs 60 and 61 - see also Chapter 25 by Vicary et al. and Chapter 8 by Gordon and Sachs in this volume.
3. The hypersensitivity reactions together with the five deaths associated with this side-effect from zomepirac (Zomax)[59].
4. The high incidence of skin reactions exhibited from fenclofenac[62].
5. The exacerbation of various inflammatory bowel diseases by potent PG synthesis inhibitors[49,62].

As will be discussed later, the very statistical bases upon which some of these decisions were made is seriously questioned. But given that there have been indications for withdrawal of these drugs, the question has to be asked why the drugs in groups 1 to 4 above have been so toxic even after clear indications of relative safety from pre-clinical studies of their toxicology and from phase I-III clinical studies? Is it because of:

1. Novel properties (both pharmacological and toxicological) inherent in some but not all structural types?

2. Associations with long plasma half-lives?
3. Lack of education of medical practitioners (e.g. monitoring of drug intake, toxic symptoms, drug interactions)?
4. New toxic properties revealed only in the elderly or diseased patient?

Some of these points will be taken up by different authors in this volume, but to date there does appear to be some evidence for all these points. Clearly, the recent concerns indicate that the use of new and existing NSAIDs will in the future require much more careful monitoring and investigation than previously.

IV. ANTIRHEUMATIC DRUGS AND FUTURE DEVELOPMENTS

The problems associated with the use of corticosteroids have been known for a relatively long time now, and thus there has been more cautious approach towards their use and attention to minimizing their side-effects and enhancing the selectivity as part of the programmes for the development of new steroids. However, as will be seen in the papers by contributors to the section on "Glucocorticoids" there is now much concern about the high incidence of aseptic bone necrosis in patients receiving even modest doses of methyl prednisolone. As indicated in these studies the pronounced dose-response effect observed in the appearance of this serious side-effect must also be of concern for the recent application of megadose prednisolone therapy.

Extensive toxicity exhibited by the so-called slow-acting antirheumatic drugs (SAARDs) e.g. D-penicillamine and the gold complexes, was considered in part at the previous meeting, but here particular attention will be devoted to new aspects (see Chapters in Part 2 in the section on "Antirheumatic and Immunoregulatory Agents"). Of special interest is the possibility that there may be genetic factors (reflected in the HLA haptotypes) underlying the predisposition towards the development of side-effects by these agents (see Chapters by Dequecker and others in that section). While development of new SAARDs is very slow, it is probably very important. The following recent summary of the state of art with the SAARDs, and commentary by one of the USA's leading rheumatologists, Professor Harry Paulus[64] is a reflection of the need for much safer and effective SAARDs:

1. Half of RA patients taking SAARDs discontinue after 1 year because of (a) toxicity, (b) lack of benefit.
2. Only 10-15% of RA patients take SAARDs after 5 years.
3. In conclusion: "We need better SAARDs that produce more reliable and sustained benefit and are tolerated during many years of treatment."

Problems which may emerge in the future with the new generation of disease-modifying immunoregulatory agents (as reviewed by Lewis and Gilman (Chapter 27), present us with a formidable task of trying to predict their possible toxicity in man from appropriate animal models of toxicity which as yet we have very little idea of being able to choose or formulate.

V. CONCLUSIONS

The main points which emerge from this review of the historical development of the untoward side-effects from anti-inflammatory and analgesic drugs are that:

1. Historically an upsurge in reports of adverse reactions to drugs always appears following their introduction.
2. The assessment of "severe" ADRs recorded in the past has been under-rated by present-day standards.
3. The upsurge in ADRs to NSAIDs recorded in recent years has been in the past related to an increase in the total numbers of drugs, but there are also special problems with the newer drugs. To discard old drugs because we are so much aware of their toxicity might in fact prove undesirable without further knowledge of the safety of the newer agents in comparison with the older traditional drugs.
4. The options to reduce the incidence of ADRs are inherently frail because the statistical basis upon which incidences of ADR has been compiled are inherently weak.
5. Comprehensive educational and scientific programmes are required to reduce the apparent high incidence of side-effects from current anti-inflammatory and anti-arthritic agents.

REFERENCES

1. Rainsford, KD and Velo, GP (eds) (1984). Side-effects of Anti-inflammatory Analgesic Drugs. Advances in inflammation Research, vol. 6. (New York: Raven Press)
2. Rainsford, KD (1984). Aspirin and the Salicylates. (London: Butterworths)
3. Longmore, G (1798). Account of fourteen men of the royal artillery at Quebec, who were nearly poisoned by drinking a decoction of certain plants. Ann Med Edin, 3, 364
4 Gross, M and Greenberg, LA (1948). The Salicylates. A Critical Bibliographic Review. (New Haven: Hillhouse Press)
5. Myers, ABR (1876). Salicin in acute rheumatism. Lancet, 2, 676
6. Anonymous (1876). Salicylic acid and salicin in acute rheumatism. Guy's Hosp Gazette, 1 (N.S.), 84
7. Maclagan, TJ (1879). The treatment of acute rheumatism by salicin and salicylic acid. Lancet, 1, 875
8. Maclagan, TJ (1879). Note on the danger attending the use of salicylic acid in acute rheumatism. Lancet, 1, 327
9. Shaw, LE (1887). Cases of haemorrhage occurring during treatment by salicylate of soda. Guy's Hosp Rep XLIV, 125
10. Buess, H and Balmer, H (1962). Carl Emil Buss (1849-1878) und die Begrundung der Salicylsäure-Therapie. Gersherus, 19, 130
11. Roche, M (1912). Acide acetyl-salicylique et de soude. Bull Gen de Therapeut Medicale Paris, 163,218
12. Douthwaite, AH and Lintott, GAM (1938). Gastroscopic observation of the

effect of aspirin and other substances on the stomach. Lancet, 235, 1222
13. Hurst, A and Lintott, GAM (1939). Aspirin as a cause of haematemesis: A clinical and gastroscopic study. Guy's Hosp Rep, 89, 173
14. Sajous, S and Hundley, P (1931). In Pierson, GM and Bortz, EL (eds) Cyclopedia of Medicine, vol II. (Philadelphia: FA Davis)
15. Franke (1903). Vergiftungercheinungen nach Aspirin. Munch Med Wochenschr, 50, 1299
16. Otto and Mayer (1903). Ueber einen weiteren Fall von Neban wirkung des Aspirins. Dtsch Med Wochenschr, 29, 123
17. Dockray, JS (1905). Some toxic effects of aspirin. Br Med J, 2, 1692
18. Killen, SJ (1911). Poisoning after samll doses of aspirin. Br Med J, 1, 476
19. Brown, A (1911). A note on a toxic effect of aspirin. Lancet, 2, 761
20. Waller, HE (1911). Toxic effect of aspirin. Lancet, 2, 916
21. Blackie, JB (1911). Toxic effect of aspirin. Lancet, 2, 1094
22. Albercrombie, PH (1911). Poisoning after small doses of aspirin. Br Med J, 1, 1314
23. Fowler, DD and Faragher, EB (1977). Drug and non-drug factors influencing adverse reactions to pyrazoles. J Int Med Res, 5 (Suppl. 1), 108
24. Davies, DS (1977). Phenylbutazone: factors influencing plasma concentrations. J Int Med Res, 5 (Suppl. 2), 15
25. Anonymous (1984). Phenylbutazone and oxyphenbutazone: time to call a halt. Drug Therap Bull, 22, 5
26. Loshak, D (1985). Anti-inflammatory drugs under fire. Lancet, 1, 40
27. Lövegren, O and Allender, E (1965). Indomethacin and peptic ulcer. Br Med J, 1, 996
28. O'Brien, WM (1968). Indomethacin: a survey of clinical trials. Clin Pharmacol Ther, 9, 94
29. Day, TK (1983). Intestinal perforation associated with osmotic slow release indomethacin capsules. Br Med J, 287, 1671
30. Hort, JF (1975). Adverse reactions to alclofenac. Curr Med Res Opin, 3, 333
31. Personal communication, Dr MEJ Billingham
32. Scherrer, RA and Whitehouse MW (eds) (1974). Anti-inflammatory Agents. Chemistry and Pharmacology, vol. 1, (New York: Academic Press)
33. Shen, TY (1981). Toward more selective anti-arthritic therapy. J Med Chem, 24, 1
34. Lombardino, JG (1978). Newer Agents for the treatment of arthritis. Ann Rep Med Chem, 13, 167
35. Rainsford, KD (1982). An analysis of the gastrointestinal side-effects of non-steroidal anti-inflammatory drugs, with particular reference to comparative studies in man and laboratory animals. Rheumatol Int, 2, 1
36. Smith, JB and Willis, AL (1971). Aspirin selectively inhibits prostaglandin production in human platelets. Nature (New Biol), 231, 235
37. Vane, JR (1971). Inhibition of prostaglandin synthesis as a mechanism of action for aspirin-like drugs. Nature (New Biol), 231, 235
38. Flower, RJ (1974). Drugs which inhibit prostaglandin synthesis. Pharmacol Rev, 26, 33
39. Vane, JR (1979). Summing-up. In Rainsford, KD and Ford-Hutchinson, AW (eds), Prostaglandins and Inflammation. Agents and Actions, Suppl AAS6. (Basel: Birkhäuser)
40. Sorkin, EM and Brogden, RN (1985). Tiaprofenic acid: a review of its pharmacological properties and therapeutic efficacy in rheumatic diseases and pain states. Drugs, 29, 208

41. Higgs, GA, Flower, RJ and Vane, JR (1979). A new approach to antiinflammatory drugs. Biochem Pharmacol, 28, 1959
42. Whittle, BJR, Higgs, GA, Eakins, KE, Moncada, S and Vane, JR (1980). Selective inhibition of prostaglandin production in inflammatory exudates and gastric mucosa. Nature, 284, 271
43. Hunter, JO, Alun-Jones, V, Shorthouse, M and Bold, JM (1985). Effect of tiaprofenic acid and indomethacin on prostaglandin levels in the human stomach and duodenum. XVIth International Congress of Rheumatology, Sydney, Australia, F9
44. Peskar, BM, Weiler, H and Meyer Ch (1984). Inhibition of prostaglandin production in the gastrointestinal tract by anti-inflammatory drugs. In: Rainsford, KD and Velo, GP (eds), Side-effects of Anti-inflammatory Analgesic Drugs. p.39 (New York: Raven Press)
45. Boughton-Smith, NK and Whittle, BJR (1984). Stimulation and inhibition of prostacyclin formation in the gastric mucosa and ileum in vitro by anti-inflammatory agents. Br J Pharmacol, 78, 173
46. Rainsford, KD, Fox, SA and Osborne, DJ (1984). Comparative effects of some non-steroidal anti-inflammatory drugs on ultrastructural integrity and prostaglandin levels in the rat gastric mucosa: relationship to drug uptake. Scand J Gastroentol, 19 (Suppl. 101), 55
47. Rainsford, KD, Fox, SA and Osborne, DJ (1985). Relationship between drug absorption, inhibition of cyclooxygenase, and lipoxygenase pathways, and development of gastric mucosal damage by non-steroidal anti-inflammatory drugs in rats and pigs. In: Bailey, JM (ed), Prostaglandins, Leukotrienes, and Lipoxins. p.639 (New York: Plenum Press)
48. Kitchen, AE, Dawson, W, Rainsford, KD and Cawston, T (1985). Inflammation and mode of action of anti-inflammatory drugs. In: Rainsford, KD (ed.), Anti-inflammatory and Antirheumatic Drugs, vol. I, p. 21. (Boca Raton, Florida: CRC Press)
49. Del Favero, A (1983). Antirheumatic analgesics and drugs used in rheumatoid arthritis and gout. In: Dukes, MNG and Elis, J (eds), Side Effects of Drugs Annual, vol. 7. (Amsterdam: Exerpta Medica), p. 104
50. Taggart, HMcA and Alderdice, JM (1982). Fatal cholestatis jaundice in elderly patients taking benoxaprofen. Br Med J, 284, 1372
51. Hindson, C, Daymond, T, Diffey, B and Lawlor, F (1982). Side-effects of benoxaprofen. Br Med J, 284, 1368
52. Various authors (1982). Side-effects of benoxaprofen. Br Med J, 284, 1782
53. Lasagna, L (1984). Techniques for ADR Reporting. In: Detection and Prevention of Adverse Drug Reactions (Centre for the Study of Drug Development, Tufts University), p. 146
54. Wiskemann, A (1981). Photosensibilisierung durch Benoxaprofen. Arzneim-Forsch, 31, 730
55. Anonymous (1984). Lilly closing out Oraflex clinicals after increased liver cancer incidence. FDC Reports, 2 January 1984
56. Del Favero, A (1984). Anti-inflammatory analgesics and drugs used in rheumatoid arthritis and gout. In: Dukes, MNG (ed.) Side Effects of Drug Annual, vol. 8 (Amsterdam: Exerpta Medica), p. 100
57. Anonymous (1983). Flosint's UK PL Suspended. Scrip, No. 856, 1
58. Anonymous (1983). Review, Scrip, Nos. 857 and 858, 16
59. Anonymous (1984). Flosint data sheet revised in Italy. Scrip, No. 863, 4
60. Fok, KH, George, PJM and Vicary, FR (1985). Peptic ulcers induced by piroxicam. Br Med J, 290, 117
61. Vrhovac, B (1984). Anti-inflammatory analgesics and drugs used in gout. In: Dukes, MNG (ed.), Meyler's Side Effects of Drugs, 10th edn. (Amsterdam:

Elsevier, p. 1984
62. Langman, MJS, Morgan, L and Worrall, A (1985). Use of anti-inflammatory drugs by patients admitted with small or large bowel perforations and haemorrhage. Br Med J, 290, 347
63. Anonymous (1984). Scrip, No. 912, 19
64. Paulus, HE (1985). Slowly acting anti-rheumatic drugs (SAARD's) rarely improve the outcome of rheumatoid arthritis patients. XVIth International Congress of Rheumatology, Sydney, Australia, R35

2
Epidemiology in the United Kingdom of adverse drug reactions from non-steroidal anti-inflammatory drugs

JCP Weber
Association of the British Pharmaceutical Industry
Lately of Medicines Division, Department of Health, London, UK

CONTENTS

I. INTRODUCTION

Anyone who examines the lists of suspected adverse drug reactions (ADRs) available on request by doctors, hospital pharmacists and pharmaceutical companies from the Medicines Division of the United Kingdom Department of Health, will become aware that drugs of similar therapeutic group often produce quite different numbers of reports of ADR. One obvious reason for this is that some drugs are prescribed much more frequently than others. However, even after due allowance is made for this, sometimes considerable differences remain.

Side-effects of Anti-inflammatory Drugs. Rainsford, KD and Velo, GP (eds)
Part 1: Clinical and Epidemiological Aspects. (Lancaster: MTP Press)

II. ADVERSE REACTIONS REPORTING

A. Constancy of reporting

It is sometimes thought that the voluntary reporting of ADR is a very variable and haphazard procedure, and that no comparative information, or indeed little information at all other than the fact that this or that ADR is suspected to have occurred, can be derived from it. The data are certainly "soft", but in the chapter I shall try to show that such assumptions are by no means necessarily valid.

B. Factors influencing reporting rate

When a new drug is marketed it is not uncommon for the total number of ADR reports it produces to rise to a peak at about 2 years after marketing, and thereafter to decline[1]. This decline is due to a reduction in the reporting of clinically mild or trivial reactions. The more serious ADR, such as haematemesis, perforation of peptic ulcers, blood dyscrasias, etc. are reported from year to year in quite a constant manner. It is common knowledge that the number of reports received represent only a fraction of the ADR actually occurring, and this is due principally to the small proportion, perhaps 15-20%, of available doctors who report[2]. The important point is that the number of reports for a given drug is unlikely to show any prolonged increase or decrease on a previously established trend by chance alone and in the absence of some causative factor.
The types of change found in practice, and their possible reasons are quite few and can be listed thus:

Prolonged rise.	Increased patient exposure. Introduction of new dosage form with ADR potential.
Transient rise.	Journal article or warning from regulatory agency.
Prolonged fall.	Decreased patient exposure.

C. Prescriptions and ADR reports

It is often assumed that ADR report totals are proportional to prescriptions. This is in fact seldom true. ADR reports are often quoted comparatively for several drugs as so many per million prescriptions. Because of non-proportionality the rate per million prescriptions varies with the total number of prescriptions upon which the calculation is based such estimates should therefore state this total. They are liable to be misleading if compared with estimates for other similar drugs derived from different prescription totals. Statistical comparison of the two proportions for two drugs using ADR reports as numerator and prescriptions as denominator is more accurate if very large differences are demonstrable, as in the paper previously quoted[1]. Even this method is ultimately based on proportionality though, so what is needed is a reasonably accurate estimate of ADR report totals at specific prescription totals which are the same for two or more drugs to be compared. It is then entirely legitimate to calculate the (continuity-corrected if necessary) normal variate of the difference between the proportions to estimate statistical significance.

III. LOG-LINEAR TREND ANALYSIS

This method has been fully described elsewhere[3]. Briefly, if the cumulative totals of ADR reports (ΣR) be plotted against the cumulative prescription totals (ΣP) at suitable intervals (usually yearly, but shorter intervals can be used if the data are available) the resulting equation is of the type:

$$\Sigma R = m \log_e \Sigma P + c$$

where m is the regression coefficient and c the intercept of the curve on the ordinate. These curves are usually convex upwards, but any type, passing through a linear relationship to a convex-downwards curve, can occur depending on the relation between reporting rate and prescribing rate. Since curves are less easy to use than linear plots they are best converted to linear form by using the logarithm of ΣR. The equation thus becomes:

$$\log_e \Sigma R = m \log_e \Sigma P + c$$

The equations should be based on at least four points. They provide a useful estimate of trend where the correlation coefficient (r) is at least 0.95. In this event the "measure of confidence" (r^2), representing the pure mathematical relationship between the dependent and independent variables is at least 90%. The method can thus provide:

1. a means of interpolating calculated values of ΣR at any chosen value of ΣP;
2. a means of (cautious) extrapolation to any specific value of ΣP;
3. a means by which a prolonged change in trend can be signalled;
4. a means by which large constant or increasing differences in ΣR for two or more similar drugs at identical prescription totals can be noted.

A. Constancy of trends

Confining the method to situations where $r \geq 0.95$ is a guarantee of considerable accuracy in the estimate of ΣR. Such situations are in practice frequently encountered. It may be wondered how often such a trend calculated over 4 or 5 years, is representative of other periods in the marketing of the drug. Equation parameters for indomethacin for three separate 5-year periods in its marketing life in respect of reports of gastrointestinal haemorrhage or perforation (R_g) are set out in Table 1. The equations show some slight increase in reporting rate relative to prescribing rate during the first of the 5-year periods. However, this is only sufficient to produce an excess of eight reports in 4 million prescriptions and does not indicate a significant difference in trend. The two remaining equations, covering a 10-year period, are almost identical, indicating no change in trend during that period either. A similar situation exists for ibuprofen, another non-steroidal anti-inflammatory drug (NSAID) marketed for a sufficiently long time to make it a suitable subject for investigation of methodology.

Table 1 Equation data (indomethacin) for three 5 year periods

Period	m	c	r	r^2 (%)
1968-72	0.735	-7.85	0.998	99.6
1973-77	1.090	-13.58	0.998	99.6
1978-82	1.036	-12.67	0.999	99.8

If the reporting trends for R_g for these drugs are constant, it should be possible to forecast from the equations for 1973-77 what cumulative totals of these reports would be expected for the years 1978-82, given, with hindsight, a knowledge of the cumulative prescription totals for those years. It should be noted that true prospective forecasting in relation to a particular point in time is much more difficult because it requires a reasonably reliable estimate of the number of prescriptions likely to have been written during the period intervening.

Table 2 presents an accuracy-testing forecast where the actual number of prescriptions during the test period was known. It demonstrates the good correspondence between the observed and estimated values of ΣR_g, thus confirming the constancy of the trend over a long period. The 90% confidence intervals of the estimates are also given in the table. Although they are not particularly helpful when a specific trend is under consideration they demonstrate the absence or presence of significant differences between the individual values of the trends for two drugs at the 10% significance level. A preferred method of estimating the significance of such differences, as has already been mentioned, is by calculation of the continuity-corrected normal variate at identical prescription totals using the two separate equations for the respective drugs. For indomethacin the equation parameters are given in Table 1, for 1973-77, and for that period for ibuprofen they were: $m = 0.826$, $c = -9.35$ and $r = 0.96$.

It must be emphasized that, in Table 2, we are dealing with cumulative totals of R_g, so that the totals of 122 and 58 respectively for indomethacin and ibuprofen against the year 1978 indicate that this was the total number of reports from the beginning of the comparison period, i.e. from the end of 1973. This gives a mean number per year for indomethacin of about 22, and for ibuprofen of about 12. The respective means for the test period are approximately 18 and 13 per year. Since the prescription totals were not very greatly different it comes as no great surprise that the 90% confidence intervals for the two drugs overlap, indicating no significant differences in prescription-related reporting rates, a fact that may surprise some physicians. It should perhaps be noted that the data for indomethacin relate only to standard dosage forms, i.e. they do not include any type of slow-release form. The reasonably close correspondence of the point-estimates derived from the 1973-77 data with the observed totals is to be noted.

Table 2 Observed and point-estimates of Reports of Gastrointestinal haemorrhage and ulceration, ΣR_g, for 1978-82 calculated from equations based on 1973-77

	INDOMETHACIN			IBUPROFEN		
Year	Observed	Estimated	90% CI	Observed	Estimated	90% CI
1978	122	119	100-141	58	65	32-133
1979	142	142	120-166	70	78	36-137
1980	160	163	138-193	85	91	40-209
1981	172	181	152-216	95	103	44-241
1982	189	195	165-236	110	116	48-279

The rate of voluntary reporting of suspected ADR in the United Kingdom increased sharply by a factor of about three from 1977 onwards[2], and it might be thought this might interfere with the reporting trends estimated at different periods of time. However, as with the two drugs used as examples, individual drugs are not in themselves responsible for the increase, which is an overall effect of the large influx on to the market of many new products between 1976 and 1982, including especially NSAIDs.

IV. USE OF THE METHOD

It cannot be too strongly stressed that log-linear trend analysis is essentially a monitoring and signalling system which does not give any indication of the incidence or prevalence of ADR. Its results cannot therefore be compared directly with those of prospective clinical studies, although it is extremely difficult to carry out such studies in regard to the more severe adverse reactions due to the huge numbers of patients likely to be needed. The method does give an estimate of the concern of prescribing doctors about particular ADRs. The greater the concern, the more consistently will reports be made.

When the method is used to detect a change in trend it must be seen to produce results consistently outside the confidence limits of the previous trend and not to be confined to a single observation.

Table 3 Estimated number of reports of GI haemorrhage or perforation at various prescription totals

	100,000	200,000	500,000	1,000,000	2,000,000
Piroxicam	3	34	64	102	163
Azapropazone	3	7	21	46	102
Ketoprofen	7	11	25	43	75
Diflunisal	14	19	29	41	56
Fenbufen	4	6	13	23	39
Naproxen	3	5	11	19	34
Diclofenac	1	3	6	12	24
Ibuprofen	1	2	4	8	14
Sulindac	3	4	6	9	13
Indomethacin*	≤1	≤1	2	4	9
Flurbiprofen	<1	<1	2	3	4
Phenylbutazone	<1	<1	1	2	4

*Only standard (i.e. non-slow-release dosage forms). Numbers underlined are extrapolated.

A suspicion of a marked upward change necessitates the repetition of testing at shorter intervals, e.g. quarterly, or even monthly if the requisite data are available. Assurance of increased reporting of one drug in comparison with another of the same therapeutic group and for the same ADR should not be claimed unless the appropriate proportions are significantly different at a probability level of at least 1% at several prescription totals. The differences will usually be seen to increase as the totals rise.

V. APPLICATION TO NSAIDs

The method has been applied to the epidemiology of three groups of ADR from various NSAIDs. They are gastrointestinal haemorrhage or perforation (Table 3), aplastic anaemia or agranulocytosis (Table 4) and hepatic ADR (Table 5).

In these tables the calculated ADR cumulative totals at various hypothetical prescription totals are presented to demonstrate constant differences in reporting trends for different adverse reactions and different drugs. Ranking has been done at one prescription level only in each table, i.e. 2 million, 8 million and 3 million, respectively, in order to be able to present the data in logical order. Square brackets have been used to indicate proportions not significantly different from each other. It will be seen that reports are sometimes so few that no consistent trend occurs.

Table 4 Estimated number of reports of serious blood dyscrasias at various prescription totals

	$.5x10^6$	$1x10^6$	$2x10^6$	$3x10^6$	$5x10^6$	$8x10^6$
Phenylbutazone	4	9	16	24	38	59
Naproxen	1	2	5	8	15	26
Piroxicam	0	1	3	6	11	22
Azapropazone	3	5	8	11	16	22
Flurbiprofen	2	3	4	6	8	12
Indomethacin[a]	1	2	3	4	6	8
Ibuprofen	1	1	2	3	4	5
Sulindac[b]	2	4		No reliable trend		
Diclofenac[b]	0	0	3	No reliable trend		
Fenbufen[b]	2	No reliable trend				
Diflunisal[b]	0	0	4	No reliable trend		

[a]All dosage forms included.
Numbers underlined are extrapolated.
[b]Values shown are observed values at very approximate prescription totals.

In such situations it can be concluded either that the reports are not true drug-related adverse reactions or that the reaction is extremely rare.

Table 5 Estimated number of reports of hepatic ADR at various prescription totals

	500,000	100,000	2,000,000	3,000,000
Sulindac	5	14	37	65
Diclofenac	4	9	24	40
Fenbufen	5	10	21	31
Diflunisal	2	4	7	10
Phenylbutazone	1	1	4	9
Piroxicam	2	4	6	8
Indomethacin*	<1	<1	<1	2
Ibuprofen	<1	<1	<1	<1
Flurbiprofen		No trend		
Azapropazone		No trend		
Naproxen		No satisfactory trend		1

* All dosage forms.
Numbers underlined are extrapolated.

REFERENCES

1. Weber, JCP (1984). Epidemiology of adverse reactions to nonsteroidal anti-inflammatory drugs. In: Rainsford, KD and Velo, G (eds), Advances in Inflammation Research, vol 6. (New York: Raven Press), p. 1
2. Spiers, CJ, Griffin, JP, Weber, JCP, Glen-Bott, M and Twomey, C (1984). Demography of the U.K. adverse reactions register of spontaneous reports. Health Trends, No. 3, 16:49
3. Weber, JCP (1986). Mathematical models in adverse drug reaction assessment. In: D'Arcy, PF and Griffin, JP (eds), Iatrogenic Diseases. (London: Oxford University Press) (In press)

Discussion

Anonymous I think you mentioned that there was one drug that caused a lot more ADR's, that didn't fall into the usual logarithmic pattern of the straight line and there were one or 2 drugs that perhaps fell underneath that line.

Dr Weber Well the top drug there as you've probably noticed when the table was up was in fact piroxicam but I can't really add anything to that. I would like to say that in fact what I am describing here is essentially methodology and that if one is in fact going into reasons why, then there are a whole lot of things which have to be taken into consideration which are non-mathematical which involve clinical medicine, pharmacology, philosophy and a number of other things which I suspect that Professor Inman will be talking about later on in the programme.

3
Assessment of adverse reactions to NSAIDs: pre- and post- marketing

EF Barker
Anti-inflammatory Drug Group, Division of Oncology and Radiopharmaceutical Drug Products, Office of Drug Research and Review Center for Drugs and Biologics, Food and Drug Administration, Bethesda, Maryland, USA

CONTENTS

Side-effects of Anti-inflammatory Drugs. Rainsford, KD and Velo, GP (eds)
Part 1: Clinical and Epidemiological Aspects. (Lancaster: MTP Press)

I. INTRODUCTION

The discovery process associated with the introduction of a new drug into medical practice is one of characterizing the effects of the drug in terms of risks and benefits. I discuss here the process of discovering the risks of new drugs, specifically NSAIDs, both pre-marketing and post-marketing, as they have evolved in our group at the FDA (Food and Drug Administration).

The critical assessment of the risks of drugs begins during controlled clinical trials. By the time of approval for marketing in the US, sufficient patients have been studied so that adverse reactions occurring in 1% or more of the patients studied can generally be identified. Notice two important qualifications: one is the patients studied. Their results are applicable to the patient population with the indication for which the drug will be approved, but there have been selection criteria for the studies which make the results directly applicable only to a subset of patients with the indication; generally those patients with classical uncomplicated disease, otherwise in good health and on only a limited number of other drugs. The other important qualification is that only common reactions, i.e. those occurring at 1% and above, can generally be identified with the number of patients studied during the IND/NDA process.

The risks of rarer reactions, and risks to patients with complications of their basic disease or with other conditions, or who are on multiple drugs, are discovered after approval and during extended use by practitioners. During the IND/NDA process the FDA and drug companies are moving towards doing studies in patient populations who, a priori, might be expected to have a higher risk of a reaction. This, however, is usually a confirmatory rather than a discovery stεp in the process.

For this discussion of the pre-approval phase I would like to divide the discussion into two parts. One deals with numerator issues and the other with denominator concerns.

The numerator problems which occur during the IND/NDA process are:

(A) Distinction between "events" and "adverse reactions".
(B) Use of drop-outs for ADRs as equated with "serious" or "significant".
(C) Impact of lack of uniformity in reporting events.
(D) Impact of lack of uniformity in terminology.
(E) Importance of being able to consolidate terms.
(F) Importance of being able to count patients only once.
(G) Importance of being able to link ADRs with other patient data.

II. NUMERATOR CONCERNS

A. Distinction between "events" and "adverse reactions"

The frequency of events is obviously much greater than that of reactions clearly attributable to drug effects. Establishing causal association between the event and the intake of drug is facilitated when there are multiple similar reports and when there is positive rechallenge. Even these considerations may, however, be misleading.

In acute-dose analgesic studies, particularly in postoperative pain, sleepiness/drowsiness/sedation are the most frequently reported events and occur in up to 30% of subjects. These events appear to reflect the level of analgesia rather than drug toxicity despite the fact that they are frequent and recur in the same patients.

Comparison of rates of events reported in the placebo group is critical in assessing whether use of the drug enhances the frequency of background events, or in some terminology "causes" the problem. We do not subtract the placebo rate from the active treatment rate as we feel that the latter reflects more nearly the risks of that particular event in clinical practice, and this is the frequency used in devising the package insert. An interesting facet of acute analgesic studies, is the much higher frequency of headaches in the placebo group than in the active treatment group. This could be interpreted as a direct analgesic effect on headache, or an effect of the drug in lowering the frequency of naturally occurring secondary headaches in painful states.

B. Use of drop-outs for ADRs "serious" or "significant"

It has been usual to use drop-out rates as indicators of serious or significant events. These rates have been useful particularly in comparison of treatment groups, which have been matched on important variables at baseline.

A full and clear description of these events is encouraged, as these descriptions provide an essential basis for assessment of drug-relatedness. However, under the best of circumstances in less than 10% do the reports allow a categorization of "definite" or "remote", and one is left with more than half of the remaining being "possible" and the rest "probable".

C. Lack of uniformity in reporting events

This is an important factor in inter- and intra-study variation. Clear definition of reportable events set forth in the protocol prior to the initiation of the study helps dissipate this frequently uninterpretable source of variation. Large variations found between investigators probably reflect a lack of systematized classification of events rather than differences in the populations at test, or true differences in the frequency of events.

D. Lack of uniformity in terminology

This is an important source of confusion and possible underestimation of risk. The description and definition of dermatological events seems particularly susceptible to this problem. Again clear definition of diagnostic categories would appear essential to ensure more consistency in reporting.

One can underestimate by several-fold the occurrence of a reaction if it is reported under different terms by different investigators. That is why we need to look at reactions across studies to see if the same reaction is being reported under different terms by another investigator.

E. Consolidation of terms

This issue is related to the terminology problem. It may be more of a problem in interpreting non-domestic clinical trials where terms not generally used in the same way are used to describe events. Unless there is clear definition of terms as used in the country of origin, the reports may be confusing rather than helpful. This represents a loss of useful safety data.

Unless the terms used to describe events in both domestic and foreign trials are fully defined, consolidation between trials and investigators is difficult, and specific risks may be underestimated or undetectable.

F. Importance of being able to count patients only once

Different reactions tend to emerge in different time patterns. Some, such as common upper gastrointestinal events, appear early - almost immediately - and may persist throughout drug exposure; others are delayed, such as changes in liver function tests which emerge after 3-4 months of dosing. Still others such as peptic ulcer occur at low but consistent frequency across the duration of exposure.

Subjects who develop dyspepsia usually continue in the study. While they are in the study, dyspepsia, if it persists, is noted at the time of each visit where it will be counted as a new event or emergent symptom at each time point resulting in serious overestimation of this reaction. We feel it important that any single event in any single patient be counted only once.

G. Importance of being able to link ADRs with other patient data

In order to attempt to look for risk factors we need to be able to compare demographic terms; concurrent diseases, concurrent medications, laboratory data, etc. We may request clinical summaries of patients with a particular reaction if the incidence seems unusual in some way. CRF as such are designed for punch key operators; the clinical summaries we request are for physician review.

All of the above need to be available for placebo patients and positive control drugs as well as the new drug which is being reviewed for approval.

III. DENOMINATOR SUBSETS

The denominator considerations during the IND/NDA phase are:

(A) Demographic subsets, i.e. age, sex.
(B) Disease subsets, i.e. indications, other diseases, other medications.
(C) Dosage subsets, i.e. amount, time to first occurrence of ADRs.
(D) Investigator subsets.

A. Demographic subsets

Demographic data are essential to the determination of increased susceptibility of specific patient population groups to drug effects, e.g. nephrotoxic effects of NSAIDs. If it is not possible to assess the impact of demographic subsets, then important risks limited to or occurring predominantly in specific patient groups will be lost or missed. Thus the implication of the observation for the prescriber or drug user will not be articulated.

B. Disease subsets

NSAIDs are currently used and tested in an increasing variety of clinical conditions. Risks associated with use vary not only with the primary indication but also in the presence of coexisting disease and the concurrent use of other medications. This is of special concern in the elderly patient. Up until recently this group has not been considered appropriate or desirable for enrolment in controlled clinical studies, with rigorous entrance criteria. In the US currently we are attempting to specifically study the elderly to see if the normal decrease in renal function and changes in metabolism in general may alter their handling of drugs they are likely to use.

We do not believe that most drugs will be precluded in this population, but rather that the dose will need to be adjusted, and/or that additional precautions, such as ensuring adequate hydration, must be observed. These cautions or restrictions are critical considerations in devising appropriate labels.

C. Dosage subsets

Both the dosage and time to first occurrence of the ADR are important. Some reactions appear clearly dose-dependent and may be mitigated or avoided by clear definition of the appropriate dose. Others are dependent on duration of exposure.

Some, such as acute gastrointestinal ulceration, appear related to neither, and cannot be specifically avoided by lowering the dose and shortening the exposure. There are some NSAIDs with prohibitively narrow therapeutic indices, and these products rarely reach final approval.

D. Investigator subsets

One of the largest sources of variation in the frequency of reports is that occurring between investigators. The inclusion of placebo and positive control treatment groups is essential for reasonable assessment of investigator effect on the rate of reactions. There is investigator difference which is not obviated by clear definition of terms in the protocol, or of the population in the study, but appears related to differences in investigators' perception of events. From such data we define for the package insert an incidence rate for events which appear causally related to treatment.

After a drug is marketed, spontaneous reporting of events is the most important source of new data. This system provides information on rarer, unexpected, events, late or latent events, and reactions specific to population not examined during pre-marketing controlled clinical trials. Factors influencing these reports will be discussed as numerator and denominator factor considerations.

IV. POST-MARKETING NUMERATOR PROBLEMS

The numerator problems which occur after marketing are shown in Table 1, and discussed below.

Table 1 Numerator considerations - post-marketing

(1)	Factors which affect reporting: "Newness" (e.g. Weber curve) Literature reports Package insert Other factors (liability concerns)
(2)	Documentation: Discharge summaries Laboratory reports including normal ranges Unusual features which lead to identification of risk factors
(3)	Problems of getting from terms to cases: Culling out duplicate reports Getting follow-up information

A. Factors which affect reporting

Obviously irregularity of reporting is a major problem. Some factors influencing the rate of reporting are well described.

1. The newness of the drug

We, as well as others (see Chapter 2 by Weber, in this volume), have observed a peaking of reports for the first 2-3 years of marketing, with rather impressive fall-off after this time. We do not think this reflects a change in underlying rate of reactions. The shape of the fall-off curve may vary, and currently for one product the fall-off is much slower than anticipated. It is unclear whether this reflects a true difference in frequency of events for that particular agent or whether it is reflective of the global increase in reports for all agents.

2. Literature reports

It seems clear that initial reports of a new adverse reaction to a drug further stimulate reports if the reaction is drug-related and not rare. There is, however, an initial period after the initial report when it is not clear whether it is "real" or a chance occurrence.

3. Package insert

We feel that listing of reactions in the package insert may inhibit some reports; however this is not all together clear. In the US we have a section in the adverse reaction section which lists uncommon reactions where the causal relationship of the reaction to the drug is not known. We hope this will stimulate reports of "good cases". We only put reactions in this section when we have had a number of reports (more than 7-10) but none are clearly drug-related. Another section of the adverse reaction section lists the uncommon reactions where we will list a reaction if we only have one report with a very good causal relationship, usually a rechallenge. We would like to encourage physicians to send in additional reports on the reactions which are uncertain.

4. Liability concerns

It appears that some physicians, or perhaps their lawyers, feel that reporting a reaction to a drug may decrease the physician's responsibility for the reaction in terms of liability suits. It is not very clear how often this is a factor but it does appear to be increasingly influential.

B. Documentation

Documentation is rarely complete, and in fact is rarely adequate. In a recently prepared summary of data on 767 serious upper gastrointestinal (UGI) cases from the Voluntary Reporting System for 10 approved NSAIDs we found that age was not reported in 32%, sex not reported in 19%, whether or not hospitalization was required was not reported in 41%, history of previous UGI disease unreported in 75%, dose unreported in 33%, duration of treatment in 40%, whether or not other drugs were used in 48%, whether other medical conditions were present were unreported in 68%.

Lack of adequate documentation limits the usefulness of the

report and hinders identification of underlying risk factors or detection of features unique to the patient or that reaction.

C. Problems of getting from terms to cases

We find it essential to cull out duplicate reports, probably the most persistent cause of misinterpretation; an essential task which is tedious and unrewarding. This is intimately associated with the previous category of documentation. Poor documentation of cases, particularly absence of basic demographic data, prevents elimination of reports which are duplicated or even in triplicate. Follow-up information is rarely provided so final outcome, except in fatal cases, is usually unknown.

V. DENOMINATOR PROBLEMS

Finally, the post-marketing denominator problems are shown in Table 2, and discussed below.

Table 2 Denominator considerations - post marketing

(1)	What to use, i.e. total prescriptions, new prescriptions, patients exposed, patient days of exposure
(2)	What to compare, i.e. relative rates, relative percentages of specific reactions to all reported reactions

A. Which to use

It is clear that when frequencies of ADRs are tabulated by any system wide variations can occur depending on the denominator chosen, e.g. there may be different rates for new prescriptions, compared to rates for patient days of exposure. It is unclear which rates of reactions most closely express the risk to a patient on treatment. Possibly they are each of interest and the risks attendant upon use of a drug vary under different circumstances. We tend to look at the effect of different denominators as part of our effort to understand the data.

B. What to compare

Relative rates have been the rates most commonly used up until now, and they are those generated by most systems. Variations in rates in different studies commonly reflect variations in the denominators chosen, rather than real differences.

The post-marketing voluntary reporting system has weaknesses which are unappealing to epidemiologists, and they are exploring other databases, like large HMOs and state Medicaid databases. They agree voluntary reporting is good for generating signals of potential problems but they feel it is not very good for trying to analyze or understand them. So far, however, with few exceptions, whenever we in the FDA have a problem to solve, our most useful database - not only for signalling but for understanding the signal - has been the individual cases physicians have reported to us. Its great strength is that it covers the entire population of use, and presents a reasonable sample of that use.

This has been an overview of what we are doing today in the risk assessment of NSAIDs and an overview of some of the limitations of the systems. It is felt that the state of the art in ADR evaluation is not as good as efficacy evaluation, but that it is evolving rapidly. We hope the system will become increasingly more focused, but there is a lack of clear definitions and the meaning of the data is occasionally unclear, the true incidence or true relative risk continue to be elusive. We feel that public and professional interest and concern will inevitably compel further refinements in both the pre-marketing and post-marketing assessments.

Discussion

Dr A Herxheimer, UK I think there's one point in your denominator consideration which might be added and that is the protocol subsets, because there are possibilities for different protocols for studying a drug listed in an adverse reaction which could be quite different when you rely on spontaneous reports or ask direct questions and so on, so I would add that as a 5th point on your slide.

Dr Barker I'm sorry, I don't understand what you wanted me to do.

Dr Herxheimer Add to your slide of denominator considerations.

Dr Barker Oh yes, clearly, yes, the experimental model in which the drug is tested will to some extent determine those ulcer incidences.

Dr Herxheimer I don't mean the experimental model, I mean the method by which the adverse reactions is elicited.

Dr Barker But even with the same method there will be enormous variations and in the most recent NSAID's that we reviewed, there was a common protocol for the assessment of adverse reactions. Multi-investigator trials with a relatively small number of investigators and the rate of reporting of upper GI reactions varied between investigators from 5% to 90% with a common protocol.

Dr M Znaminowska, Canada One of your denominator considerations you said, is that each patient should be only counted once for each adverse affect. Would you enlarge on it? I would have a problem with this I think. One given adverse reaction reported at different times of a time frame, if it was in the study would, I think, perhaps have a different meaning. Also one symptom can represent many syndromes. I would have a problem with this as a general rule.

Dr Barker We made certain decisions to do things in certain ways, because we thought they gave us the best estimate of risks to individual patients. This grew out of the observation that many patients who are subjects in studies, develop particularly relatively mild GI effects early on, but they're not severe enough to drop out of the study. They can continue in the study with a low level (nausea, dyspepsia). It seemed unwise for us to count this as a new case or new emergence syndrome symptom at each time point. That is why we're trying to count each patient only once.

Dr Znaminowska What if you had the same side-effect reported with increasing severity?

Dr Barker If that happened they usually drop out of the study, and we do consider those as much more indicative of serious events. What happened was, our system was being overloaded with mild reactions which did not inhibit subjects continuing in the trials.

Dr Bernard, USA Dr Barker, how do you account for the side-effects that may occur in patients in clinical trials before they receive the clinical drugs in these trials?

Dr Barker Do you mean the reactions which may occur in the placebo?

Dr Bernard Dr Ridenberg once described adverse - non drug reactions and often in our clinical trials we do not account for those mild side-effects which we attribute to those drugs only after they've been received in the clinical trial, because we don't document them at base line. How can we better account for them before we attribute them to drug exposure?

Dr Barker I really don't know. The use of comparison treatment groups is the most useful way, but they are often misleading as I think I described in the beginning, particularly for secondary background phenomenon. Disease subsets are going to elicit certain number of background events which may be counted as adverse reactions separating them from those events from what are due to drugs is clearly difficult. The placebo group is one that is most commonly used to separate the difference.

4
Incidence of serious side-effects from non-steroidal anti-inflammatory drugs (NSAIDs) in the USA

H Jick
Boston Collaborative Drug Surveillance Program, Boston University Medical Center, Boston, USA

CONTENTS

I. INTRODUCTION

Any discussion of the problem of toxicity from NSAIDs should be viewed in the context of the use of drugs in general and NSAIDs in particular. Excluding for the moment aspirin, which is still probably the most extensively used NSAID, it is apparent from available data that the use of NSAIDs is enormous. There is little doubt that tens of millions of people in the world use these drugs every day.

According to available information over 750 million dollars was spent on analgesics obtained from drug stores and hospitals in the USA in 1982. Close to 19 million prescriptions were filled for ibuprofen alone. Information available to the BCDSP from Group Health Cooperative (GHC) of Puget Sound, a health maintenance

Side-effects of Anti-inflammatory Drugs. Rainsford, KD & Velo, GP (eds)
Part 1: Clinical and Epidemiological Aspects. (Lancaster: MTP Press)

organization in Seattle, Washington, with about 280,000 members, shows that 82% of all members filled at least one prescription at a local GHC pharmacy in 1981 and the average number of prescriptions filled per member was 7.5. In 1981 alone, there were over 18,000 prescriptions filled for indomethacin, over 12,000 for phenylbutazone, over 22,000 for ibuprofen, over 10,000 for aspirin-containing drugs and thousands for the newer NSAIDs.

It is against the background of the massive exposure to these drugs that the problem of serious NSAID-induced illness must be evaluated.

II. EVALUATION OF NSAID-INDUCED SIDE-EFFECTS

Well-documented case reports leave little doubt that NSAIDs can cause a large variety of serious illnesses including liver, kidney, bone marrow, skin and CNS disease[1-35]. In addition, severe allergic reactions to NSAIDs have been well documented[28]. The critical question is thus not whether serious toxicity can be caused by NSAIDs, but rather how often each NSAID causes them.

The answer to this question requires formal studies which are able to quantify risks on a drug-specific basis. The method which is best suited to accomplish this task is the follow-up or cohort study. In such a study a group of people who are exposed to particular drugs are followed up after first receipt of the drug(s) to determine the frequency of occurrence of certain adverse effects. In some instances a comparable group of people who do not use the drug(s) under study are also followed up. It is possible, in principle, to obtain from such studies risks for certain illnesses attributable to a particular drug.

When adverse effects are reasonably common and the effect occurs shortly after a drug is started, follow-up studies are feasible and many such studies have been reported[36].

On the other hand, for most commonly used drugs, the risk of serious drug-induced disease is very low and quantification of risk would require the follow-up of very large numbers of users. The problem is compounded if the drug-induced illness occurs only after chronic use, since the cohort study would have to continue for years.

Considering the expense and difficulties involved in performing long-term cohort studies of the many drugs of interest, it is not surprising that until recently, when a major technological advance has occurred, few long-term follow-up studies of users of particular drugs have been performed and quantification of serious adverse effects of NSAIDs have not been available.

III. NEW DEVELOPMENTS

Recently, a major new development has provided for a remarkable advance in our ability to quantify the problem of drug-induced illnesses caused by NSAIDs as well as other drugs. This development relates to the availability of large automated databases which include information on all outpatient drug exposures and hospitalizations in large defined populations. Such databases already exist in the US Medicare-Medicaid systems, in various health maintenance organizations, in the province of Saskatchewan and elsewhere. Under proper conditions they provide for the long-term follow-up study of many drugs at relatively low cost.

A. Puget sound studies

Our research group has for many years been utilizing information from Group Health Cooperative of Puget Sound (GHC), a consumer-owned health maintenance organization in Seattle, Washington, founded in 1947[37]. GHC currently serves more than 300,000 people in western Washington. The plan provides comprehensive prepaid medical coverage for outpatient care, drugs and hospital services. Between 1976 and 1982 about 90% of prescriptions were filled at no charge. Among the remainder, some were provided at a reduced cost or at the cost prevailing in the local community. Over-the-counter drugs are available at the pharmacies and are dispensed after receipt of a prescription. Members are admitted to hospitals maintained by the cooperative in the Seattle area[37].

1. Methodology

Information on all discharges from GHC hospitals has been recorded and placed on computer files by the Commission on Professional and Hospital Activities-Professional Activity Study (CPHA-PAS) in Ann Arbor, Michigan, since 1972. This information includes hospital discharge diagnoses, surgical procedures performed and routine demographic data. The CPHA-PAS records provide for ready identification of persons with particular illnesses. As of the end of 1983 there was information on over 300,000 GHC hospitalizations recorded on computer files.

In July 1975 the cooperative began to computerize records of all prescriptions filled in its regional outpatient pharmacies. This process was completed by 1 July 1976. Of some 1000 women interviewed in previous studies of this population, 98% stated that they routinely used the GHC pharmacies to fill their prescriptions[2-4]. In 1981, 82% of members filled at least one prescription at local GHC pharmacies. Over 50% of members filled at least one prescription for an over-the-counter drug during 1981. Thus, the drug-use records (which includes dates, dosage and number of dosage units dispensed) of virtually all members are accessible in machine-readable form and can be linked readily to hospitalization data. As of the end of 1983 over 10 million original prescriptions had been recorded in the computer files. Based upon review of the original clinical records and interview of members we have found this information to be highly accurate.

The Group Health resource has the critical advantage that clinical records are readily available so that the details of each case history may be easily obtained and reviewed. This is particularly important in studies of certain rare drug-induced illnesses since discharge diagnoses alone are insufficient to determine the nature of the disease present in a given individual.

We have completed and published a number of follow-up studies of NSAIDs utilizing the GHC resource[38-40]. The sizes of the cohorts of NSAID users have varied a bit from study to study, but they generally encompass more than 40,000 people who received phenylbutazone, more than 30,000 who received indomethacin, more than 20,000 who received ibuprofen and many thousands who used some of the the newer NSAIDs.

2. Principal findings

We have identified no recipients of these drugs who developed NSAID-attributable renal disease[38] or blood disorders[39] serious enough to require hospitalization. Hospitalization for stomach bleeding (in people under 65 years of age) has been rare[40]; the maximum attributable risk we estimate to be less than one per million person-days at risk.

In other reviews of the GHC data resource we have found no hospitalizations for Stevens-Johnson syndrome or anaphylaxis among NSAID users. We are currently reviewing the data for cases of drug-induced liver disease requiring hospitalization and have as yet found no cases attributable to NSAIDs.

Based on the experience at GHC we have concluded that serious toxicity caused by NSAIDs (other than aspirin) is quite uncommon. There are a number of important caveats to this conclusion. The most important is that our experience with many of the newer NSAIDs is thus far relatively small, and we do know that rates for certain drug-induced illnesses vary among the different NSAIDs. We shall continue to examine the data from GHC with great interest as the experience with the newer NSAIDs becomes larger.

It should also be emphasized that our results apply to illnesses which require hospitalization. Those which are treated out of hospital would be missed, and the extent of this problem is unknown to us.

We have completed studies relating to aspirin which involved other data resources available to us[41,42]. These studies have indicated that gastric bleeding serious enough to cause hospitalization in persons with no prior history of upper gastrointestinal disease is attributable to daily aspirin use at an annual rate of about 15 per 100,000 daily users. The rate of gastric ulcer attributable to daily aspirin use in this study was 10 per 100,000 person-years at risk.

Finally we have reported on observational studies of the relation of regular aspirin use to hospitalization for acute myocardial infarction[42]. These studies revealed a strong negative association between the two.

IV. CONCLUSIONS

In summary, it is well documented that NSAIDs can cause serious illness. At the same time, the use of these drugs is very large.

Experience from a health maintenance organization in Seattle, Washington, USA, indicates that NSAID-caused serious illness is quite rare among users of the drugs prescribed there.

REFERENCES

1. Buscaglia AJ, et al. (1984). Pulmonary infiltrates associated with naproxen. J Am Med Assoc, 251, 65
2. Quinn, JP (1984). Eosinophilic meningitis and ibuprofen therapy. Neurology, 34, 108
3. Klein, SM and Khan, MA (1983). Hepatitis, toxic epidermal necrolysis and pancreatitis in association with sulindac therapy. J Rheumatol, 10, 512
4. Heymann, WR et al. (1984). Naproxen-induced lichen planus. J Am Acad Dermatol, 10, 299
5. Baker, LRI et al. (1984). Mefenamic acid-induced interstitial nephritis and renal failure. Postgrad Med J, 60, 82
6. Whittaker, SJ et al. (1982). Case report. Sulindac hepatotoxicity. Gut, 23, 875
7. Boike, SC et al. (1983). Zomepirac-related acute renal failure. Drug Intell Clin Pharmacol, 17, 56
8. Warren, SE and Mosley, C (1983). Zomepirac-associated renal failure and tubular dysfunction. J Am Med Assoc, 249, 396
9. Nader, DI and Schillaci, RF (1983). Pulmonary infiltrates with eosinophilia due to naproxen. Chest, 83, 280
10. Thomsen, BS and From, A (1983). Acute renal failure possibly associated with fenoprofen therapy. Arthritis Rheum, 26, 234
11. O'Sullivan, M et al. (1983). A case of toxic epidermal necrolysis secondary to indomethacin. Br J Rheumatol, 22, 47
12. Schwartz, JI and Maura, RJ (1983). Severe depersonalization and anxiety associated with indomethacin. South Med J 76, 679
13. Whelton, A et al. (1983). Sulindac and renal impairment. J Am Med Assoc, 249, 2892
14. Frais, MA et al. (1983). Piroxicam-induced renal failure and hyperkalemia. Ann Intern Med, 999, 129
15. Hughes, JA and Sudell, W (1983). Hemolytic anemia associated with naproxen. Arthritis Rheum, 26, 1054
16. Martin, RL et al. (1983). Fatal pemphigus vulgaris in a patient taking piroxicam. N Engl J Med, 309, 795
17. Lee, RP et al. (1983). Ibuprofen: a severe systemic reaction. Can Med Assoc J, 129, 854
18. Kapoor, A (1983). Reversible gynecomastia associated with sulindac therapy. J Am Med Assoc, 252, 2284
19. Hall, RI et al. (1983). Enteritis and colitis associated with mefenamic acid. Br Med J, 287, 1182
20. Hamburger, J and Potts, AJC (1983). Non-steroidal anti-inflammatory drugs and oral lichenoid reactions. Br Med J, 287, 1258
21. Sprung, DJ (1982). Sulindac causing a hypersensitivity reaction with peripheral and mediastinal lymphadenopathy. Ann Intern Med, 97, 564
22. Mease, PJ et al. (1982). Zomepirac, interstitial nephritis and renal failure. Ann Intern Med, 97,454
23. Hynd, R et al. (1982). Neutropenia and pseudomonas septicemia after sulindac therapy: case report. Military Med 147, 768

24. Lockhart, JM (1982). Tolmetin-induced thrombocytopenia. Arthritis Rheum, 25, 1144
25. Ford MJ, and Prescott, LF (1982). Phenylbutazone pericarditis. Scot Med J, 27, 252
26. Asherov, J et al. (1982). Diplopia following ibuprofen administration. J Am Med Assoc, 248, 649
27. Memon, AN (1982). Pancreatitis and sulindac. Ann Intern Med, 97, 139
28. Driver, PS et al. (1982). Anaphylactic-like reactions to zomepirac. Drug Intell Clin Pharmacol, 16, 616
29. Giroux, Y et al. (1982). Cholestatic jaundice caused by sulindac. Can J Surg, 25, 334
30. Ashraf, M et al. (1982). Aplastic anemia associated with fenoprofen. Br Med J, 284, 1301
31. Aaron TH and Muttitt ELC (1982). Reactions to acetylsalicylic acid. Can Med Assoc J, 126, 609-611
32. Schimizzi, GF et al. (1982). Severe reversible thrombocytopenia associated with meclofenamate. Arthritis Rheum, 25, 359
33. Goebel, KM and Mueller-Brodman, W (1982). Reversible overt nephropathy with Henoch-Schonlein purpura due to piroxicam. Br Med J, 284, 311
34. Ballas, ZK and Danta, SJ (1982). Sulindac-induced aseptic meningitis. Arch Intern Med 142, 165
35. Gabrielson, TO et al. (1981). Drug-induced bullous dermatosis with linear IgA deposits along the basement membrane. Acta Dermatovenes, 61, 439
36. Cohen, MR (1977). A compilation of abstracts and an index of articles published by the Boston Collaborative Drug Surveillance Program. Hospital Pharmacy, 12, 455
37. Jick, H, Madsen, S, Nudelman, PM, Perera, DR and Stergachis, A (1984). Postmarketing follow-up at Group Health Cooperative of Puget Sound. Pharmacotherapy, 4, 99
38. Fox, DA and Jick, H (1984). Nonsteroidal anti-inflammatory drugs and renal disease. J Am Med Assoc, 251, 1299
39. Danielson, DA, Douglas, SW III, Herzog, P, Jick, H and Porter, JB (1984). Drug-induced blood disorders. J Am Med Assoc, 252, 3257
40. Jick, H, Feld, AD and Perera, DR (1986). Certain nonsteroidal anti-inflammatory drugs and hospitalization for upper gastrointestinal bleeding. Pharmacotherapy (In press)
41. Levy, M (1974). Aspirin use in patients with major upper gastrointestinal bleeding and peptic-ulcer disease. A report from the Boston Collaborative Drug Surveillance Program, Boston University Medical Center. N Engl J Med, 290, 1158
42. Jick, H and Miettinen, OS (1976). Regular aspirin use and myocardial infarction. Br Med J, 1, 1057

Discussion

Dr G Ehrlich, USA You have interesting data and I think also with the combination of the first 3 papers and perhaps that to be continued by Prof O'Brien later, they point up one of the quanderies we're facing, because first of all we're dealing with numbers here. Now you're dealing with the patients in an HMO who, it could be argued, are being treated better or being surveyed better or at least attract a group of people who are less likely to develop problems. They certainly don't tell us about the person who is admitted to Belview - the alcoholics and people of this sort, who probably are at greater risk. Second of all, given that you have a special population, they are beginning to point to the individual, the rare individual, who develops special problems and I think that's the one we need to know. When June Frese and I did a book on prognoses we found that it was extremely easy to develop prognostic criteria for populations. It was extremely difficult to extrapolate from this for the risk of a particular person and obviously it's much more important to know which one is going to develop meningitis, which one is going to develop the eosinophilic pulmonary disease, which one is going to develop the rare blood dyscrasia even if these don't show up in the total numbers and they still don't point us to the individual at risk which is after all what we are ultimately going to be after.

Prof Jick Right George, this gives me an opportunity to say something that I've said at least 5000 times!!!! before, this will be 5001!!!!, and I hope you all appreciate that the state of knowledge in the adverse reaction area is really rudimentary at best. We have primarily relied on spontaneous reports in the past, and we all know the limitations of that. It's our objective in these studies and I think one we really have to keep in mind, if we're not going to make a lot of mistakes and waste a lot of money. What we're trying to do is advance the state of knowledge a bit beyond where we are to start with, which is very low indeed and we are beginning to presume to answer all questions for all men. My guess, if you wanted a guess, was for the 1 in 100,000 persons who has been unlucky enough to get a blood disorder through some drug there is no way anyone is going to be able to predict that. What we're trying to do is to provide a framework in which these matters can be looked at in a formal sense where some reasonable quantification begins to become available and can be believed and interpreted by individuals who are very concerned in this area. So our objectives are really quite limited, George, and we hope that we are helping our little bit to push us forward somewhat, toward the great Heaven where all information and all truth is known.

5
Trends and patterns in adverse drug reactions to non-steroidal anti-inflammatory drugs reported in Sweden

BE Wiholm*,, M Myrhed* and E Ekman***
*Department of Drugs, National Board of Health and Welfare, Uppsala, Sweden
**Department of Clinical Pharmacology, Karolinska Institute, Huddinge Hospital, Huddinge, Sweden

CONTENTS

I. INTRODUCTION

Adverse reactions (ADRs) from analgesics have since many years been of concern to drug regulatory agencies. This is partly due to their widespread use. In Sweden the total sales of non-narcotic analgesics ammounts of 240 million so called defined daily doses (DDD) per year which is sufficient for a continuous treatment of 7 to 8% of the population (Figure 1).

During the last few years a substantial number of new non-steroidal anti-inflammatory drugs (NSAIDs) have been introduced internationally, some of which e.g. benoxaprofen and zomepirac rather quickly had to leave the market because of alleged serious adverse effects. Most of these drugs were never approved for marketing in Sweden. Still the number of NSAIDs (excluding salicylates) has increased from three to ten during the last 15 years and their use has also been tripled (Figure 2). The grounds for the withdrawal of benoxaprofen and zomepirac have been questioned and it has been implied that they were based on

Side-effects of Anti-inflammatory Drugs. Rainsford, KD and Velo, GP (eds)
Part 1: Clinical and Epidemiological Aspects. (Lancaster: MTP Press)

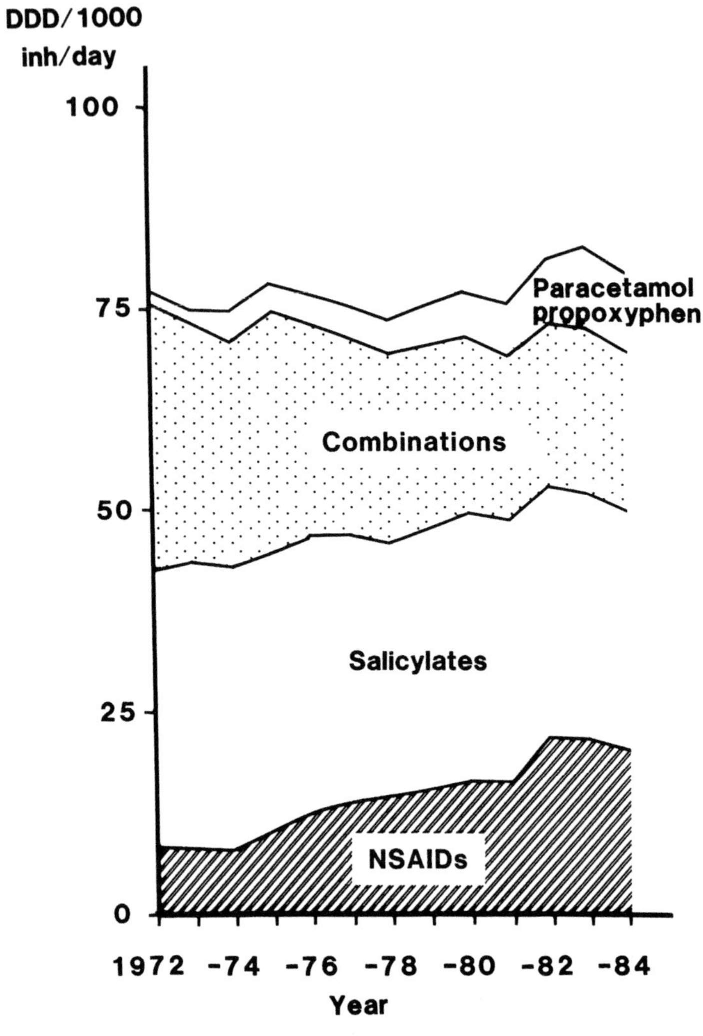

Figure 1 Sales of non-narcotic analgesic drugs in Sweden expressed as the number of defined daily doses per 1000 inhabitants per day.

the number rather than the incidence of ADRs[1]. In Sweden, drug consumption can be established from several sources, which can be used as indirect estimates of the exposed population. Under certain conditions it is therefore possible to get relatively good estimates of the incidence of reported ADRs.

Here we present trends and patterns of ADRs reported for NSAIDs in relation to sales and prescription data. The salicylates are not considered and the presentation is confined to preparations registered in Sweden (Table 1).

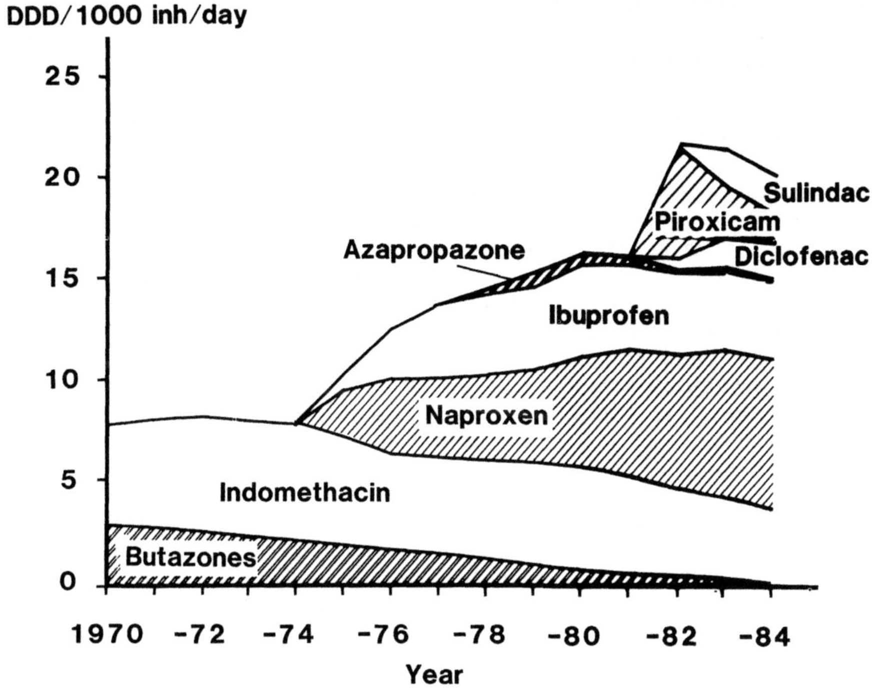

Figure 2 Sales of non-steroidal anti-inflammatory drugs excluding salicylates in Sweden expressed as the number of defined daily doses per 1000 inhabitants per day. The total sales in 1984 was sufficient for the contir.uous treatment of 2% of the population (166,000 patients).

Table 1 Non-steroidal anti-inflammatory drugs available in Sweden

Generic name	Year of first licence	Defined daily dose (DDD) (mg)
Phenylbutazone	Feb 1956	300
Oxyphenbutazone[a]	Sep 1963	300
Indomethacin	May 1965	100
Ibuprofen	Mar 1975	800
Naproxen	Mar 1975	500
Azapropazone	Jan 1978	750
Diclofenac	Dec 1981	100
Piroxicam	Dec 1981	20
Sulindac	Oct 1982	200

[a] oxyphenbutazone was withdrawn from the market by the manufacturer in July 1984

II. MATERIALS AND METHODS

A. Adverse reactions

In Sweden, a system for the monitoring of spontaneous reports of ADRs was set up in 1965, and is now a part of the Department of Drugs of the National Board of Health and Welfare. The ADR Section is since 1985 operated by three physicians, two pharmacists and an assistant. The senior physician is also secretary of the Swedish Adverse Drug Reactions Advisory Committee (SADRAC) which is chaired by the Head of the Department of Drugs and which has several clinical specialists appointed.

For the first 10 years reporting was voluntary, but from 1975 it has been compulsory to report suspected reactions that are fatal or otherwise serious as well as new and unexpected reactions.

There is a special form for reporting but letters and copies of medical records are also accepted. For most of the serious cases and all the fatal ones complete copies of the full medical case records, laboratory investigations etc. are requested.

A preliminary evaluation of the cause-effect relationship is made by the physicians of the ADR section. This classification is further discussed by a working party of SADRAC on a monthly basis and finally settled by the full Committee which meet quarterly. In this presentation only reactions which have been classified as having a possible or probable causal relationship by SADRAC are considered.

B. Drug sales and prescription registers

For an evaluation of the risk/benefit ratio of drugs it is also important to know to what extent different drugs are used, on what indications and to whom they are prescribed. During the last ten-year period various drug-oriented registers have been established which are useful in providing these important background data.

C. Wholesale level

Total drug sales statistics are available since 1965 and computerized since 1972. These statistics show the total amount of every drug sold from each pharmacy and can be expressed in volume, monetary terms or so called defined daily doses (DDD). The DDD is a technical unit of measurement and equals the estimated average daily dose for grown ups when the drug is used on its main indication[2]. The number of DDDs sold per 1000 inhabitants per day is a useful but gross measure of drug consumption in the population. For comparisons with ADRs the total number of DDDs (in millions) per year is a more appropriate measure. The DDDs for the drugs considered in this presentation are shown in Table 1.

D. Prescription level

Since 1974 a random sample of 1/288 prescriptions is picked out in the pharmacies. Information about age and sex of the patient, the name, amount and daily dosage of the drug is coded and computerized. From this survey the average or median prescribed daily dose can be calculated by age and sex. The number of prescriptions per 1000 inhabitants and year is used as an estimate of the prescribing pressure on the population.

Since 1978 the Diagnosis and Therapy Survey has been run in collaboration between the drug industry, the National Corporation of Swedish Pharmacies, the Swedish Medical Association and the National Board of Health and Welfare. In this survey a random sample of physicians each week register all prescriptions on special forms which also state the indication for each drug treatment. Data from these three registers are published annually[3].

III. RESULTS

A. Number of reports

The annual number of ADR reports has gradually increased from 160 in 1965 to 2800 in 1984. The number of reports concerning NSAIDs has increased stepwise with the introduction of new products on the market (Figure 3). In 1982 there was a remarkable increase up to 300 reports when diclofenac, piroxicam and sulindac were introduced. The majority of these reports concerned gastrointestinal problems and skin reactions to piroxicam. In that year NSAIDs accounted for 15% of all reports in contrast to a previous average of 4-7%. Up to 1985 a total of 1855 reports of adverse reactions to NSAIDs have been received by SADRAC. The number of reports to the different substances between 1970-84 are shown in Table 2.

Table 2 Number of reports and adverse reactions with a possible or probable association to NSAIDs in Sweden since 1970[a]

	Period	Number of Reports	Number of Reactions	Number of Fatal cases
Phenylbutazone	1970-84	133	177	6
Oxyphenbutazone	1970-84	308	441	6
Indomethacin	1970-84	290	368	16
Naproxen	1975-84	227	291	2
Ibuprofen	1975-84	160	192	3
Azapropazone	1978-84	98	124	1
Diclofenac	1982-84	70	92	1
Piroxicam	1982-84	322	388	2
Sulindac	1982-84	110	154	1
Total[b]		1691		38

[a] This time period was chosen because sales data for the corresponding years were available

[b] This is less than the sum of all the above because in some cases more than one preparation had a possible causal relation

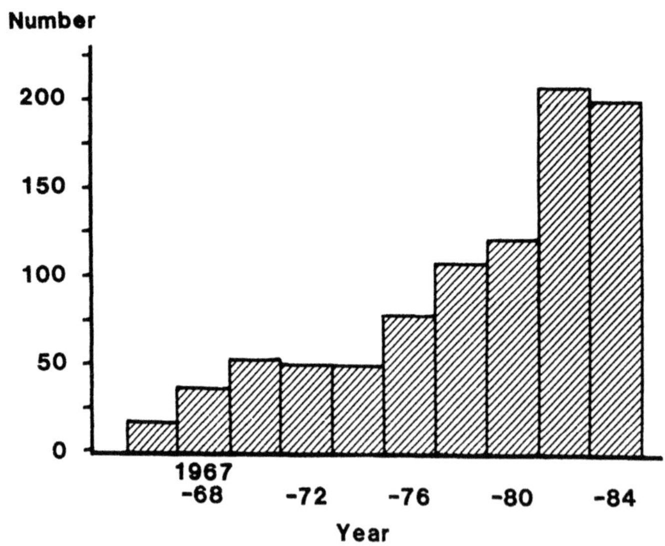

Figure 3 Number of reports of suspected adverse reactions to NSAIDs in Sweden 1965-84. The drugs concerned are those shown in Table 1. To decrease chance fluctuations the average number for two years are shown, e.g. 1965 +1966 etc.

B. **Adverse reaction profiles**

Fig.4(a)

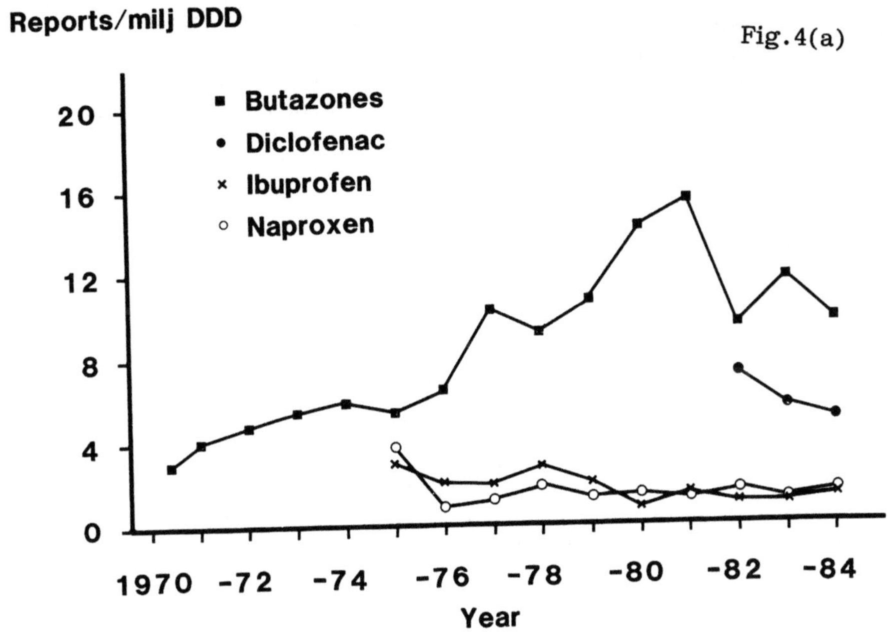

Fig.4(b)

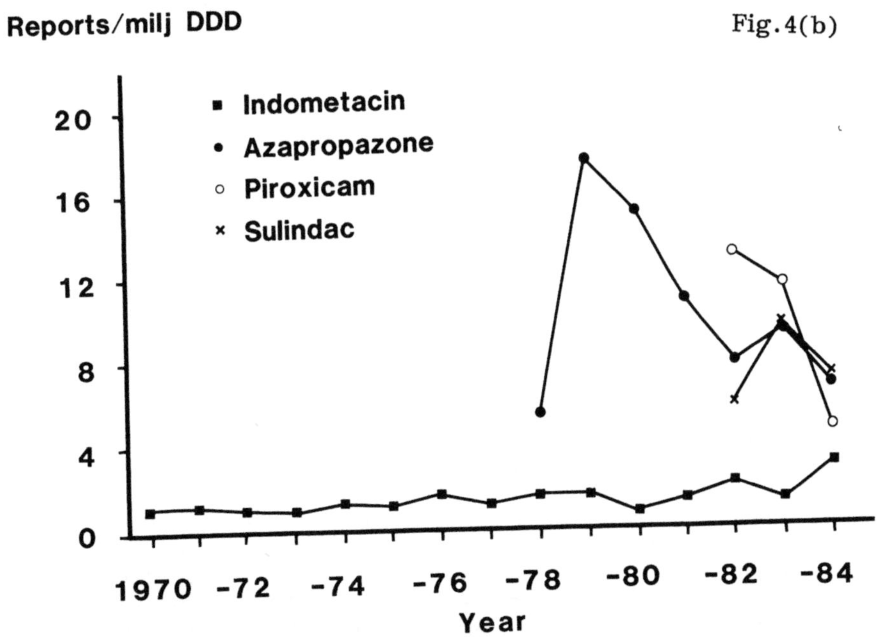

Figure 4(a & b) The pattern of adverse reactions by system organ classes reported to NSAIDs in Sweden 1970-84.

The patterns of reactions reported for the different NSAIDs have some features in common e.g. gastrointestinal ulcers which probably depend on a common mechanism of action, and skin reactions some of which - like photosensitivity might be related to physiochemical properties of the drugs. More interestingly there are distinct differences in the ADR-profiles between the different NSAIDs (Figure 4(a,b)). For the oldest products the butazones (phenylbutazone, oxyphenbutazone) sialoadenitis (n=68) and parotitis (n=66) seems to be a special feature. Pancreatitis has also been reported to be connected to the butazones in 15 out of 16 cases.

The highest proportion of blood dyscrasias is reported for indomethacin, the butazones and naproxen but severe reactions like pancytopenia and aplastic anaemia constitutes a higher percentage of the blood dyscrasias reported for the butazones than for the others. For indomethacin, CNS-reactions (28%) are prominent. Confusion in elderly patients dominates (33 cases) but there are also reports describing hallucinations (n=6), psychotic reactions (n=4) and epileptic convulsions (n=5).

Reports of visual disturbances including reversible decreases in visual acuity and asthmatic reactions stand out in the profile reported for ibuprofen; skin reactions - especially photosensitivity - for azapropazone and hepatic reactions for sulindac.

As previously mentioned gastrointestinal reactions are a prominent feature in the profile of all the NSAIDs but especially so for piroxicam. This is especially true for gastric and duodenal ulcers, which will be analysed in detail below. Ulcers and perforations in the lower intestinal tract however has almost exclusively been reported to occur during indomethacin treatment.

Other rare reactions reported for the NSAIDs have been eosinophilic pneumonia 16 (butazones 15), vasculitis 8, and exacerbation of systemic lupus erytomatodes 3. Ulcerative colitis has also been reported to have been activated or triggered off by NSAID treatment in rare cases. In 3 out of a total of 5 cases indomethacin has been suspected.

C. ADRs in relation to sales and prescriptions

The incidence of adverse reaction reports in relation to the sales varies markedly both between the different drugs and over time (Figure 5a, b). For the butazones there was a steady increase in reported incidence from 1970-1981, which is in contrast to that for indomethacin, naproxen and ibuprofen. This may partly be explained by frequent discussions about phenylbutazone and oxyphenbutazone associated ADRs in Sweden.

For the newer drugs the general level of reporting seems to be higher than for the older ones (except the butazones). There are also more or less pronounced peaks in the reported incidence during the first or second year of marketing. Such phenomena make overall comparisons between different drugs difficult to evaluate. The average incidence of all reports between 1975-84 varies between 1.4 and 15.2 per million DDD which correspond to 0.5-5.6 per 1000 patient years if the DDD is assumed to be correct

(Table 3). This low incidence mainly reflects a vast under-reporting of minor reactions. For severe and potentially life threatening reactions under-reporting is probably less prominent.

Table 3 Reported incidence of adverse reactions to non-steroidal anti-inflammatory drugs in Sweden

	Total number of reports per		
Generic name (time period)	DDD x 10^6	1000 DDD years	100,000 prescriptions
Phenylbutazone (1975[a]-84)	5.1	1.9	6
Oxyphenbutazone (1975-84)	15.2	5.6	22
Indomethacin (1975-84)	1.4	0.5	6
Naproxen (1975-84)	1.4	0.5	9
Ibuprofen (1975-84)	1.5	0.6	11
Azapropazone (1978-84)	12.7	4.6	67
Diclofenac (1982-84)	5.5	2.0	24
Piroxicam (1982-84)	11.2	4.1	69
Sulindac (1982-84)	8.2	3.0	85

[a] Time period limited by availability of prescription data

Table 4 Reported incidence of liver reactions in Sweden

Generic name	Time period	Number of reports	Incidence per 100,000 DDD years
Sulindac	1982-84	25	75
Oxyphenbutazone	1970-84	30	37
Diclofenac	1982-84	10	30
Azapropazone	1978-84	4	19
Phenylbutazone	1970-84	18	18
Piroxicam	1982-84	8	10
Indomethacin	1970-84	30	5
Naproxen	1975-84	18	4
Ibuprofen	1975-84	6	2

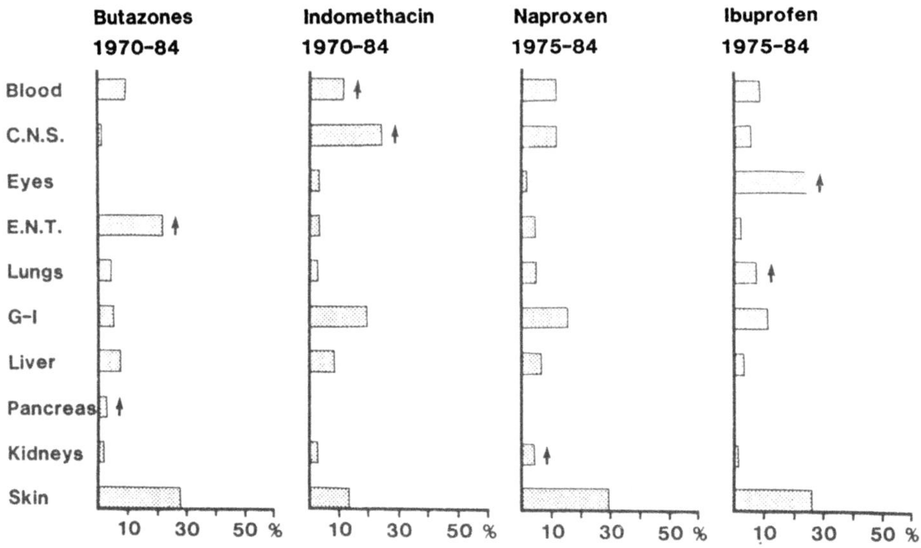

Figure 5(a) Number of reports of adverse drug reactions from NSAIDs per million defined daily doses (DDD) sold in Sweden (1970-84): butazones (phenylbutazones + oxyphenbutazone), diclofenac, ibuprofen, naproxen

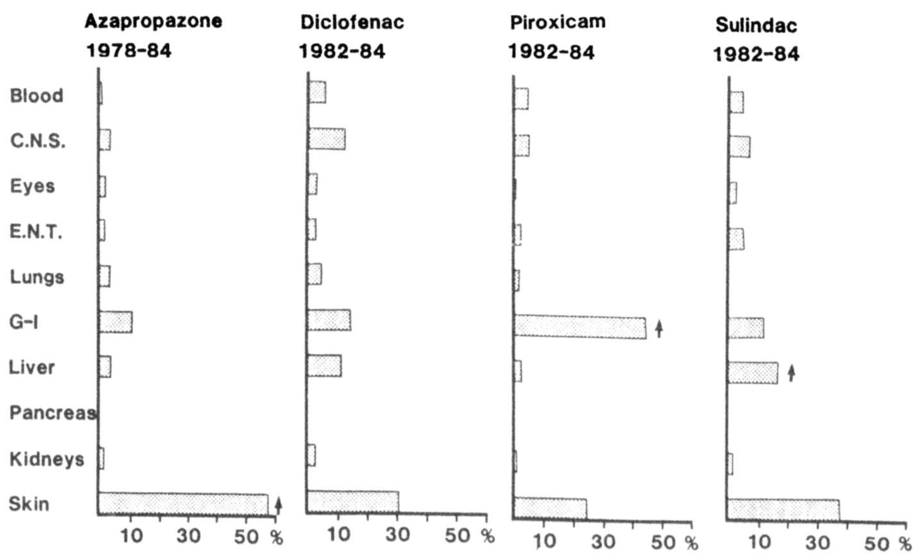

Figure 5(b) Indomethacin, azapropazone, sulindac, piroxicam.

Sulindac has the highest incidence of reported liver reactions with 75 cases per 100,000 treatment years (Table 4). This may be connected to the fact that sulindac is a pro-drug which undergoes pharmacodynamic activation during its metabolism and that there is extensive enterohepatic recirculation.

The Stevens-Johnson syndrome and toxic epidermal necrolysis are very rare but severe skin reactions which occur in about 10 cases per million inhabitants per year in Sweden. Oxyphenbutazone has the highest reported incidence with 21 cases per 100,000 treatment years (Table 5). Also sulindac, phenylbutazone and piroxicam may increase the risk for these diseases while the reported incidence for naproxen, indomethacin and ibuprofen are close to the spontaneous incidence.

Table 5 Reported incidence of the Stevens-Johnson's syndrome and toxic epidermal necrolysis in Sweden

Generic name	Time period	Number of reports	Incidence per 100,000 DDD years
Oxyphenbutazone	1970-84	17	21
Sulindac	1982-84	3	9
Phenylbutazone	1970-84	7	7
Piroxicam	1982-84	3	4
Naproxen	1975-84	5	1
Indomethacin	1970-84	4	0.7
Ibuprofen	1975-84	1	0.3
Azapropazone	1978-84	-	-
Diclofenac	1982-84	-	-

Blood dyscrasias also occur very infrequently. Aplastic anaemia has been reported to have a yearly incidence of 2 cases per million inhabitants[4], while agranulocytosis and thrombocytopenia occurs in 9 and 59 cases per million inhabitants per year in Sweden[5,6]. The reported incidence is highest for oxyphenbutazone (Table 6) and lowest for ibuprofen. No cases have been reported for azapropazone which may be related to its low use (Figure 2).

The reported incidences of gastrointestinal ulcers are depicted in Table 7. Apparently piroxicam seems to carry a high risk for inducing such complications. However these data are very complicated to interpret and evaluate and may serve as a samplecard of possible bias encountered in spontaneous reporting systems and thus form a good basis for a methodological discussion.

Table 6 Reported incidence of blood dyscrasias in Sweden

Generic name (time period)	Total No. of reports	Incidence per 100,000 DDD years			
		Agranulocytosis penia	Thrombocyto-	Pancytopenia	Total
Oxyphenbutazone (1970-84)	29	16	15	5	35
Diclofenac (1982-84)	5	6	9	-	15
Phenylbutazone (1970-84)	14	2	5	7	14
Piroxicam (1982-84)	7	1	8	-	9
Sulindac (1982-84)	2	3	3	-	6
Naproxen (1975-84)	20	1	3	0.2	5
Indomethacin (1970-84)	26	1	3	0.5	4
Ibuprofen (1975-84)	4	0.3	0.7	0.3	1
Azapropazone (1978-84)	-	-	-	-	-

Table 7 Reported incidence of gastrointestinal ulcers and bleedings in Sweden

Generic name	Total number	Incidence per 100,000 DDD years			
		Ulcers		Bleedings unsp.	Total (n)
		Uncompl.	Bleed. & perf.		
Piroxicam	118	75	47	28	151
Azapropazone	7	5	28	9	42
Sulindac	5	3	9	3	15
Phenylbutazone	11	-	1	10	11
Oxyphenbutazone	7	1	1	6	9
Indomethacin	22	1	2	2	5
Diclofenac	1	-	3	-	3
Ibuprofen	3	-	0.7	0.3	1

IV. DISCUSSION

The annual number of ADRs reported to the NSAIDs have increased with time and the total number (n=1855) is now quite sub stantial. The number of severe - and even fatal reactions (Table 2) are obviously high enough to be of concern - especially in a small country such as Sweden with only 8 million inhabitants. Moreover there seems to be product related, qualitative as well as quantitative, differences in adverse effects.

In order to evaluate the implications of these reports it is of vital importance to have good knowledge about the size and demographic characteristics of the population exposed to various drugs as well as the rate of reporting.

When related to the sales expressed as the number of DDDs or 1000 treatment years the total frequency of reports is low (Table 3). In fact it is many orders of magnitude lower than what is seen in controlled clinical trials or in hospital surveillance schemes[7]. However, the total rate of reporting is probably very low in spontaneous reporting systems. In one study of consecutive patients admitted to a department of infectious disease only 13% of all ADRs fulfilling the Swedish reporting criteria were actually reported[8].

For certain types of severe reactions the reporting has been found to be better, e.g. blood dyscrasias 20-40% and the Stevens-Johnson's syndrome 20%[5,6,9]. Even with this degree of under-reporting the incidence of NSAID induced blood dyscrasias and severe cutaneous reactions seems to be low. Agranulocytosis has been estimated to occur in 0.3-0.6% of patients treated with anti-thyroid drugs[10], and in a survey of patients discharged from hospitals in Stockholm anti-thyroid drugs, sulphonamides and phenothiazides were much more common than NSAIDs as suspected inducers of agranulocytosis[6]. The reported incidence of thrombocytopenia from thiazides in Sweden has been calculated to be 1 in 47,000 patients which is in the same order of magnitude as that seen here from the modern NSAIDs[5]. The reported incidence of pancytopenia from acetazolamide is 1 in 18,000 patient years and from co-trimoxazole 3 per 100,000 10-day courses. The Stevens-Johnson's syndrome is also much more commonly induced by penicillins and sulphonamides than by NSAIDs[9,11]. Unfortunately no studies have been performed concerning the reporting rate of gastrointestinal ulcers or liver reactions.

The incidence of reported ADRs also depends on the choice of denominator (Table 3). Firstly, the relation between the DDD and the average prescribed daily dose (PDD) varies from 1 : 1 for piroxicam (DDD = PDD = 20 mg) to 1 : 1.5 for ibuprofen (DDD = 800 mg, PDD = 1200 mg). The incidence of ADR reports for ibuprofen is thus increased by 50% if the PDD is used as a denominator instead of the DDD.

Secondly the ranking of the reported incidences varies for some drugs if the number of prescriptions is used as a denominator instead of the number of DDDs (Table 3). This may be related to differences in use between the drugs. Some of these are more oftenly than others used for short periods (Table 8) e.g. for sport injuries, acute gout or menstrual pains. It is interesting to note that the ranking of the NSAIDs in Sweden in almost every instance agrees with that reported from the UK using numbers of prescriptions as a denominator in both countries[12].

For drugs which are mainly used for short treatment courses, the number of prescriptions may better relate to the actual number of exposed patients than the number of DDDs. For chronic treatments the number of patient years estimated from the number of PDDs sold may on the other hand be a more adequate denominator than number of prescriptions.

The general increase in reporting makes comparisons between different time periods difficult. The initial peaks in the reporting during the first years after marketing also complicate comparisons.

Table 8 Average number of defined daily doses per prescription of NSAIDs in Sweden

Generic name	Estimated[a] number of DDDs/prescription Range of averages 1976, 1978, 1980, 1982
Oxyphenabutazone	15 - 20
Indomethacin	40 - 45
Diclofenac	40 - 45
Azapropazone	45 - 55
Naproxen	60 - 70
Ibuprofen	65 - 80
Piroxicam	70 - 80
Sulindac	90 - 100

[a] Calculated by dividing total sales by total number of prescriptions after correction for sales to hospitals.

From Figures 4a and b can clearly be seen that there is a selection in the types of reactions which get reported e.g. there must be a clear over-representation of blood dyscrasias. In general, idiosyncratic reactions seem to be over-represented. If this kind of selective reporting also operates differently for different drugs is not known. It is plausible to asssume that there may be an over-representation of reports for special reactions which have been linked to a certain drug in the literature e.g. blood dyscrasias from the butazones. Also, already from the beginning (1975) toxic amblyopia was mentioned in the Swedish product information (physicians desk reference) as a rare adverse effect of ibuprofen. However, reports of photosensitivity from azapropazone were received already during the first year of marketing (1978) but was not incorporated in our product information until 1981. Moreover, nothing has been published about azapropazone induced photosensitivity in the literature available to general practitioners in Sweden until 1984[13,14]. This indicates that signals of true differences can be picked up.

The evaluation of eventual differences in the tendency to induce gastrointestinal ulcers is especially complicated. Surgeons are notoriously low reporters and in fact the majority of the reports of ulcers and bleedings do not come from those who primarily take care of the complication. This may increase the risk of clustering effects. It is obvious that under-reporting is more marked for the older drugs where these effects are well-known and expected, and that the reported incidences are to be regarded as a minimum. The observed differences between piroxicam, sulindac and diclofenac which all came on the market at about the same time (1982) may in part be explained by differences in the marketing strategies. Piroxicam was heavily marketed as an extremely well tolerated drug and for sulindac the pro-drug concept was stressed. This may have led physicians to try these new products on patients who were known to have "sensitive stomachs". Later when the problems arose - which ought to have been foreseen - these physicians felt cheated by the product and the marketing and thus reported extra vigorously. The experience from Belgium, Norway and the UK could also be explained by this[12,15,16].

It is however also possible that piroxicam carries a substantial potential to elicit peptic ulcers in the way it is used today. Piroxicam has a long half-life (average 30 hours) which means that prostaglandin synthesis may be inhibited around the clock even with a once daily drug intake[17]. Moreover, the metabolism varies at least 5-fold with some individuals having a half-life of piroxicam of more than 100 hours. As 85% of all patients in Sweden are prescribed a standard dose of 20 mg/day those with slow metabolic rate will achieve high steady-state concentrations of the drug and may be at special risk for developing peptic ulcers.

The frequency of peptic ulcers have been reported to increase from about 1% in patients treated with 20 mg/day up to 7.5% in those receiving 40 mg daily[18].

A scientifically valid comparison of the relative potency of the various NSAIDs to elicit symptomatic peptic ulcers can however only be made by a simultaneous comparison in a formal epidemiological study which also take other confounding risk factors into consideration.

V. CONCLUSION

Spontaneous ADR-reporting systems are mainly suited for the generation of signals. However by analysis of these reports in relation to sales and prescription data much additional information can be gained. These data must however always be interpreted with care and often be complemented with in depth studies. NSAIDs can give rise to a wide variety of serious adverse reactions but in general these reactions seem to be rare. There seem to be quantitative as well as qualitative differences among the NSAIDs in the occurrence of these rare reactions. The validity of these observed differences should be tested in formal epidemiological studies.

1. Inman, WHW (1984). Risks in medical intervention. PEM News, 2, 16-36
2. Nordic Statistics on Medicines 1978-80, Part I, p. 79. Nordic Council on Medicines, Box 607, S-751 25 Uppsala, Sweden
3. Statistisk sammanställning 1979-84. (Introduction and codes in English). National Corporation of Swedish Pharmacies, S-105 14 Stockholm, Sweden
4. Levy, M, Slone, D, Shapiro, S, et al (1983). The design of a study of the drug etiology of agranulocytosis and aplastic anemia. A report from the International Agranulocytosis and Aplastic Anemia Study. Eur J Clin Pharmacol, 24, 833
5. Böttiger, LE, Westerholm, B (1973). Drug induced blood dyscrasias in Sweden. Br J Med, 3, 339
6. Arneborn, P, Palmblad, J (1982). Drug-induced neutropenia in the Stockholm area 1973-78. Acta Med Scand, 212, 289
7. Miller, RR and Greenblatt, DJ (1976). Drug Effects in Hospitalized Patients Wiley Biomedical Publishing Co.
8. Britton, S, and Jourp-Rönström, C (1981). Vådan av vård III: Anmälan av biverkan från personal och patienter. Läkartidningen, 78, 1670
9. Böttiger, LE, Strandberg, I and Westerholm, B (1971). Drug-induced febrile mucocutaneous syndrome. Acta Med Scand, 190, 455-63
10. Cooper, DS, Goldminz, D, Levin, AA et al (1983). Agrnaulocytosis and antithyroid drugs. Annals of Internal Medicine, 98, 26
11. Wiholm, B-E. Unpublished observations from the Swedish system
12. Weber, JCP (1984). Epidemiology of adverse reactions to non-steroidal anti-inflammatory drugs. In: Rainsford, KD and Velo, GP (eds), Side effects of anti-inflammatory analgesic drugs, p. 1. (New York: Raven Press)
13. Anonymous (1976). Information on Adverse Reactions. Jpn Med Gazette, 13, 9
14. Swedish Adverse Reaction Advisory Committee (1984). Photosensitivity - a survey of reported cases with a view to the approaching season. SADRAC Bulletin, 42, 1. (Sweden: Department of Drugs)
15. Laake, K, Kjeldaas, L, and Borchgrevink, CF (1984). Side effects of piroxicam (Feldene). Acta Med Scand, 215, 81
16. Meyer, P and Thijs, I (1985). Peptic ulcers induced by piroxicam. Br Med J, 290, 789
18. Brogden, RN, Heel, RC, Speight, TM and Avery, GS (1984). Piroxicam. A Reappraisal of its Pharmacology and Therapeutic Efficacy. Drugs, 28, 292

Discussion

Dr U Rensing, Switzerland I noticed that when comparing Butazolodine and indomethacin over the years, there was a much higher reporting on adverse reactions with Butazotatone in the later years. Do you have any explanation for that, for these are both drugs that have been in use for many years in your country and yet you see a difference in reporting?

Dr Wiholm: Well, actually, being a religious man, I believe this is because it might be differences between the drugs or at least physicians worry more about treating people with phenylbutazone than they do with indomethacin.

Dr Rensing The second question related to this. You've always compared different time periods when comparing different drugs, so all these say, temporal correlations, to the knowledge of medicine in medicine, come into action here?

Dr Wiholm Yes, they do.

Dr Rensing So these data might be greatly distorted?

Dr Wiholm These data might be greatly influenced by, for instance, the lack of the novel reporting for the older drugs, you know, drugs which were introduced long before we started the system of continuous reporting. They will lack the initial reporting. If you look at the number of reports for pancytopenia and mucocutanous syndromes and effects like that, the rate of reporting is rather constant over the years and I think that might then mean that we get a fairly stable proportion of all cases.

Dr KD Rainsford, UK Could it be that there's some relationship to the absolute usage that is completely independent of the factors which you talked about such as doctor or patient awareness and so forth? It seems to be that if you take the top league of your drugs they are sulindac, azapropazone and piroxicam if we're to believe that in GI and some other side-effects, but they're also in the high usage bracket and could it be that the statistical incidence is somehow or other better revealed by uping the numbers in the denominator?

Dr Wiholm Azapropazone is not used appreciably, so that the total number of daily defined doses sold are only 7 million as compared to many hundreds of millions defined daily doses of indomethacin and about, well I don't really remember, I think it's 14 or 16 million defined daily doses sold of piroxicam. So that might not be, but the patient selection is important. The wider the use of a drug, the larger the risk would be that I choose the wrong patient.

Professor K Brune, FRG May I ask you, the pharmacologist is almost somewhat puzzled to see that the active metabolite of a compound turns out to be much more dangerous than the parent compound, so I would like you to explain a little bit now the usage of phenylbutazone and oxyphenbutazone in Sweden and why that oxyphenbutazone appears so much more toxic than phenylbutazone in your data?

Dr Wiholm I have wondered about that myself and I would like to return this with a question. Does all the phenylbutazone become oxyphenbutazone and only oxyphenbutazone or is there also another metabolic pathway because I thought maybe if you give the same amount in milligrams, you might actually give more oxyphenbutazone when you use it per se, but I don't know this.

Professor Brune: Well, this certainly is a complex aspect and we could have a full little meeting on that, but basically the other metabolites appear to be less effective in terms of anti-inflammatory effect, so I think the only point you could make is that your active dosage of oxyphenbutazone may be slightly higher under some circumstances, but I would rather search for this phenomena by the indications which are assigned to oxyphenbutazone or phenylbutazone in your country.

Dr Wiholm I think that's the more important explanation too, because oxyphenbutazone was used for sports injuries where it was used for shorter periods of time. The actual number of defined daily doses per prescription is only 18 for oxyphenbutazone and is much more for phenylbutazone, so phenylbutazone was used for longer periods of time, but that doesn't explain it because then it means you are treating a younger and healthier population with oxyphenbutazone and still we see more reactions reported to it.

6
Rare adverse reactions to non-steroidal anti-inflammatory drugs

WM O'Brien
Division of Rheumatology,
Department of Internal Medicine,
University of Virginia Hospital,
Charlottesville, VA 22908, USA

CONTENTS

Side-effects of Anti-inflammatory Drugs. Rainsford, KD & Velo, GP (eds)
Part 1: Clinical and Epidemiological Aspects. (Lancaster: MTP Press).

I. INTRODUCTION

This chapter attempts to survey the rare adverse reactions caused by non-steroidal anti-inflammatory drugs (NSAIDs). I shall summarize all the reported reactions to NSAIDs (a detailed review with 491 references is published elsewhere[1]), and suggest any unusual reactions to individual drugs by comparing each drug with the accumulated experience with other NSAIDs over the past 20 years. After the withdrawals of both benoxaprofen (Oraflex, Opren) and zomepirac (Zomax), and the recent disquieting reports of serious skin reactions[2] and gastrointestinal bleeding[3-5] with piroxicam (Feldene) and its relabelling, this review is indeed timely. The appearance of the problems after extensive testing and regulatory review, and after wide public exposure and numerous reactions suggest society does not have methods for adequately assessing the safety of new drugs. Sulindac (Clinoril) is of special interest, since it causes two rare but unusual reactions - agranulomatous hepatitis and acute pancreatitis - and also since it possibly may have less renal toxicity than other NSAIDs.

Three general types of adverse reactions can occur. First the elderly are intolerant of NSAIDs with long half-lives. They have old tired enzymes and old tired kidneys. As a result, drugs may accumulate, resulting in toxicity. Age has always been the major risk factor identified in studies of adverse reactions.

A second type of reaction is due to the direct effects on prostaglandin synthesis. Mucus production protects the stomach and its production is stimulated by prostaglandins[6,7]; thus any drug which inhibits their production is likely to be ulcerogenic at least to some degree. When mild renal failure is present (it may be clinically inapparent), prostaglandin secretion produces renal vasodilation preserving renal blood flow; prostaglandin inhibitors thus may precipitate renal failure in the diseased individual. The situation is worsened if the individual is taking potassium-retaining diuretics and potassium supplements, a scenario which may lead to rapid hyperkalaemia and even death.

Drugs such as tolmetin, ibuprofen, diclofenac and ketoprofen, because of their short half-lives of 1-2 hours, might have a less enduring effect than the more slowly metabolized and excreted NSAIDS. Piroxicam (half-life of 32 hours) should be used with caution in the elderly.

A third mechanism is pure idiosyncrasy: the rare but perhaps fatal reaction which would be difficult to detect in clinical trials involving 1000 or 2000 subjects. The most feared reactions are hepatocellular necrosis, aplastic anaemia and anaphylaxis. Even after prolonged marketing, significant fatal idiosyncrasies may not be detectable by statistical study of large registries. The anaesthetic halothane obviously caused hepatic necrosis and could be demonstrated to do so by giving small test doses to anaesthesiologists who were sensitive to the drug[8].

II. DETECTING SIDE-EFFECTS

The recent withdrawals from marketing of two NSAIDs - benoxaprofen in the summer of 1982 and zomepirac sodium in the spring of 1983 - raise the question of how efficiently the medical establishment evaluates and responds to adverse drug reports (ADRs). There have been suggestions, particularly in the Oraflex (benoxaprofen) case, that the Food and Drug Administration failed to detect serious problems which perhaps should have kept the drug from ever being marketed. I would argue that many of the flaws shown in the FDA's handling of benoxaprofen are typical of those seen in drug registries, and that it is time to realize that published case reports by physicians are distinctly the best means of detecting previously unknown drug toxicities, especially if these side-effects are rare or unusual.

Registries undoubtedly have a useful role in drug surveillance: because of their size they can help to indicate the overall incidence of previously detected ADRs. (In Sweden, for example, figures compiled by the Adverse Drug Reactions Committee[9,10] show unmistakably that phenylbutazone and oxyphenbutazone are the most common causes of drug-related aplastic anaemia). However, for picking up previously unknown adverse effects registries are inadequate, for several reasons:

1. Despite their claims of thoroughness, even the largest registries in fact are handicapped by under-reporting of adverse reactions, both by manufacturers to the FDA (e.g. about 30 known benoxaprofen fatalities were not reported when the drug was approved in April 1982[11]) and by physicians to the UK Committee on Safety of Medicines (CSM); e.g. only 15% of women who died of thromboembolism while taking oral contraceptives were reported to the CSM[12].
2. Registries collect inadequately detailed, often superficial, data. For instance, Inman's data on benoxaprofen, collected by the Drug Surveillance Research Unit at the University of Southampton[13,14] lumped hepatic reactions under the general

heading of "gastrointestinal" and thus effectively missed them. Similarly, a recent report from the Boston Collaborative Drug Surveillance Program on the renal effects of non-steroidals[15] failed to pick up the sometimes serious effects of these drugs. Indeed, post-marketing surveys generally tend to detect no new toxicities[16].

3. When registries do collect useful data, they too often fail to analyze it profitably. In a 1982 general review of the FDA's system[17] the General Accounting Office found that a large proportion of adverse reactions reported to the FDA effectively get buried in an inefficient computerized recording system. More specifically, a Congressional subcommittee report[18] provides clear evidence that the FDA failed to take advantage of data already in its system when it decided to approve the sale of Oraflex.

For all of these reasons, registries are inadequate for detecting new adverse reactions. Certainly there are also some shortcomings in individual case reports: some fail to provide sufficient detail to shed full light on specific adverse reactions and it is admittedly impossible to estimate reliably the incidence of a given adverse reaction on the basis of isolated cases[19]. Despite these limitations, however, case reports clearly give fuller and more timely information about ADRs which have not turned up in pre-marketing clinical trials. If there is any doubt, we need only look at either the Oraflex story, in which Taggart's[20] and other case reports played the central role in showing the drug's life-threatening hepatorenal toxicity, or the Zomax story, in which, again, individual reports of anaphylactoid reactions to the drug led the manufacturer to discontinue sales. The lessons suggested by the histories of these two non-steroidals are convincingly confirmed by Venning's study[21]: for the twenty most important adverse reactions observed in Great Britain since thalidomide, the yellow card system failed to provide early warning in every case; by contrast, 19 of the 20 reactions were first noted in published case reports.

III. COMMON SIDE-EFFECTS

A. Gastrointestinal side-effects

The gastrointestinal (GI) side-effects of anti-inflammatories are well known. They cause two major problems: diffuse gastritis and discrete ulcers, both gastric and duodenal. Diffuse gastritis, while it does occur with several of the non-steroidals introduced in the past 20 years, is not a major problem with any of them. It is, however, a major problem with aspirin. The recent study of Silvoso and his associates at Missouri[22] indicates the seriousness of this problem. In patients on chronic aspirin therapy, 17% had gastric ulcers, 40% had gastric erosions, and 76% gastric erythema. Ulcers occurred even with buffered and enteric-coated aspirin. The real question is whether aspirin is well tolerated as a long-term agent, and the answer is clearly "no".

The second major GI side-effect of NSAIDs is discrete ulceration. It would appear that, even in the absence of medication, the incidence of peptic ulceration is higher (perhaps by a factor of 3 or 4) in rheumatoid arthritics than in other patient populations[23]; RA seems clearly to be a disease in which there is already a propensity to ulcerate. In early studies of indomethacin in the treatment of RA, gastric ulceration occurred particularly at higher doses. This type of side-effect appears also with all the other NSAIDs but is relatively rare in actual practice. To put the problem in perspective: at 20 mg/day of prednisone given for 2 years, the incidence of gastric ulceration in rheumatoid arthritics is about 25%[24-26]; with indomethacin doses above 150 mg/day given for 2 years, the rate of ulceration is less than 2%[27]. One might even note that, since the spontaneous rate of ulcer formation in the general population is about 1% per year, the rate seen with indomethacin is no greater than that seen spontaneously. On the other hand, most spontaneous ulcers are duodenal, while about two-thirds of those induced by indomethacin and the other NSAIDs are gastric[27].

The problem may be more acute in the elderly; in one geriatric unit 33 of 531 admissions were due to GI bleeding, and 17 were related to the use of NSAIDs[28]. One NSAID appears to have a high incidence of acute GI bleeding i.e. piroxicam. This is demonstrated both in animal data and in data from series of case reports[3,4] and national registries[5].

While some NSAIDs might have a slightly lower profile than others in terms of GI ulceration, none has been shown to be substantially lower in the incidence of these side-effects than others. Sulindac is a pro-drug and since it is inactive might have fewer gastric side-effects. Surveys in American Medicaid patients indicate that it is just as ulcerogenic as other non-steroidals.

B. Renal "side-effects"

All of the NSAIDs, but particularly fenoprofen, have been reported to cause acute interstitial nephritis. The reports are few and the reaction is obviously a rare one. The occasional NSAID-caused interstitial nephritis occurs suddenly and as an idiosyncrasy. It is often characterized by eosinophils in the renal parenchyma and can usually be reversed if the drug is promptly discontinued. An important clue to the presence of this sort of lesion is the presence of eosinophiluria.

The situation is quite different, however, in the individual with compromised renal function. In such patients, prostaglandins may be produced at an unusually high rate in order to achieve renal vasodilation and thus increase renal blood flow and prevent renal failure. If such patients receive non-steroidal therapy, the inhibition of the prostaglandins, which provide the only mechanism available to perfuse the kidneys, may precipitate sudden renal failure. This reaction is due to the inhibition of renal prostaglandin production and, rather than being an adverse effect, is a physiological effect. With the decrease in renal function, hyperkalaemia may also occur. Finally, inhibition of renal prostaglandins may cause a rare hyporeninaemic hypoaldosteronism. Four major reviews have appeared[29-32].

An encouraging development was the report by Bunning and Barth[33] that three patients who developed azotaemia on naproxen or ibuprofen did not do so when briefly exposed to sulindac. Workers in Rome[34] reported sulindac has less effect on renal blood flow and prostaglandins in 1-week trials than did ibuprofen. Mitnich[35] questioned Bunning and Barth's conclusions, since the trials of sulindac were run under different conditions than the original exposure to other NSAIDs. Whelton and his associates reported a case of severe renal failure due to sulindac[36]. Finally a Danish group failed to confirm that sulindac differed from naproxen in its effects on prostaglandins or renin in a 2-week trial in patients with thiazide-treated heart failure[37]. Thus, it seems likely that sulindac has less renal effects than other NSAIDs, but more careful studies may shed further light in this confusing but important area.

C. Enterohepatic recirculation and diarrhoea

The enterohepatic recirculation of certain of the non-steroidals may also have adverse consequences. These occur particularly with indomethacin, sulindac and mefenamic acid. Indomethacin will produce diarrhoea in about 5% of patients receiving it [38-40], and has also been know to cause ileal[41] and jejunal ulceration[42,43]. The worst problems occur with mefanmic acid, which may produce very severe diarrhoea and even steatorrhoea[44,45]. This can occur in up to 30% of patients and can promptly be averted by discontinuing the drug.

D. Headaches

Many indoles, including serotonin, have central nervous system (CNS) activity; perhaps it is not surprising that high doses of indomethacin, which is chemically similar to serotonin, can induce severe, even disabling headaches[27,46]. Such severe headaches are not usually seen with the other NSAIDs, though virtually all of them may occasionally cause drowsiness or dizziness.

IV. RARE ADVERSE REACTIONS

A. Dermatological adverse reactions

1. Erythema multiforme and its variants

Most of the dermal side-effects seen with the non-steroidals are fairly mild; but an extremely serious one, erythema multiforme, has also been described on a number of occasions. The outcome of this reaction can be fatal. A particularly severe variant of erythema multiforme, Stevens-Johnson syndrome, involves also stomatitis and conjunctivitis; the fatality rate in this syndrome is 6 to 25%[47]. Almost all of the non-steroidals have been reported to cause erythema multiforme[2,48,49].

The two once-a-day NSAIDs (piroxicam and benoxaprofen) introduced in 1982 seem to cause a higher incidence of these serious dermal reactions. In its brief time on the market benoxaprofen was implicated in at least 11 cases of erythema multiforme. In addition, a recent report from the spontaneous adverse reaction reporting system of the American Academy of Dermatology[2] noted that, of 33 cases of non-photosensitivity vesiculobullous reactions reported with various non-steroidals, 29 were associated with piroxicam. Overall, this report estimates that serious dermal reactions occur more frequently with benoxaprofen and piroxicam than with any other NSAIDs recently or currently marketed in the United States.

2. Photosensitivity reactions

A significant number of the non-steroidals, especially some of the phenylpropionic acids, have been reported to cause photosensitivity reactions of various sorts. Laboratory studies[50,51] indicate that minor phototoxic reactions, involving immediate erythema and, in most cases, urticarial weals, may occur in sun-exposed areas of patients taking piroxicam, naproxen and tiaprofenic acid. A similar reaction, involving a bullous erythematopapular eruption of sun-exposed areas of the skin, has been noted in eight Swiss patients taking carprofen[52]; two of these cases required hospitalization and treatment with systemic steroids. Again, as in the case of more serious dermatological reactions, the once-a-day non-steroidals may cause a disproportionate number of photosensitivity reactions. Benoxaprofen caused an unusual photo-allergy which may have occurred in all patients receiving the drug[53], as well as a bullous dermatitis in sun-exposed areas of the skin[54]. There have been more than 65 reported cases of similar reactions to piroxicam[2,55] - "photosensitivity eruptions"[55] which in most cases involved vesicles or bullae. These reactions have been rare with diclofenac.

3. Miscellaneous dermatological reactions

The most common cutaneous reaction to aspirin is urticaria, which may be caused in aspirin-sensitive patients or exacerbated (apparently on a dose-related, non-allergenic basis) in about 25% of patients with chronic urticaria[56-58]. (Unlike asthmatic attacks in aspirin-sensitive patients, this reaction does not appear to be due to prostaglandin inhibition[57]). The other non-steroidals may also cause urticaria, especially in aspirin-sensitive patients. Benign morbilliform eruptions (not erythema multiforme) may occur at high doses with most if not all of the phenylalkanoic acids.

B. Musculoskeletal adverse reactions

1. Aseptic necrosis

Several investigators have suggested that long-term indomethacin therapy might cause aseptic necrosis of the hip[59], but this has not been substantiated. In the published cases it is possible, if not likely, that the osteonecrosis had been present before the drug was started. To the extent that the condition did worsen during indomethacin therapy, it is possible that the drug, by relieving pain, enabled the patients to be more active and that the additional movement was responsible for the joint damage[60]. This appears to be a "pseudo" -adverse reaction!

C. Pulmonary adverse reactions

1. Asthma in aspirin-sensitive patients

Somewhere between 2% and 20% of adult asthmatics[61] (and a smaller portion of asthmatic children) have an unusual syndrome, marked by nasal polyps and hypersensitivity to aspirin, which apparently involves a general lack of prostaglandins[62,63]; even without exposure to aspirin this syndrome may become progressively worse. If such asthmatics do take aspirin, they may experience rhinitis, wheezing and/or bronchospasm[64], which in some cases may be fatal.

In the past two decades evidence has grown that such hypersensitivity reactions to aspirin are dependent not on immunological mechanisms, but simply on the inhibition of prostaglandins. Consequently, laboratory tests [65-68] have shown that if affected individuals (especially those who are also intolerant of iodides[69]) are exposed to any of the non-steroidal agents they may experience immediate bronchial constriction.

2. Acute pulmonary oedema

In the past 30 years a number of cases have been described of salicylate intoxication producing pulmonary oedema, usually in patients who are heavy smokers[70]. The reaction has not been seen in patients taking other NSAIDs.

3. Diffuse pulmonary infiltrates

Several of the non-steroidals have been reported to cause a hypersensitivity pneumonitis. Presenting symptoms have usually included fever, non-productive cough, wheezing and rales. X-ray usually reveals diffuse bilateral infiltrates, virtually every case described in detail has also shown eosinophilia in the blood or sputum or both. In the three cases in which it was performed, lung biopsy revealed thickening of the alveolar walls and inflammatory infiltrate, whether of monocytes and polys[71], of lymphocytes, histiocytes and eosinophils[72] or of epithelioid granulomas[73]. Of the 11 patients in whom such reactions have been noted, the only fatality[74] appeared to result primarily from hepatic involvement. The other 10 patients recovered either after simple withdrawal of non-steroidal therapy or following treatment with corticosteroids.

4. Possible reactivation of latent tuberculosis

At least one case[75] has been described in which a patient's latent pulmonary tuberculosis may have been reactivated by treatment with ibuprofen plus indomethacin suppositories. Later reports from the same clinic[76,77] suggest that this problem may occur with most if not all of the non-steroidals.

5. Anaphylaxis

Anaphylaxis has been described with virtually all of the non-steroidals. The largest number of published case reports involve zomepirac sodium which was at least withdrawn from the market by the manufacturer in 1983. The true nature of this "anaphylactoid" reaction is not known, but it may not be mediated by IgE. It differs in one crucial respect from true anaphylaxis: it is distinctly less severe and has rarely proved to be fatal. It must again be emphasized that the reaction can occur with any NSAID[78]. Of those patients who have been investigated very intensively (before the reaction), several have had low levels of complement and extractable nuclear antigens. Since the syndrome resembles hereditary angioneurotic oedema, it is possible that these drugs induce similar symptoms in individuals who are inherently susceptible.

6. Febrile reactions

Six patients treated with ibuprofen - five of them either for lupus erythematosus[79,80] or mixed connective tissue disease[74], the other for dental pain[81] - have had a generalized reaction characterized by fever, abdominal pain, nausea and vomiting and elevated hepatic enzymes; biopsy in two of these cases revealed fatty changes in the liver. Some of these patients also had other sorts of symptoms, including headache, rash and joint and muscle pain. With a single exception (a patient with bilateral pleural effusions and serious hepatic changes who died in shock and respiratory failure[74]) all of these patients recovered after treatment with steroids and, in one case[81], intensive care for hypoxaemic respiratory failure. This reaction may be unique to ibuprofen, and I know of no cases due to other NSAIDs.

7. Drug-induced lupus-like syndrome

Both phenylbutazone[82] and ibuprofen[83] have been reported to induce a lupus-like syndrome. This is evidently a hypersensitivity reaction, involving fever and a diffuse erythematous rash, as well as generalized myalgia and arthralgias. The immunofluorescent test for antinuclear antibodies was positive in both of these cases, and the direct Coombs' test in one[83]. One of the two cases[82] also involved renal complications (proteinuria and haematuria). In a related phenomenon, oxyphenbutazone has been reported to cause the lupus erythematosus cell phenomenon and thrombocytopenia[84].

8. Vasculitis

The induction of cutaneous vasculitis is another peculiar allergic reaction. It seems to be extremely rare, but a number of cases were observed nine times.

9. Other generalized reactions

A single case of peripheral and mediastinal lymphadenopathy associated with sulindac has been described[85], in a patient who also developed erythema multiforme. The lymphadenopathy reversed when sulindac was withdrawn, but recurred with rechallenge. Some investigators[86] have suggested that at least one non-steroidal, indomethacin, might decrease the ability of a patient to respond to infection, and at least one child treated for juvenile RA[87] did develop a severe haemorrhagic case of chickenpox, despite the fact that she received no steroids. On the whole, however, the animal evidence that indomethacin increases susceptibility to infection is unconvincing, and occasional cases such as that of haemorrhagic varicella may well be coincidental to NSAID therapy.

D. Cardiovascular adverse reactions

The non-steroidals probably have little direct effect on the prostaglandins involved in the functioning of the heart or coronary circulation. In animals, aspirin, indomethacin and ibuprofen, when given intravenously in huge doses (at 300 times the usual oral blood levels), have been shown to make the myocardium more sensitive to ouabain[88]. Likewise, huge intravenous doses of indomethacin (at 50 times the usual oral blood levels) in humans with arteriosclerosis produce weak catheter evidence of vasoconstriction, but no clinical evidence of angina or ST segment changes[89]. On the other hand, Golding[90] reported preliminary evidence suggesting that indomethacin may aggravate myocardial ischaemia, and thus perhaps anginal pain, in some patients. For most patients, however, it seems unlikely that the usual oral doses of indomethacin or other NSAIDs will produce such side-effects.

The most significant cardiovascular effects of the non-steroidals are likely to result not directly from the inhibition of prostaglandins in the heart itself, but indirectly, from the inhibition of circulating prostaglandins. Researchers at Harvard have recently shown that, in patients with severe congestive heart failure - especially those with hyponatraemia - indomethacin decreases cardiac output, presumably by reducing levels of circulating prostaglandins[91]. In such patients, any non-steroidal might exacerbate congestive heart failure.

E. Haematological adverse reactions

The majority of the most serious adverse reactions to the non-steroidals are idiosyncratic reactions, and among these some of the most severe are blood dyscrasias. Fortunately these reactions appear to be extremely rare, especially in view of the widespread and long-term use of many of these drugs.

1. Aplastic anaemia

The most feared of the blood dyscrasias certainly is aplastic anaemia; the mortality rate in drug-induced cases is usually of the order of 67%[92]. Although it is often difficult to be certain of a direct causal link between the ingestion of a particular drug and the appearance of aplastic anaemia (especially with patients who are taking several drugs which may depress the marrow), there is good evidence for individual cases of aplastic anaemia with all NSAIDs: 13 case reports with 21 cases, of which 14 were fatal. In registries of drug reactions, however, neither aspirin nor any of the newer non-steroidals appear as leading causes of aplastic anaemia, supporting my contention that these are extremely rare reactions.

2. Pure red cell aplasia

An extremely rare pure red cell aplasia has been described on five occasions with NSAIDs. One must be cautious in interpreting these reports, since the same condition can occur spontaneously as in immunological phenomena in rheumatoid arthritis.

3. Effects on thrombocytes

a. Inhibition of platelet function - Of the non-steroidals, aspirin has distinctly the most striking and long-lasting effects in inhibiting platelet aggregation and, in some patients, prolonging bleeding time. While the newer NSAIDs inhibit aggregation only for the few hours during which they remain in the bloodstream, the effects of aspirin may last 12-15 days. Moreover, because aspirin affects the hepatic synthesis of vitamin K, its effects on bleeding time are considerably more complex than those of the other non-steroidals. Not surprisingly, then, virtually any of the newer agents, especially those with short half-lives, appear to be safer than aspirin for use in haemophiliacs, though clearly they should be administered to such patients only with careful monitoring[93]. As a result of their effects on platelet function, virtually all of the non-steroidals may rarely cause clinical bleeding of varying severity.

b. Thrombocytopenia - Rare cases of thrombocytopenia, some of them severe, have been described with many of the non-steroidals: 35 cases with indomethacin, including five fatalities[94]; as well as isolated cases with other NSAIDs.

4. Neutropenia

An isolated neutropenia or agranulocytosis, which can rarely be fatal, has also been observed with several of the non-steroidals. Recent evidence suggests that NSAID-induced neutropenia is rare indeed: a Swedish survey[95] found only 0.07 cases per million tablets sold in the case of indomethacin, a rate approximately 1/60 that found with penicillamine. Neutropenia seems to be notably more rare with the newer NSAIDs, but has been noted in about a dozen case reports.

5. Haemolytic anaemia

At least seven cases of autoimmune haemolytic anaemia have been reported with mefenamic acid and three cases with ibuprofen, three cases with naproxen[96-98] and two cases with diclofenac[99]. The reaction, which has not to our knowledge been observed with the other non-steroidals, certainly appears to be rare[100], but can be severe.

Considering the widespread use of NSAIDs, the incidence of haematological reactions is quite rare. With limitations on the use of phenylbutazone, haematological reactions to NSAIDs are very infrequent, but should blood counts be monitored? I was unable to find a single case report in which monitoring either detected or improved the care of the patient. Blood counts could be normal a few days before the reaction occurred.

a. Stomatitis and sialadenitis - Stomatitis may occur with virtually any of the non-steroidals; if such ulcers persist the patient should be changed to another NSAID. A number of patients have experienced sudden, mumps-like swelling of the salivary (usually parotid) glands.

Phenylbutazone[101,102] and oxyphenbutazone[103] have also been found to cause thyroid enlargement, occasionally striking, and hypothyroidism. Though two other NSAIDs, diclofenac and fenclofenac, are structurally rather similar to tetraiodothyronine, they appear to have no effect on thyroid function[104].

b. Oesophageal injury - Two recent studies[105,106] have suggested that the non-steroidals may cause benign oesophageal stricture, especially in patients with gastro-oesophageal reflux, perhaps by inhibiting the production of mucosal prostaglandins. In one survey[106], 49% of patients hospitalized for benign oesophageal stricture had been prescribed NSAIDs in the preceding year, as against only 12% of controls. In the other[105], of 70 patients hospitalized for benign oesophageal stricture, 22 had "regularly consumed" non-steroidals, versus only 10 of 70 matched controls ($p < 0.02$). In the latter study, eight different NSAIDs were recorded as having been taken regularly; the three most frequently named (aspirin, indomethacin and ibuprofen) are the three most widely prescribed.

There have also been three case reports of frank oesophageal ulceration associated with indomethacin therapy[107-109]. All three patients had taken a low dose of indomethacin (mean 83.3 mg/d, only 50 mg/d p.o.) for a short period (mean 2.5 weeks); one nontheless bled to death[108]. This problem appears to be particularly likely to occur in the elderly, bed-ridden patients, in whom prolonged contact of the drug with the oesophageal mucosa can obviously produce severe injury.

Pancreatitis has been reported as a complication of sulindac in several instances[110-114] and of indomethacin at least once[115]. This may be a result of the intensive enterohepatic recirculation which causes the pancreas to be continuously exposed to the drug. Although such episodes of pancreatitis may be quite severe, they can again be averted by discontinuing therapy.

c. Lower gastrointestinal (GI) complications - In patients with a history of lower bowel disease it appears that virtually any of the non-steroidals may reactivate the disease. Ibuprofen has caused flares in quiescent ulcerative colitis in at least three cases[116-118]; indomethacin has led to acute perforations of sigmoid diverticula in two patients with no recent history of GI symptoms[119]; and naproxen has caused one patient with diverticulitis to bleed and another to perforate[116]. One recent survey compared 268 patients with colonic or small bowel perforations, and found twice as much NSAID consumption as in matched controls; 64 had taken these drugs, suggesting that the problem might be more common than previously thought[120].

F. Hepatic adverse reactions

1. "Transaminitis"

In the area of idiosyncratic reactions involving the liver, the problem of "transaminitis" has been well described. As we know, patients on aspirin therapy frequently develop elevations in the serum transaminase[121,122], and the same phenomenon occurs with many if not all of the other non-steroidals. On biopsy this turns out to be not inflammation of a laboratory test, as the misnomer "transaminitis" implies, but a mild form of hepatitis. Biopsy reveals anatomical lesions in the liver, often minor, but with infiltrates of monocytes[123,124]; electron microscopy has also shown ultrastructural changes in the hepatocytes[125]. Clinically, transaminitis is in most cases a nuisance, perhaps necessitating withdrawal of non-steroidal therapy, rather than a serious adverse effect.

2. Hepatitis

Aspirin is unique among the NSAIDs in its effects on the liver, particularly its alteration of hepatic synthesis of vitamin K, a change which in turn may prolong prothrombin time. A significant number of cases have been reported of salicylate-induced hepatitis - at least 11 since 1977. Two patients on diclofenac died with hepatitis, both being only possibly related to the drug. Only one case has ever been published implicating diclofenac[126] and, considering the widespread use of the drug, this may be no more than the background "noise" of unrelated non-A, non-B hepatitis.

In considering hepatitis caused by most of the non-steroidals, several points stand out. First, the reaction appears to be extremely rare; only 34 case reports of which I am aware, only a handful of cases involving even such widely used agents as indomethacin and ibuprofen. Second, hepatitis induced by most NSAIDs seems clearly to be a hypersensitivity reaction. This is suggested by the fact that many of the cases have occurred within 2-12 weeks of the initiation of therapy, and by the fact that at least a third of the patients involved in these cases also had other organ involvement, whether dermal[114,127-130], pulmonary[74,130], haematological[98,129,131,132] or renal[98]; about half of the patients had fever. Finally, the mortality rate in most NSAID-induced hepatitis has been comparatively moderate: six deaths in 35 cases (17.1%). This low mortality differs drastically with other instances of drug-induced hepatitis, again suggesting these may be examples of incidental viral infections rather than true drug reactions.

Finally, it seems likely that the hepatitis which occurred with benoxaprofen was not an idiosyncratic allergic reaction at all, but a direct toxic effect resulting from drug accumulation. Several facts point to this conclusion: the greater frequency of hepatitis with benoxaprofen (at least 14 published cases in less than 2 years of marketing); the fact that, in the published cases, the reaction usually occurred, not early in therapy, but after several months of treatment; and the fact that it struck elderly patients so heavily (mean age of the 14 patients in the published cases was 75.9 year). Benoxaprofen had an unusually long half-life, more than 100 hours in older people; such patients, especially those given the full therapeutic dosage, almost surely accumulated the drug in their systems and suffered the direct cytotoxic effects, both in the liver and in the renal tubules, of what were in effect overdoses. Histological evidence - extensive bile plugging of the cholangioles and eventually hepatocellular necrosis - suggests that the insoluble glucuronide of benoxaprofen directly injured the liver. As a result of all of these unusual facts, the mortality rate in the 14 published benoxaprofen cases was 78.6%, and the drug was understandably withdrawn from marketing.

G. Miscellaneous genitourinary adverse reactions

At high doses some of the non-steroidals can produce a chemical cystitis; this may occur, for instance, with zomepirac, but can easily be avoided by forcing fluids.

H. Central nervous system (CNS) adverse reactions

1. Aseptic meningitis

Some individuals may be inherently susceptible to the side-effects of the non-steroidal agents. There have been 14 case reports of aseptic meningitis induced by NSAIDs; the great majority of these cases have involved ibuprofen. In humans the reaction, which has been reproduced by challenges with a single tablet of ibuprofen, is usually manifested by headache, fever and chills, mental confusion and nuchal rigidity, with more generalized arthralgia, conjunctivitis and lymphadeonpathy in some cases; the cerebrospinal fluid typically shows elevated leukocyte counts (in some cases almost entirely neutrophils) and, usually, elevated protein levels, but with no evidence of infection. In all of the published cases thus far, the reaction has reversed after discontinuation of non-steroidal therapy - despite the fact that in one case[133] the reaction also involved acute pancreatitis, pneumonitis and parotitis, and in another[134] also involved acute renal failure with tubular necrosis.

2. Ocular adverse reactions

Ocular reactions to the non-steroidals have likewise been both rare and generally reversible. Most of the accounts of such reactions have involved indomethacin and ibuprofen - perhaps not surprisingly, since these are the two most widely used of the newer NSAIDs. Surveys of ocular reactions, however, involving a total of nearly 900 patients, have found no such ocular side-effects - a fact which suggests that they must be quite rare. Moreover, patients treated with ibuprofen do not show macular degeneration such as is seen in some treated with antimalarials.

3. Miscellaneous CNS reactions

It has long been known that hearing impairment and even permanent deafness may be caused by chronic use of aspirin and other salicylates[135,136]. Rare causes of transient loss of hearing have been noted with indomethacin[137,138], phenylbutazone and ibuprofen[139].

In the area of psychological effects, the clinician should be alert to the fact that the non-steroidals may have subtle effects on mentation. Especially at high doses, the drug can depress mental function in older patients[140]. Indomethacin may cause severe, even suicidal depression in some patients[138]. There have also been several reports of acute psychosis following the administration of indomethacin. Finally, two clinicians have noted eight cases of cognitive dysfunction (forgetfulness, inability to concentrate and/or depression) in elderly patients, four of which may have been associated with naproxen and four with ibuprofen[141].

I. Overdosages

Accidental overdosages of the non-steroidals have been reported very rarely. This may be due to the presence of a kind of built-in safety mechanism: the drugs are gastric irritants, and large doses might be expected to induce vomiting. Even if large amounts of these drugs were kept down, one would expect adverse reactions to be relatively mild, since most of them have relatively simple excretion mechanisms and would likely be quickly cleared by the kidney. For most of these drugs it appears that, once the albumin binding sites are saturated, the free drug is rapidly excreted. The importance of non-linear pharmacokinetics is well demonstrated experimentally for naproxen[142,143], and in failure in suicide attempts with the drug. But benoxaprofen, with linear pharmacokinetics, results in fatalities with overdoses.

J. Drug interactions

Drug interactions involving the non-steroidals appear to be relatively rare. The most likely interactions are probably those with diuretics and antihypertensives. In patients receiving beta-blockers, such as propranolol, the concomitant use of indomethacin (perhaps of any prostaglandin inhibitor) may cause the blood pressure to rise[144]. In patients on thiazide diuretics, especially furosemide, indomethacin may blunt the diuretic effect of the thiazides[144], thus exacerbating congestive failure and hypertension. In some patients the combined use of indomethacin and triamterene (a weak, potassium-sparing diuretic) may lead to reversible acute renal failure[145]. In addition, all of the non-steroidals, by means of their effects on prostaglandins, can cause an acute decrease in renal blood flow and a sudden, even lethal, rise in potassium levels. The physician should certainly exercise caution in prescribing (and diligence in observing the patient on) any NSAID concurrently with any beta-blocker or diuretic. While the short half-life of diclofenac makes it less likely to cause renal side-effects, the best course is obviously to proceed cautiously in any elderly patient with impaired renal function who is receiving antihypertensives.

Most of the non-steroidals are tightly bound to albumin and might theoretically produce problems when given with anticoagulants or oral antidiabetics. It appears that other NSAIDs are bound at different sites on albumin and are much less likely to cause such interactions[146,147]. In particular, several studies have indicated that some NSAIDs - ibuprofen[148], naproxen and tolmetin[146], all with relatively short half-lives and presumably less avid albumin binding - can safely be given to patients on at least some anticoagulants. The obvious advice to the physician is that, if a non-steroidal is to be prescribed to a patient also taking an anticoagulant, oral antidiabetic or any drug which is tightly bound to albumin, caution should be exercised.

Lithium has been widely used to treat depression, and there is evidence that its effects may be accentuated by non-steroidals, perhaps especially indomethacin[149,150]; patients given both lithium and other NSAIDs (e.g. ibuprofen) have experienced such symptoms as nausea and drowsiness[149]. Since lithium may also be used to treat the neutropenia of Felty's syndrome, it would be well to keep in mind that there could be potential interactions.

Probenecid decreases the excretion of indomethacin[151] and naproxen[152] and, in fact, has been used therapeutically to increase blood levels of some NSAIDs in hopes of preventing the severe morning stiffness of rheumatoid arthritis. It should be used with caution with any of the non-steroidals.

V. DISCUSSION

The major question of safety in treating rheumatic diseases is this: what are we trying to avoid? Is it the minor adverse reaction, such as gastritis, or the rare idiosyncrasy? We presumably do not want a drug which is totally free of side-effects if the price of such safety is a loss of therapeutic potency. If the drug works and the side-effect is (like gastritis) easily detected by the physician, it may well be acceptable to both the patient and the physician. Either an attempt can be made to tolerate the side-effect (for example, if the non-steroidal causes oedema but is effective therapeutically, the oedema can be treated with thiazide); or, if the side-effect is seriously bothersome (for example, severe dyspepsia), the drug can be discontinued and another non-steroidal substituted for it.

This, I think, is the central clinical point to make concerning the most frequent adverse reaction to all the non-steroidals, ulceration. In practical terms we are not seeking a drug that is wholly free from this side-effect. If the patient is carefully monitored after the drug is prescribed, the symptoms of gastric distress are readily apparent, and the drug may (and of course should) be promptly discontinued. In uncontrolled trials of indomethacin in which the patients were seen frequently; under those circumstances less than half of 1% developed ulcers[27]. Thus if the physician carefully observes the patient, the problem of ulceration can be minimized.

When we turn to the rare, idiosyncratic side-effects, these occur with such statistical infrequency that there is no reasonable way to plan to avoid them. Some of them, however, can be fatal - obviously a very serious medical (and medical-legal) problem. The best that can be done, practically speaking, is for the physician to be knowledgeable about the possible rare reactions, alert to detect one should it occur, and quick to discontinue the drug in that case.

VI. CONCLUSIONS

Excluding the most frequent kind of problems seen with the non-steroidal anti-inflammatory drugs or NSAIDs - gastritis, peptic ulceration and renal effects - published reports indicate that these drugs cause a wide variety of rare adverse reactions. The most serious of these are hypersensitivity reactions: blood dyscrasias (aplastic anaemia, thrombocytopenia, agranulocytosis, haemolytic anaemia), erythema multiforme and hepatitis. Aseptic meningitis and anaphylactoid reactions may affect patients with underlying immunological abnormalities; urticaria, bronchospasm and proto-colitis may affect aspirin-sensitive patients. Other unusual reactions include several kinds of bullous dermatitis, febrile reactions, pneumonitis, oesophageal ulceration, parotitis, pancreatitis, and neurological or psychological effects. Age is the major risk factor in such reactions, and the problems of using NSAIDs with long half-lives in the elderly are emphasized.

REFERENCES

1. O'Brien, WM and Bagby, GF (1985). Rare adverse reactions to nonsteroidal anti-inflammatory drugs. J Rheumatol, 12, 13, 347
2. Stern, RS and Bigby, M (1984). An expanded profile of cutaneous reactions to nonsteroidal anti-inflammatory drugs: reports to a specialty-based system for spontaneous reporting of adverse reactions to drugs. J Am Med Assoc, 252, 1433
3. Ward, K and Weir, DG (1982). Piroxicam and upper gastrointestinal haemorrhage. Ir Med J, 75, 10
4. Fok, KH, George, PJM and Vicary, FR (1985). Peptic ulcers induced by piroxicam. Br Med J, 290, 117
5. Laake, K, Kjeldaas, L and Borchgrevink, CF (1984). Side-effects of piroxicam (Feldene): a one-year material of 103 reports from Norway. Acta Med Scand, 215, 81
6. Robert, A, Nezamis, JE, Lancaster, C and Hanchar, AJ (1979). Cytoprotection by prostaglandins in rats: prevention of gastric necrosis produced by alcohol, HCl, NaOH, hypertonic NaCl, and thermal injury. Gastroenterology, 77, 433
7. Bolton, JP, Palmer, D and Cohen, MM (1978). Stimulation of mucus and non-parietal cell secretion by the E-2 prostaglandins. Dig Dis Sci, 23, 359
8. Subcommittee on the National Halothane Study of the Committee on Anesthesia, National Academy of Sciences-National Research Council. Summary of the national halothane study: possible association between halothane anesthesia and postoperative hepatic necrosis. J Am Med Assoc, 197, 775
9. Bottiger, LE, Nordlander, M and Strandberg, I (1974). Deaths from drugs: an analysis of drug-induced deaths reported to the Swedish Adverse Drug Reaction Committee during a five-year period (1966-1970). J Clin Pharmacol, 14,401
10. Bottiger, LE (1977). Phenylbutazone, oxyphenbutazone and aplastic anaemia. Br Med J, 2, 265
11. The Regulation of New Drugs by the Food and Drug Administration: The New Drug Review Process (1982). Hearings before a Subcommittee of the Committee on Government Operations, House of Representatives, Ninety-seventh Congress, Second Session, August 3 and 4, 1982, Washington, DC: US Government Printing Office, pp. 1-688
12. Inman, WH and Vessey, MP (1968). Investigation of deaths from pulmonary, coronary, and cerebral thrombosis and embolism in women of childbearing age. Br Med J, 2, 193
13. Inman, WHW (1982). First results of post marketing surveillance study from the University of Southampton (unpublished manuscript). Southampton, England, 26 February, pp. 1-4

14. Inman, WHW (1982). Prescription-event monitoring: a preliminary study of benoxaprofen and fenbufen (unpublished manuscript). Southampton, England, pp. 1-33
15. Fox, DA and Jick, H (1984). Nonsteroidal anti-inflammatory drugs and renal disease. J Am Med Assoc, 251, 1299
16. Coles, LS, Fries, JF, Kraines, RG and Roth, SH (1983). From experiment to experience: side effects of nonsteroidal anti-inflammatory drugs. Am J Med, 74, 820
17. US General Accounting Office (1982). Report to the Secretary of Health and Human Services: FDA Can Further Improve Its Adverse Drug Reaction Reporting System. Washington, DC: HRD-82-37, pp. i-iv, 1-28
18. Fourteenth Report by the Committee on Government Operations together with Additional Views (1983). Deficiencies in FDA's Regulation of the New Drug "Oraflex", Washington, DC: US Government Printing Office, pp. 1-26
19. Venulet, J, Blattner, R, von Bulow, J and Berneker, GC (1982). How good are articles on adverse drug reactions? Br Med J, 1, 252
20. Taggart, HM and Alderdice, JM (1982). Fatal cholestatic jaundice in elderly patients taking benoxaprofen. Br Med J, 284, 1372
21. Venning, GR (1983). Identification of adverse reactions to new drugs (in five parts). Br Med J, pp. 286, 199, 289, 365, 458, 544
22. Silvoso, GR, Ivey, KJ and Butt, JH (1979). Incidence of gastric lesions in patients with rheumatic disease on chronic aspirin therapy. Ann Intern Med, 91, 517
23. Bowen, R Jr, Mayne, JG, Cain, JC, et al (1960). Peptic ulcer in rheumatoid arthritis and relationship to steroid treatment. Proc Staff Meet Mayo Clin, 35, 537
24. Berntsen, CA and Freyberg, RH (1961). Rheumatoid patients after five or more years of corticosteroid treatment: a comparative analysis of 183 cases. Ann Intern Med, 54, 938
25. Bunim, JJ (1958). Critical evaluation of synthetic steroids in the treatment of rheumatoid arthritis. Arch Int Am Rheumatol, 1, 464, 82
26. Kammerer, WH, Freyburg, RH and Rivelis, AL (1958). Peptic ulcer in rheumatoid arthritis patients on corticosteroid therapy. Arthritis Rheum, 1, 122
27. O'Brien, WM (1968). Indomethacin: a survey of clinical trials. Clin Pharmacol Ther, 9, 94
28. Davies-Caradoc, TH (1984). Nonsteroidal anti-inflammatory drugs, arthritis, and gastrointestinal bleeding in elderly in-patients. Age Ageing, 13, 295
29. Henrich, WL (1983). Nephrotoxicity of nonsteroidal anti-inflammatory agents. Am J Kidney Dis, 2, 478
30. Clive, DM and Stoff, JS (1984). Renal syndromes associated with nonsteroidal anti-inflammatory drugs. N Engl J Med, 310, 563
31. Stillman, MT, Napier, J and Blackshear, JL (1984). Adverse effects of nonsteroidal anti-inflammatory drugs on the kidney. Med Clin North Am, 68, 371
32. Garella, S and Matarese, RA (1984). Renal effects of prostaglandins and clinical adverse effects of nonsteroidal anti-inflammatory agents. Medicine (Baltimore), 63, 165
33. Bunning, RD and Barth, WF (1982). Sulindac: a potentially renal-sparing nonsteroidal anti-inflammatory drug. J Am Med Assoc, 248, 2864
34. Ciabattoni, G, Cinotti, GA, Pierucci, A, et al (1984). Effects of sulindac and ibuprofen in patients with chronic glomerular disease. Evidence for the dependence of renal function on prostacyclin. N Engl J Med, 310, 279
35. Mitnick, PD (1983). Sulindac and renal failure. J Am Med Assoc, 250, 34
36. Whelton, A, Bender, W, Vaghaiwalla, F, Hall-Craggs, M and Solez, K (1983).

Sulindac and renal impairment. J Am Med Assoc, 249, 2892
37. Svendsen, UG, Gerstoft, J, Hansen, TM, Christensen, P and Lorenzen, IB (1984). The renal excretion of prostaglandins and changes in plasma renin during treatment with either sulindac or naproxen in patients with rheumatoid arthritis and thiazide treated heart failure. J Rheumatol, 11, 779
38. Coste, F, Delbarre, F, Cayla, J, et al (1965). L'indomethacine en rhumatologie. Presse Medicale, 73, 1673
39. Kelly, M (1966). Treatment of 193 rheumatic patients with indomethacin, a new antirheumatic drug. J Am Geriatr Soc, 14, 48-55
40. Donnelly, P, Lloyd, K and Campbell, H (1967). Indomethacin in rheumatoid arthritis: an evaluation of its anti-inflammatory and side effects. Br Med J, 1, 69-75
41. Shack, ME (1966). Drug induced ulceration and perforation of the small bowel. Ariz Med, 23, 517
42. Somogyi, A, Kovacs, K and Selye, H (1969). Jejunal ulcers produced by indomethacin. J Pharm Pharmacol, 21, 122
43. Sturges, HF and Krone, CL (1973). Ulceration and stricture of the jejunum in a patient on long-term indomethacin therapy. Am J Gastroenterol, 59, 162
44. Marks, JS and Gleeson, MH (1975). Steatorrhea complicating therapy with mefenamic acid. Br Med J, 4, 442
45. Chadwick, RG, Hossenbocus, A and Colin-Jones, DG (1976). Steatorrhea complicating therapy with mefenamic acid. Br Med J, 1, 397
46. Thompson, M and Percy, JS (1966). Further experience with indomethacin in the treatment of rheumatic disorders. Br Med J, 1, 80-3
47. Chanda, JJ and Callen, JP (1978). Erythema multiforme and the Stevens-Johnson syndrome. South Med J, 71, 566
48. Dubois, A, Malbos, S, Chevreau, P, Hansel, S and Janbon, C (1982). Erytheme polymorphe et syndrome de Stevens-Johnson apres traitement par diflunisal. Nouv Presse Med, 11, 606
49. O'Sullivan, M, Hanly, JG and Molloy, M (1983). A case of toxic epidermal necrolysis secondary to indomethacin. Br J Rheumatol, 22, 47
50. Cirne de Castro, JL, Diffey, BL, Pal, B and Daymond, TJ (1984). Phototoxic reactions to nonsteroidal anti-inflammatory drugs (an exchange of letters). Br J Rheumatol, 23, 155
51. Diffey, BL, Daymond, TJ and Fairgreaves, H (1983). Photoxic reactions to piroxicam, naproxen and tiaprofenic acid. Br J Rheumatol, 22, 239
52. Merot, Y, Harms, M and Saurat, JH (1983). Photosensibilisation au carprofene (Imadyl), un nouvel anti-inflammatoire non steroidien. Dermatologica, 166, 301
53. Diffey, B and Hindson, H (1982). Side effects of benoxaprofen. Br Med J, 284, 1630
54. DuVivier, A (1982). Bullous dermatitis associated with benoxaprofen. Lancet, 1, 47
55. Stern, RS (1983). Phototoxic reactions to piroxicam and other nonsteroidal anti-inflammatory agents. N Engl J Med, 309, 186
56. Moore-Robinson, M and Warin, RP (1967). Effect of salicylates in urticaria. Br Med J, 4, 262
57. Settipane, GA (1983). Adverse reactions to aspirin and related drugs. In: Rainsford, KD and Velo, GP (eds), Side-Effects of Anti-inflammatory/Analgesic Drugs. (New York: Raven Press), pp. 189-201
58. Bailin, PL and Matkaluk, RM (1982). Cutaneous reactions to rheumatological drugs. Clin Rheum Dis, 8, 493
59. Ronningen, H and Langeland, N (1979). Indomethacin treatment in

osteoarthritis of the hip joint: does the treatment interfere with the natural course of the disease? Acta Orthop Scand, 50, 169
60. Arora, JS (1968). Indomethacin arthropathy of hips. Proc R Soc Med, 61, 669
61. Aaron, TH and Muttitt, ELC (1982). Reactions to acetylsalicylic acid. Can Med Assoc J, 126, 609
62. Samter, M and Beers, RF (1968). Intolerance to aspirin: clinical studies and consideration of its pathogenesis. Ann Intern Med, 68, 975
63. Samter, M and Beers, RF (1967). Concerning the nature of intolerance to aspirin. J Allergy Clin Immunol, 40, 281
64. Settipane, GA, Chafee, FH and Klein, DE (1974). Aspirin intolerance: II. A prospective study in an atopic and normal population. J Allergy Clin Immunol, 53, 200
65. Smith, AP (1971). Response of aspirin-allergic patients to challenge by some analgesics in common use. Br Med J, 2, 494
66. Szczeklik, A, Gryglewski, RJ and Czerniawska-Mysik, G (1977). Clinical patterns of hypersensitivity to nonsteroidal anti-inflammatory drugs and their pathogenesis. J Allergy Clin Immunol, 60, 276
67. Szczeklik, A, Gryglewski, RJ, Czerniawska-Mysik, G and Zmuda, A (1976). Aspirin-induced asthma: hypersensitivity to fenoprofen and ibuprofen in relation to their inhibitory action on prostaglandin generation by different microsomal enzymic preparations. J Allergy Clin Immunol, 58, 10
68. Fisherman, EW and Cohen, GN (1978). Hypersensitivity to five non-steroidal anti-inflammatory agents: ibuprofen, fenoprofen, indomethacin, naproxen and tolmetin. Ann Allergy, 41, 75
69. Fisherman, EW and Cohen, GN (1976). Ibuprofen (Motrin) hypersensitivity in intrinsic and extrinsic allergic patients. Ann Allergy, 37, 353
70. Walters, JS, Woodring, JH, Stelling, CB and Rosenbaum, HD (1983). Salicylate-induced pulmonary edema. Radiology, 146, 289
71. Fein, M (1981). Sulindac and pneumonitis. Ann Intern Med, 95, 245
72. Nader, DA and Schillaci, RF (1983). Pulmonary infiltrates with eosinophilia due to naproxen. Chest, 83, 280
73. Lebacq, EG and Desmet, V (1977). Sarcoid granulomas associated with phenylbutazone treatment. Mt Sinai J Med (NY), 44, 778
74. Bravo, JF, Jacobson, MP and Mertens, BF (1977). Fatty liver and pleural effusion with ibuprofen therapy. Ann Intern Med, 87, 200
75. Brennan, M (1980). Activation of latent tuberculosis by nonsteroidal anti-inflammatory agents. Can Med Assoc J, 122, 400
76. Brennan, M (1982). Latent tuberculosis and anti-inflammatory agents. Can Med Assoc J, 126, 21
77. Tomasson, HO, Brennan, M and Bass, MJ (1984). Tuberculosis and nonsteroidal anti-inflammatory drugs. Can Med Assoc J, 130, 275
78. O'Brein, WM and Bagby, GF (1983). Anaphylactoid reactions to nonsteroidal anti-inflammatory drugs. In: Rainsford, KD and Velo, GP (eds), Side Effects of Anti-inflammatory/Analgesic Drugs. (New York: Raven Press), pp. 203-207
79. Mandell, B, Shen, HS and Hepburn, B (1976). Fever from ibuprofen in a patient with lupus erythematosus. Ann Intern Med, 85, 209
80. Sonnenblick, M and Abraham, AS (1978). Ibuprofen hypersensitivity in systemic lupus erythematosus. Br Med J, 1, 619
81. Lee, RP, King, EG and Russell, AS (1983). Ibuprofen: a severe systemic reaction. Can Med Assoc J, 129, 854
82. Farid, N and Anderson, J (1971). S.L.E.-like reaction after phenylbutazone. Lancet, 1, 1022
83. Bar-Sela, S, Levo, Y, Zeevi, D, Slavin, S and Eliakim, M (1980). A lupus-like syndrome due to ibuprofen hypersensitivity. J Rheumatol, 7, 379

84. Handley, AJ (1971). Thrombocytopenia and L.E. cells after oxyphenbutazone. Lancet, 1, 245

85. Sprung, DJ (1982). Sulindac causing a hypersensitivity reaction with peripheral and mediastinal lymphadenopathy. Ann Intern Med, 97, 564

86. Jacobs, JC (1971). Sudden death in arthritic children receiving large doses of indomethacin. J Am Med Assoc, 199, 182

87. Rodriguez, RS and Barbabosa, E (1971). Haemorrhagic chicken pox after indomethacin. N Engl J Med, 285, 690

88. Wilkerson, RD and Glenn, TM (1977). Influence of nonsteroidal anti-inflammatory drugs on ouabain toxicity. Am Heart J, 94, 454

89. Friedman, PL, Brown, EJ, Gunther, S et al (1981). Coronary vasoconstrictor effect of indomethacin in patients with coronary-artery disease. N Engl J Med, 305, 1171

90. Golding, D (1970). Angina and indomethacin. Br Med J, 4, 622

91. Dzau, VJ, Packer, M, Lilly, LS, Swartz, SL, Hollenberg, NK and Williams, GH (1984). Prostaglandins in severe congestive heart failure: relation to activation of the renin-angiotensin system and hyponatremia. N Engl J Med, 310, 347

92. Bottiger, LE and Westerholm, B (1972). Aplastic anaemia: II. Drug-induced aplastic anaemia. Acta Med Scand, 192, 319

93. McIntyre, BA, Philp, RB and Inwood, MJ (1978). Effect of ibuprofen on platelet function in normal subjects and haemophiliac patients. Clin Pharmacol Ther, 24, 616

94. Cuthbert, MF (1974). Adverse reactions to non-steroidal antirheumatic drugs. Curr Med Res Opin, 2, 600

95. Arneborn, P and Palmblad, J (1982). Drug-induced neutropenia - a survey for Stockholm 1973-1978. Acta Med Scand, 212, 289

96. Hughes, JA and Sudell, W (1983). Hemolytic anemia associated with naproxen. Arthritis Rheum, 26, 1054

97. Jensen, K (1976). Bivirkninger af naproksen. Ugeskr Laeger, 138, 3284

98. Patmas, MA, Wilborn, SL and Shankel, SW (1984). Acute multisystem toxicity associated with the use of nonsteroidal anti-inflammatory drugs. Arch Intern Med, 144, 519

99. Ciucci, AG (1979). A review of spontaneously reported adverse drug reactions with diclofenac sodium (Voltarol). Rheumatol Rehabil Suppl, 2, 116

100. Korsager, S, Sorensen, H, Jensen, OH and Falk, JV (1981). Antiglobulin-tests for detection of auto-immunohaemolytic anaemia during long-term treatment with ibuprofen. Scand J Rheumatol, 10, 174

101. Kleint, V (1971). Kropfbildungen mit mechanischen storfolgen unter phenylbutazon. Deutsch Gesundheitswesen, 26, 1057

102. Vermeulen, A and Schoot, JB van der (1972). De invloed van fenylbutazon op de schildklier. Ned Tijdschr Geneeskd, 116, 369

103. Lane, RJM, Clark, F and McCollum, JK (1977). Oxphenbutazone-induced goitre. Postgrad Med J, 53, 93

104. Fowler, PD, Crook, PR and Hothersall, TE (1982). Diclofenac sodium and thyroid function tests. Rheumatol Rehabil, 21, 42

105. Heller, SR, Fellows, IW, Ogilvie, AL and Atkinson, M (1982). Non-steroidal anti-inflammatory drugs and benign oesophageal stricture. Br Med J, 285, 167-8

106. Wilkins, WE, Ridley, MG and Pozniak, AL (1984). Benign stricture of the oesophagus: role of non-steroidal anti-inflammatory drugs. Gut, 25, 478

107. Gardies, A, Gevaudan, J, LeRoux, C, Cornet, C, Warnet-Duboscq, J and Viguie, R (1978). Ulcere iatrogene de l'oesophage. Nouv Presse Med, 7, 1032

108. Agdal, N (1979). Drug-induced oesophageal damage: a review and report of a

fatal case of indomethacin-induced ulceration. Ugeskr Laeger, 141, 3019
109. Bataille, C, Soumagne, D, Loly, J and Brassinne, A (1982). Oesophageal ulceration due to indomethacin. Digestion, 24, 66
110. Mallory, A and Kern, F (1980). Drug-induced pancreatitis: a critical review. Gastroenterology, 78, 813
111. Goldstein, J, Laskin, DA and Ginsberg, GH (1980). Sulindac associated with pancreatitis. Ann Intern Med, 93, 151
112. Siefkin, AD (1980). Sulindac and pancreatitis. Ann Intern Med, 93, 932
113. Memon, AN (1982). Pancreatitis and sulindac. Ann Intern Med, 97, 139
114. Klein, SM and Khan, MA (1983). Hepatitis, toxic epidermal necrolysis and pancreatitis in association with sulindac therapy. J Rheumatol, 10, 512
115. Guerra, M (1967). Toxicity of indomethacin: report of a case of acute pancreatitis. J Am Med Assoc, 200, 552
116. Schwartz, HA (1981). Lower gastrointestinal side effects of nonsteroidal anti-inflammatory drugs. J Rheumatol, 8, 952
117. Rampton, DS and Sladen, GE (1981). Relapse of ulcerative proctocolitis during treatment with non-steroidal anti-inflammatory drugs. Postgrad Med J, 57, 297
118. Walt, RP, Hawkey, CJ and Langman, MJS (1984). Colitis associated with non-steroidal anti-inflammatory drugs. Br Med J, 288, 238
119. Coutrot, S, Roland, D, Barbier, J, Van Der Marcq, P, Alcalay, M and Matuchansky, C. (1978). Acute perforation of colonic diverticula associated with short-term indomethacin. Lancet, 2, 1055
120. Langman, MJS, Morgan, L and Worrall, A (1985). Use of anti-inflammatory drugs by patients admitted with small or large bowel perforations and haemorrhage. Br Med J, 290, 347
121. Seaman, WE and Plotz, PH (1976). Effect of aspirin on liver tests in patients with RA or SLE and in normal volunteers. Arthritis Rheum, 19, 155
122. Russell, AS, Sturge, RA and Smith, MA (1971). Serum transaminases during salicylate therapy. Br Med J, 2, 428
123. Rich, RR and Johnson, JA (1973). Salicylate hepatotoxicity in patients with juvenile rheumatoid arthritis. Arthritis Rheum, 16, 1-9
124. Seaman, WE, Ishak, KG and Plotz, PH (1974). Aspirin-induced hepatotoxicity in patients with systemic lupus erythematosus. Ann Intern Med, 80, 1
125. Iancu, T and Elian, E (1976). Ultrastructural changes in aspirin hepatotoxicity. Am J Clin Pathol, 66, 570
126. Dunk, AA, Walt, RP, Jenkins, WJ and Sherlock, SS (1982). Diclofenac hepatitis. Br Med J, 284, 1605
127. Kammerer, J, Sabardeil, S, Rumeau, JL, Salson, A and El Hage, A (1982). Hepatite au sulindac: une observation avec revue des trois precedentes. Gastroenterol Clin Biol, 6, 712
128. Sternlieb, P and Robinson, RM (1978). Stevens-Johnson syndrome plus toxic hepatitis due to ibuprofen. NY State J Med, 78, 1239
129. Smith, FE and Lindberg, PJ (1980). Life-threatening hypersensitivity to sulindac. J Am Med Assoc, 244, 269
130. Park, GD, Spector, R, Headstream, T and Goldberg, M (1982). Serious adverse reactions associated with sulindac. Arch Intern Med, 142, 1292
131. Stempel, DA, and Miller, JJ (1977). Lymphopenia and hepatic toxicity with ibuprofen. J Pediatr, 90, 657
132. Hartmann, H, Fischer, G and Janning, G (1984). Prolonged cholestatic jaundice and leukopenia associated with piroxicam. Z Gastroenterol, 22, 343
133. Ruppert, GB and Barth, WF (1981). Ibuprofen hypersensitivity in systemic lupus erythematosus. South Med J, 74, 241
134. Treves, R, Gastine, H, Richard, A et al (1983). Responsabilite de

l'ibuprofen dans une meningite aseptique et une insuffisance renale aigue au cours d'un lupus erythemateux dissemine. Rev Rhum Mal Osteoartic, 50, 75
135. Myers, EN, Bernstein, JM and Fostiropolous, G (1965). Salicylate ototoxicity. N Engl J Med, 273, 587
136. Miller, RR (1978). Deafness due to plain and long-acting aspirin tablets. J Clin Pharmacol, 18, 468
137. Taylor, KPA and Rothermich, NO (1973). Deafness and hand tremor with indomethacin. J Am Med Assoc, 226, 1471
138. Robinson, R (1965). Indomethacin in rheumatic disease: a clinical assessment. Med J Aust, 1, 266
139. Ajodhia, JM and Dix, MR (1976). Drug-induced deafness and its treatment. Practitioner, 216, 561
140. Anderson, RJ, Potts, DE, Gabow, PA, Rumack, BH and Schrier, RW (1976). Unrecognized adult salicylate intoxication. Ann Intern Med, 85, 745
141. Goodwin, JS and Regan, M (1982). Cognitive dysfunction associated with naproxen and ibuprofen in the elderly. Arthritis Rheum, 25, 1013
142. Goodwin, JF (1964). Some physiological implications of gold in serum and urine concentrations in chrysotherapy. J Mich St Med Soc, 63, 437
143. Runkel, R, Forchielli, E, Sevelius, H, Chaplin, M and Segre, E (1974). Nonlinear plasma level reponse to high doses of naproxen. Clin Pharmacol Ther, 15, 261
144. Watkins, J, Abbott, EC, Hensby, CN, Webster, J and Dollery, CT (1980). Attenuation of hypotensive effect of propranolol and thiazide diuretics by indomethacin. Br Med J, 281, 702
145. Favre, L, Glasson, P and Vallotton, MB (1982). Reversible acute renal failure from combined triamterene and indomethacin. Ann Intern Med, 96, 317
146. Ascione, FJ (1978). Oral anticoagulants with aspirin alternatives. Drug Therapy, 8, 63
147. Shah, SJ, Bhandarkar, SD and Satoskar, RS (1984). Drug interaction between chlorpropamide and non-steroidal anti-inflammatory drugs, ibuprofen and phenylbutazone. Int J Clin Pharmacol Ther Toxicol, 22, 470
148. Duckert, F (1975). The absence of effect of the antirheumatic drug ibuprofen on oral anticoagulation with phenprocoumon. Curr Med Res Opin, 3, 556
149. Ragheb, M, Ban, TA, Buchanan, D, Frolich, JC (1980). Interaction of indomethacin and ibuprofen with lithium in manic patients under a steady-state lithium level. J lin Psychiatry, 41, 397
150. Frölich, JC, Leftwich, R, Ragheb, M, Oates, JA, Reimann, I and Buchanan, D (1979). Indomethacin increases plasma lithium. Br Med J, 1, 1115
151. Brooks, PM, Bell, MA and Sturrock, RD (1974). The clinical significance of indomethacin-probenecid interaction. Br J Clin Pharmacol, 1, 287
152. Runkel, R, Mroszczak, E, Chaplin, M, Sevelius, H and Segre, E (1978). Naproxen-probenecid interaction. Clin Pharmacol Ther, 24, 706

Discussion

Dr KD Rainsford, UK Your approach to the problem of ADR reporting leads however to questions particularly about the value you would attach to case reporting per se because this seems to be the vexed question, especially when contrasted with the value of registry data. What are your feelings about that?

Prof O'Brien I think those of you concerned should refer to the paper by Venning in the British Medical Journal in 1984 where he traces the history of drug catastrophies. Of the ADRs that we're so concerned about 10 out of 20 were picked up by individual reports from physicians and only one which is the oral antidiurectic that caused acidosis that was known in the pre-clinical testing. It's just that the average physician could not handle the acidosis which this drug produced. In none of the other 20 drugs were the signals actually given by registries. I think registries are important in determining some of the numerators and denominators, but they probably have secondary importance to careful case reporting. The presentation from the US FDA indicated the inadequacies of much of the data. We've got to get better data and we've got to have better individual reports from physicians.

Dr Rainsford So your point actually is that you start first with case reports rather than registries?

Prof O'Brien Yes. For example indomethacin was used until 1976 before anyone had any idea that it or its relatives, the NSAIDs, had a major effect on renal function, which is something that is quite obvious now.

Professor C Patrono, Italy Having been involved in some of the earlier studies on sulindac on renal prostaglandin formation and renal function I would like to contrast your single case report with results of 3 control studies of sulindac versus another NSAIDs in patients with mild renal impairment which was published last year in the New England Journal of Medicine. A more recent one by Berg from Norway by which sulindac was studied in patients with severe renal inefficiency and there is even a more recent report of Zipser in UCLA in Los Angeles in patients with severe liver dysfunction and ascites. Now all of these studies demonstrate that there is no change in renal function in patients exposed to sulindac as opposed to other non-steroidals. The reason for some contradictory findings in the literature is simply related to biochemical measurements. That is, there are people who have reported sulindac reduces urinary prostaglandin excretion. Now there are numerous reasons that are related to methodology which can account for this.

Prof O'Brien I agree that those data are very important and as I said, I think the jury is still out. However a study was reported in the Journal of Rheumatology of November 1984 by some Scandinavians, (I believe they are from Copenhagen), in which they very carefully crossed patients over from sulindac to naproxin and from sulindac to ibuprofen then they reversed the sequence, and measured the urinary prostaglandins. They didn't show a difference and certainly physicians other than I have found patients with renal impairment when given sulindac did develop failure, so I personally am confused and I don't think the question is at this time answered.

Dr JG Lombardino, USA It seems obvious to me that if there's a drug catastrophy you go back into the literature and look at all the case reports and say that I have found one that would have predicted that if we looked at it. That seems obvious, but there have been, I'm sure, many other case reports that would not have been predictive, so what would be the predictive value of a single case report looking forward into the future.

Prof O'Brien I think the answer to that is that many of these reactions are unique. There are things that haven't been seen before and there are usually cluster effects. Once a single case report occurs, other case reports appear and again I can refer you to Venning. I think there is quite convincing evidence that most of the withdrawals of NSAI drugs have been triggered by individual case reports of physicians which we then confirmed by other case reports of other physicians and that the death of drugs in the last 20 years has primarily been determined by case reports and many of these case reports appearing in the British Medical Journal.

Dr H Jick, I think it's very important to get certain rudimentary facts straight in this area because it is such an important area. Our studies are formal. We do not have registers for our patients. We follow up every single case carefully for medical events and if I might speak for Bill O'Brien for a moment, his studies are also formal. He does not run a registry, he runs a formal study with as much a full follow up as he can get. Therefore these studies are quite different from the standard registries, and I think it's extremely important that we should be able to tell the difference between a registry report and a formal study in which there is a complete follow up.

Dr Wiholm, Sweden I think that Dr Venning has made a good point, that is the observation of the single physician which leads to the study of most of the rare reactions. However, he was a little bit unfair to the registries, because most of the 20 reactions he described, actually were described before there were any registries or spontaneous reporting. More than half of these were in this group so that's a bit unfair to say that this spontaneous reporting couldn't have picked those up. Also, at least in Sweden, we take in the full case reports, the full hospital records of all severe and fatal cases, so that we have all the information. It might be that we do not publish enough of our findings so that the literature seems inadequate.

7
Pyrazolone-induced agranulocytosis: an epidemiological evaluation

Micha Levy
Clinical Pharmacology Unit,
Department of Medicine A,
Hadassah University Hospital,
Jerusalem 91-120, Israel

CONTENTS

I. INTRODUCTION

Hundreds of drugs have been alleged to cause agranulocytosis. Specifically with regard to pyrazolones, a causal relationship has been demonstrated by rechallenge, and by transfusion studies. However, the magnitude of the risk of agranulocytosis associated with pyrazolones remained uncertain, and the quality of the available information has not improved appreciably over the past 50 years. It consists of series of case reports, letters to the editor and notes to agencies monitoring adverse reactions. Most cases have involved multiple drug exposures, and attribution to a specific drug has usually been based on informal ad hoc judgments as to which one was responsible, since no specific diagnostic procedure is available and intentional rechallenge is ethically unacceptable. Such ad hoc judgments are often biased in implicating drugs already under suspicion. In addition the inaccurate documentation of the temporal relationship between drug exposure and the event give rise to serious problems of misclassification.

Side-effects of Anti-inflammatory Drugs. Rainsford, KD and Velo, GP (eds)
Part 1: Clinical and Epidemiological Aspects. (Lancaster: MTP Press)

II. ASSESSMENT OF PREVIOUS CASE REPORTS

These problems characterize the series of cases published amongst others by Pretty et al[1], Palva and Mustala[2], Kantero et al[3], and Heimpel and Abt[4]. In none of these publications was an attempt made to measure drug exposure in a control group, and it is likely that multiple sources of bias were present. For these reasons many of the inferences drawn in these studies are of questionable validity.

Shinar et al[5], in a retrospective study of hospital records in Jerusalem over 12 years found notes that dipyrone, a commonly used analgesic-antipyretic in Israel, was taken within 1 month preceding the diagnosis by 11 cases out of a total of 48 cases. It is, however, impossible to interpret these findings without obtaining standardized information on dipyrone use from a properly selected control group. As a matter of fact, during the years 1969-76, 21% of all patients who were admitted to a medical department in the same hospital gave an unsolicited positive history of having taken dipyrone during the month before admission[6].

Agranulocytosis most commonly presents with fever and infection with subsequent hospitalization and diagnosis. It is therefore essential that drug histories be carefully timed to determine whether exposure to any specific drug took place before the onset of the first symptom of agranulocytosis. Otherwise drugs (e.g. antibiotics and analgesic-antipyretics) given for the treatment of early symptoms may wrongly be implicated as causes.

Aspirin, paracetamol and phenacetin have all appeared in the drug histories of agranulocytosis patients described in the above-cited papers, although they were not usually judged to be causal. However, they could have been, and indeed some investigators have implicated these drugs. For example, Jouet et al[7] suggested that paracetamol may account for as much as 10% of all case of agranulocytosis.

Taking into account all the complexities mentioned it is not surprising that this field has been difficult to study and that reliable data have been either lacking, or, where available, incomplete or conflicting. At present it is difficult to compare quantitatively the risks associated with various analgesic drugs. This led to the present situation in which there are conflicting judgments and regulations about the use of analgesic drugs. The one estimate of the incidence of pyrazolone-induced agranulocytosis which is constantly cited in textbooks and by regulatory agencies is that of Huguley[8], which in turn is mainly based on calculations made by Discombe[9]. It is regrettable that the rates reported by them of 0.79% to 0.86% are still cited as if these studies were reasonably valid. Huguley and Discombe based their calculations on earlier reports, the first two of which[10,11] were prompted by the primary identification of small clusters of cases, followed by secondary attempts to quantify the denominators. In a third report[12] some cases of neutropenia, none of which were considered by the investigators to be clinical agranulocytosis, were observed among patients treated for rheumatoid arthritis with a combination of aminopyrine and phenylbutazone. Without giving details Discombe reclassified two patients as cases of agranulocytosis.

The additional studies to which Discombe and Huguley referred[13-15] were not based on first identifying clusters of cases, but rather on the primary identification of denominators of pyrazolone users, a more proper approach. No cases of agranulocytosis were identified. Other investigators who have used this approach rigorously have ruled out an incidence of agranulocytosis of 1% in pyrazolone users[16].

Had the estimates of Discombe and Huguley been correct, agranulocytosis would be one of the major causes of death in countries where dipyrone is commonly used, rather than a rare disease.

A potential (if very approximate) approach to estimating the magnitude of pyrazolone-induced agranulocytosis is to measure what, if any, changes in the incidence of the disease occur following bans or restriction on the use of pyrazolones. A study[17] based on all cases of agranulocytosis admitted to hospitals in the Stockholm region up to 1978 did not reveal any change in the incidence of that condition following the banning of dipyrone in 1973. This study showed an annual incidence rate for all cases of agranulocytosis of 0.009% and a mortality rate of 11%. However, other agranulocytosis-inducing drugs may have been substituted for dipyrone and have influenced the results.

III. REGISTRY DATA

Another approach to the problem has been to tally cases reported to government adverse reaction registries. However, such registries usually do not provide reliable proof of causation or of incidence because of incomplete, selective and biased reports.

In a study of dipyrone-attributed agranulocytosis, based on reports to the Swedish Adverse Reaction Registry from 1964 to 1968, Boetiger and Westerholm estimated a rate of about one out of every 3000 dipyrone users[18]. The denominator on dipyrone consumption was estimated from sale figures limited to one area and to the years 1968-69 when dipyrone consumption was already very low.

To sum up, although experimentally pyrazolones have been shown to cause agranulocytosis, all of the studies previously carried out to date to quantitate the risk appear to be unsatisfactory.

IV. ANALYTICAL EPIDEMIOLOGICAL STUDIES

The only feasible way to properly derive estimates of the risk of pyrazolone-induced agranulocytosis is by means of analytical epidemiological studies. Because of the rarity of agranulocytosis (about 6 per million per year), the case-control method is the only one available. The requirements to be fulfilled in case-control studies are the same as in other fields of scientific research; namely, adequate quality of data, fairness of comparisons, and rigorous methods. It is necessary to compare patients who have well-defined agranulocytosis with suitably selected control subjects and to determine the rates of drug use. Other relevant factors must be taken into account. A difference in the rates of exposure between the patients and the control group is compatible with a causal inference. This approach does not depend on the evaluation of causality in the individual case.

A case-control study of drug-induced agranulocytosis, with particular emphasis on pyrazolones (including dipyrone) is now in its final stages.

The study source consisted of the entire populations of the following areas: Israel, West Berlin, Milan, Barcelona, Budapest, Sofia, Stockholm and an area around Ulm, giving a total population of 22 million. The experience of these populations between the years 1980 and 1984 constitutes the study base. In each study centre regular liaison was kept by bi-weekly telephone calls with a contact person in each of the regional hospitals to ascertain potential cases of agranulocytosis. Agranulocytosis was defined as the occurrence of unpredicted acute neutropenia with a granulocyte count of $<0.5 \times 10^9$ litre with normal red cell and platelet counts. It had to be established that the neutropenia was not due to systemic disease (e.g. infectious mononucleosis, systemic lupus erythematosus, leukaemia, malignant lymphoma). Control for the cases were patients admitted to the same hospitals for reasons unrelated to drug use. Up to four controls were matched to each case. A standard interview was administered by specially trained nurses or physicians to the cases and the controls. Detailed information was obtained about drug use, day by day for the first 7 days before admission, and week by week for the 3 weeks before that. The patients were also questioned about drug use at any time in the preceding 6 months, and in the more distant past.

Data were also collected on descriptive characteristics such as age; medical information such as history of allergy, bleeding, blood transfusion; other major illnesses; and a limited amount of data concerning exposure to chemicals and radiation.

All completed forms were sent to the Drug Epidemiology Unit of Boston University where, after a check for consistency and completeness, they were entered onto computer files. A full description of the method has been published[19].

Altogether 422 cases which met the study criteria were identified. The total incidence was 5.7 cases per million per year. It was lowest in Milan and highest in Budapest. The disease was more common in females. In both men and women the incidence increased with increasing age.

It is anticipated that the results concerning the risk and incidence of agranulocytosis in relation to the use of analgesics including dipyrone and other pyrazolone derivatives will be published by the end of 1985 (see footnote at end of Chapter).

Pending publication of the final results*, it is already clear

---

* Footnote added in Press: The results of this study have been published by International Agranulocytosis and Aplastic Anaemia Study: "Risks of Agranulocytosis and Aplastic Anaemia, First Report of the Relation to Drug Usage with Specific Reference to Analgesics", in J Am Med Assoc, 256, 1749, 1986.

that the incidence of dipyrone-induced agranulocytosis is orders of magnitude lower than that reported by Huguley[8]. Under the most extreme assumptions, namely that all cases of agranulocytosis are due to pyrazolones, the incidence of the disease attributed to these drugs would be 0.3-4.0 cases per million person-days per use[20]. Actually the risk is substantially less, as we know that pyrazolones are responsible for only a part of all cases. In addition, it is important to note that the fatality rate in cases of agranulocytosis was found to be less than 10%.

V. CONCLUSIONS

At present it is by no means clear that the balance of benefit and harm to public health would be improved by substituting alternative compounds for dipyrone. It is clear that the removal of one analgesic from the market would result in substitution by one or more of the alternatives. In practice this will primarily be paracetamol, aspirin, other non-steroidal anti-inflammatory drugs and in addition an increased use of opiates, which are not only addictives but also have their own serious side-effects and disadvantages in the treatment of specific categories of patients.

In addition some of these products have not yet been in use long enough for their ill-effects to be recognized, studied or evaluated.

REFERENCES

1. Pretty, H, Gosselin, G, Colpron, G and Lang, LA (1965). Agranulocytosis: A report of 30 cases. Canad Med Assoc J, 93, 1058
2. Palva, JP and Mustala, OO (1970). Drug-induced agranulocytosis with special reference to aminophenazone I. Adults. Acta Med Scand, 187, 109
3. Kantero, I, Mustala, OO and Palva, IP (1972). Drug-induced agranulocytosis with special reference to aminophenazone. IV. Children. Acta Med Scand, 192 327
4. Heimpel, H and Abt, C (1983). Medikamente und akute Agranulozytose. Dtsch med Wochenschr, 105, 731
5. Shinar, E and Hershko, C (1983). Causes of agranulocytosis in a hospital population: Identification of Dipyrone as an important causative agent. Israel J Med Sci, 19 225
6. Levy, M, Kletter-Hemo, D, Nir, I and Eliakim, M (1977). Drug utilization and adverse reactions in medical patients: comparison of two periods: 1965-1972 and 1973-1976. Israel J Med Sci, 13, 1065
7. Jouet, JP, Huart, JJ, Bauter, F and Goudemand, M (1980). La paracetamol, cause meconnue d'agranulocytose aigue medicamenteuse. Nouv Presse Med, 9, 1386
8. Huguley, CM (1964). Agranulocytosis induced by dipyrone, a hazardous antipyretic and analgesic. J Am Med Assoc, 189, 162
9. Discombe, G (1952). Agranulocytosis caused by amidopyrine, an avoidable cause of death. Br Med J, 1, 1270
10. Holten, C (1934). Agranulocytose. Nord Med T, 8, 1659
11. Rawls, WB (1936). The effect of amidopyrine upon the red, white and polymorphonuclear blood cells of a series of 110 patients. Am J Med Sci, 192,

175

12. Gsell, O and Muller, W (1950). Parenterale Pyramidon-Pyrazolodin-Therapie von Rheumatismus und Infekten mittels Irgapyrin. Schweiz Med Wochenschr, 80, 319
13. Simon, SD and Metz, MH (1936). Amidopyrine and circulating leukocytes; effect of prolonged administration on number and type of white blood cells. J Lab Clin Med, 21, 1154
14. Cardon, I, Comess, OH, Noble, TA and Pomaranc, MM (1958). Value of amidopyrine. Ann Intern Med, 48, 616
15. Spear, W (1962). Use of aminopyrine to control fever in Hodgkin's disease. J Am Med Assoc, 180, 970
16. Gross, R, Horstmann, H, Vogel, J and Zach, J (1967). Zur Epidemiologie und Klinik der medikamentos-allergischen Agranulozytose. Med Welt, 31, 1767
17. Arneborn, P and Palmblad, J (1982). Drug induced neutropenia - a survey for Stockholm 1973-1978. Acta Med Scand, 212, 289
18. Bottiger, LE and Westerholm, B (1973). Drug induced blood dyscrasias in Sweden. Br Med J, 3 339
19. The International Agranulocytosis and Aplastic Anemia Study (1983). The design of a study of the drug etiology of agranulocytosis and aplastic anemia. Eur J Clin Pharmacol, 4, 833
20. Shapiro, S (1984). Agranulocytosis and pyrazolones. Lancet, 1, 451

Discussion

Dr KD Rainsford, UK Is there any attempt to confirm the ingestion of the drug associated with the episode of agranulocytosis by chemical means? Has it been possible for instance that in view of the relatively long half-life of some of these drugs (e.g. phenylbutazone) it might be conceivable to establish if this has been important and at the same time perhaps the ingestion of other associated drugs as well?

Prof Levy Unfortunately not. Actually you can't measure dipyrone in biological fluids since it is hydrolysed in the GI tract and even the metabolites have a short half life, so by the time we identify the cases, which is usually 2, 4, or 5 days after the drug intake, it's impossible to measure any metabolites any longer.

Dr Rainsford Yes, but I was thinking of phenylbutazone and related drugs. What particular pyrazolones have you identified as being associated with agranulocytosis. That is have you simply studied pyrazolone-associated reactions as a group or at particular types of drugs? I'm just wondering roughly what proportions of the different individual drugs have been highlighted so far in those 400 odd cases?

Dr Levy This is exactly what I hoped I was able to explain in the methodology. The proportion of the exposures of the cases doesn't give the ranking of the risk. Only its comparison to the drug use in the controls, that enables the calculations of that fraction of each of the drugs. So if you question is, what is a fraction of the pyrazolones out of the total number of cases of agranulocytosis this information will be published in a matter of a few months.

8
Potential biases influencing interpretation of data from worldwide spontaneous ADR reports

AJ Gordon* and R Sachs**
*Pfizer International Inc, 235 East 42 Street, New York, USA
**Pfizer Pharmaceuticals, 235 East 42 Street, New York, USA

CONTENTS

I. ADR REPORTING

The collection, tabulation, interpretation and reporting of safety data on marketed drugs constitute a major function for any pharmaceutical company. This activity is particularly challenging for a multinational organization when widely used therapies such as NSAIDs are involved. While spontaneous adverse reaction reporting systems managed by companies and regulators alike might act as an alerting mechanism for unusual findings, especially rare but serious events, attempts are often made to use the same data to compare side-effect incidences between drugs. The diverse and complex medical, regulatory and socio-economic environments operating in different parts of the world often severely limit the validity of intercountry comparisons even on the same drug. For

This is an summary of the authors' presentation. A full manuscript was not submitted in time for inclusion in these proceedings.

Side-effects of Anti-inflammatory Drugs. Rainsford, KD and Velo, GP (eds)
Part 1: Clinical and Epidemiological Aspects. (Lancaster: MTP Press)

example, the relative rates of spontaneous ADR reporting based on estimated usage of piroxicam over comparable periods following introduction in Germany, the US, the UK and Sweden was 1 : 3 : 6 : 10, respectively.

II. BIASES FROM ENVIRONMENTAL FACTORS

Even more important, but less understood, these same environmental factors within a given country introduce fundamental biases or factors that can profoundly influence both the number of reported ADRs (numerator) and the measurement of drug usuage (denominator), and thereby impose severe limitations on any quantification of absolute or relative safety. Among the many important sources of biases affecting the number of side-effect reports are the methods used by companies to collect and report safety information to authorities, changes in regulations or habits within a country, and the influence of the lay and professional media, all of which will be elaborated.

III. DENOMINATOR VARIABLES

Furthermore, in addition to the effect of time on the market, (new vs. old drug), which has been documented previously, it has been shown that the amount of contact time between company representatives and physicians (a common source of ADR reporting) may vary by a factor of 2.5 between drugs. Factors affecting the denominator (the population at risk) include (a) prescription size, which can vary between drugs from an average of less than 2 weeks to nearly 4 weeks; (b) differences in compliance ranging from nearly 80% to 60% depending on regimen; (c) large differences in indications for which the drugs are used (for example, in chronic arthritis a range of 20% to 60% usage); and (d) differences in demographic characteristics such as usage in elderly patients ranging from over 40% to as little as 25%. Examples are given as to how these biases may compound each other, and how even limited correction makes apparent differences in reporting rates between drugs disappear.

IV. CONCLUSIONS

It is concluded that statistics on spontaneous ADR reports must be interpreted cautiously, since the value of anecdotal reporting may be severely compromised by failure to identify and correct for the relevant biases.

Discussion

Professor JC Roujeau, France You did not mention the possibility of under-reporting of adverse group reactions due to company pressures. Two years ago we had paper about drug-induced toxic epidermal necrolysis accepted by a major French journal. Subsequently this journal was not published because of pressures from a certain company. I was told that 1 out of 4 cases of toxic epidermal necrolysis attributed to piroxicam had been erroneously attributed. Would you comment about that?

Dr Sachs The only comment I can make is that I am not personally aware of companies preventing reports in journals, and I certainly wouldn't condone it if it happened. I don't think there is a place for interference, and journals should be independent. I should mention, though, in relation to comments of Dr O'Brien, that reporting in journals while serving a purpose also strikes me as a less efficient way of bringing things to the attention of the appropriate people rather than, for example, reporting to the local regulatory authority. I don't know the policies of most journals around the world, but in the US a letter to the editor can frequently take 6 months to get into a journal. If in fact we are looking at alerting as quickly as possible, it strikes me that, fine, send it to the journal, but by all means send it also to the regulatory body and both at the same time, rather than cause any delay.

Professor WM O'Brien, USA A nice suggestion. The general accounting office of the US government did a very careful study of what happens to adverse effects reports sent to the FDA, and something like 45% of them are lost and never entered into the computer. I have the reference to that report if anybody would like it.

Dr Nicholson, UK I accept many of the reservations you have about using ADR data and number of prescriptions as a means of estimating the incidence of adverse reactions. There is obviously a multiple basis. Can I ask if, in four different countries, the same drug has the same ranking order of prescriptions or ADRs per prescription what is the simplest hypothesis to explain those facts?

Dr Sachs I don't think it's beneficial to have a hypothesis for ranking order necessarily. I don't think ranking order is valid in any country and I think it's a mistake to use these things to rank the order. If in fact it appears suspect it's because most of the people who are ranking are not making an appropriate type of analysis to produce the ranking. My contention is that it is virtually impossible to really make an appropriate type of analysis, and moreover it's wasteful in time and energy. If there is enough noise to signal a problem then I think it is time to take over. I think in the case of the USA this is exactly what they expect to do. The epidemiology group in the USA are not concerned with ranking; they are concerned with being signalled. When they get past the signal they then go to modalities which will provide real rates, and not these severe rates which I simply don't accept have any validity.

Dr A Herxheimer, Virginia, It strikes me that what you are implying is that these comparisons are so meaningless that they don't justify any action. Also we should wait for proper perspective epidemiological studies before taking any action; that is the regulatory authorities, prescribing physicians, people who compile formularies and so on, and companies too. I think you're really saying that companies should be sent these data, and they should then get to work quietly and nothing should emerge for several years that one can rely on. Meanwhile the signal becomes unbearably bad and there are a few coffins rolling around.

Dr R Sachs I didn't mean to imply what you inferred from what I said. I am not really trying here to address what action should be taken when you see a signal. I think these are really the problems for the regulatory body. Certainly my own opinion is that if a signal is either clear enough or frightening enough, then some action has to be taken, whether it is labelling or removing a drug from the market. I think it depends on the case. What I'm saying is that if you take an action like that I don't think you should congratulate yourself on a job well done. I think it's still the responsibility of the regulatory body to determine; then once they've felt they've protected the public, which is really what we're talking about, it's their job to determine what they've really seen, not say, "well there could be something, we've taken the drug off the market and we don't have to worry about it". That I think is lazy and unscientific, and that perhaps is my feeling on this matter. I certainly don't mean to imply that we should wait until everything is tidied up.

Dr Herxheimer Could I just summarize: that is act first and ask questions afterwards.

Dr Sachs Act first and ask questions maybe, but I think if you need to act you act. I think it's the individual cases we're talking about and I don't think it's beneficial to get into a discussion right now of which case does what. But the actions are frequently clear and sometimes not so clear.

Dr AS Hicklin, UK Two questions: firstly to Dr. Herxheimer. We who have to treat patients are left in a difficult situation when a drug has been useful in a very large number of patients, but dangerous in a small number. We have a dilemma with the problem of treating them with that agent. I would be interested to know what action Dr. Herxheimer would propose for regulatory bodies to find out where they were wrong in their precipitous action, which to use his phrase "stops the coffins rolling about", to prevent themselves making the same mistake again and making life more difficult for those not yet in their coffins. The second question, which I would like to address to Prof. O'Brien, is at which stage in the process do they lose 46% of the reports. Is it before the computer or in the computer.

Dr Herxheimer I would say that in the first place it hinges upon prompt communication. I think that has really got to precede action. If action precedes communication then there is distress and confusion.

Professor O'Brien Replying to the second part of Dr. Hicklin's question. I have the manuscript which I would be glad to share with you, but reports were lost in the early stages. Those reports were "yellow cards", to use the British terminology. They're called Form 1639 to use our terminology in the USA for the FDA. Over 40% of these did not get into the computer and were lost.

Dr Rainsford The point I would like to ask you, Dr. Sachs, is what do you regard as a meaningful difference between different percentages of the kind that you've constructed essentially as what you regard problem basis for differences: for example 22-33%, 32-40%. What does this really mean?

Dr Sachs If you really have to, and if you're philosophically and morally committed to make a comparison, I think you then have to try your best. I think perhaps some of the work Dr. Weber did, where he at least picked drugs from the same group, in other words they were all, but one, introduced after 1976. He corrected for use and he looked at them for the same general period of their life cycle. I think that is a start; but what I don't believe he did was, for example, to correct for different types of use of the drug. He probably could put together some enormous linear combination where there is 10% of this, and 15% of that, and make all these corrections. The worst of all is the actual reporting ring, that's the most susceptible. Virtually every one of these is going to be positive or negative. So I think when you ultimately come up with a number I guess if you correct for everything, and say alright if we see a 10-fold difference or a 100-fold difference or a difference of magnitude or something, then we're alerted. Alternatively, if it's something so frightening or so rare or so important that we have to do something more, then we're alerted. Then we take whatever steps we have to. I don't think you can put numbers on this. In fact the point I've really been trying to make is that with these numbers (and I think somebody mentioned it before), there's a high element of witchcraft in it. They're just numbers, they're not solid numbers and they are influenced by many things, many of which we don't even understand. I didn't even go into prescribing geographical differences, things like that which can also be documented, so I really don't want to be pinned down to a magic number. I think if there is something there, generally you will at least see enough to make you interested, and that is where you have to act. Don't waste time trying to manipulate numbers that were never intended and are not suitable for this exercise.

Dr Rainsford I think actually Dr Weber has made these points in the publication of the first proceedings of this meeting, and of course it's been amplified today. Thank you.

9
Prescription-event monitoring of five non-steroidal anti-inflammatory drugs

WHW Inman and NSB Rawson
Drug Safety Research Trust,
North Croft House,
Winchester Road,
Botley,
Southampton SO3 2BX,
UK

CONTENTS

I. INTRODUCTION

For more than 20 years in the United Kingdom we have been largely dependent on spontaneous reporting of suspected adverse drug reaction (ADRs) as a means of identifying potentially dangerous problems which may not have been encountered during clinical trials. The yellow card scheme is currently the only method of monitoring which can be applied to all drugs all the time. Unfortunately, reporting has often been biased by adverse publicity or by the difficulty of distinguishing ADRs from spon-

Side-effects of Anti-inflammatory Drugs. Rainsford, KD and Velo, GP (eds)
Part 1: Clinical and Epidemiological Aspects. (Lancaster: MTP Press)

taneous events. Spontaneous reporting cannot provide estimates for the incidence of ADRs and its main use is to generate internal "signals" or "alerts" which direct attention to the need for further research. In this respect it has had some notable successes, but on one occasion it failed to identify an important problem - the practolol syndrome - not because it is a bad system but because doctors did not recognise the significance of the events they had observed.

In 1980 the Drug Surveillance Research Unit (DSRU) was set up at the University of Southampton in order to establish a second countrywide scheme complementary to the yellow card system, known as Prescription-Event Monitoring (PEM)[1-3]. This has proved to be a very effective method for gathering information on large numbers of patients and about three-quarters of all general practitioners in England are believed to have collaborated. PEM commenced in January 1982 with a pilot study of benoxaprofen and fenbufen. These two drugs were selected not because of concern about their safety, but because they were expected to produce approximately 10,000 prescriptions each month and one of them, benoxaprofen, was known to produce a high incidence of photosensitivity which could then be used as a "marker" to test the validity of the method. In March 1983 the study of these two drugs was extended and later in the same year zomepirac, piroxicam and Osmosin (indomethacin slow-release) were added.

By this time benoxaprofen had been withdrawn from the market in August 1982 following reports of hepato-renal failure which were due to overdosage of elderly patients. In March 1983 zomepirac was withdrawn after reports of a small number of cases of anaphylaxis in the United States. In September 1983 the same fate befell indomethacin in the sophisticated delivery system known as the "elementary osmotic pump formulation" (Osmosin), after reports of intestinal perforation.

II. METHODS

The methods of PEM have been described elsewhere[2,3]. Briefly, general practitioners and their patients are identified by means of photocopies of prescriptions provided by the Prescription Pricing Authority (PPA). Up to four follow-up questionnaires (green forms) are sent to each general practitioner with a request that any "events" that have been noted since the patient started to take the drug, including any that may have occurred after stopping it or changing to another treatment, should be copied from the patient's practice records. Each green form carries the following definition of an event and simple example:

> An EVENT is any new diagnosis, any reason for referral to a consultant or admission to hospital (e.g. operation, accident or pregnancy), any unexpected deterioration (or improvement) in a concurrent illness, any suspected drug reaction, or any other complaint which was considered of sufficient importance to enter in the patient's notes.

N.B. The reason for stopping treatment and changes of treatment are important events. It is also very important to establish the pattern of events which occur after the patient has stopped treatment.

Example:
A broken leg is an EVENT. If more fractures were associated with this drug they could have been due to hypotension, central nervous system (CNS) effects or metabolic bone changes.

These instructions, and the example, have proved to be a very effective and simple way of explaining the difference between ADR and event monitoring to many thousands of participating general practitioners.

Patients using non-steroidal anti-inflammatory drugs (NSAIDs) tend to be elderly and to have a high mortality. Many are admitted to geriatric or terminal care units or to old people's homes. General practitioners frequently have no records of drug treatment after admission to hospital. In many cases they were not able to give the cause or even the date of death because the patient's notes had been returned to the Family Practitioner Committee before the green forms were distributed. We have, therefore, attempted to establish the cause of death by obtaining a copy of the death certificate from the Office of Population Censuses and Surveys and, where appropriate, we have also sought permission from the general practitioner to examine the dead patient's notes, or corresponded with consultants.

Table 1 Numbers of questionnaires mailed and numbers returned for the five NSAIDs

	Benoxaprofen	Fenbufen	Zomepirac	Piroxicam	Osmosin
No. of questionnaires mailed	29,773	12,317	19,207	20,646	21,886
No. of questionnaires returned (%)	17,125 (58%)	7,019 (57%)	11,091 (58%)	14,084 (68%)	13,325 (61%)
No. of valid questionnaires returned (%)	15,100 (51%)	6,153 (50%)	9,556 (50%)	12,568 (61%)	12,265 (56%)

III. RESULTS

Altogether, 103,829 green forms were posted to general practitioners and 62,644 (60.3%) were returned. A total of 2065 (3.3%) were returned without comment; in some cases the envelopes had not been opened. Others noted that the doctor had left the practice, retired or died. A total of 3462 (5.5%) reported that the patients were no longer registered with the practice. In 1224 (2.0%) there was no record that the drug had been prescribed or taken by the patient although, of course, the patient could not have been included in the study unless a prescription had been dispensed by the pharmacist. In all, 7002 green forms (11.2%) provided no useful information. The remaining 55,642 forms provide the data described in this chapter. The distribution and returns of questionnaires are shown in Table 1.

The overall female to male ratio was two to one, increasing to about three to one in the very elderly. For benoxaprofen, fenbufen and Osmosin 64% of the patients were aged 60 or more years and the corresponding figure for piroxicam was 67% (see Table 2).

Table 2 Age distribution for the five NSAIDs (percentages)

Age (years)	Benoxaprofen (n=12,709)*	Fenbufen (n=5058)	Zomepirac (n=8560)	Piroxicam (n=9880)	Osmosin (n=10,758)
<50	15	17	31	16	17
50-59	21	19	17	17	19
60-69	28	27	20	26	27
70-79	26	25	21	28	26
80+	10	12	11	13	11

* n = Number of patients for whom age was recorded

With zomepirac, however, only 52% of the patients were over 60 and this difference is reflected in the distribution of indications shown in Table 3. Zomepirac was promoted as a general-purpose analgesic as well as an anti-inflammatory agent, and the proportion of patients with arthritis was less than half the corresponding proportion with the other four drugs. Zomepirac had been used significantly more frequently for conditions such as prolapsed intervertebral disc, headache or dysmenorrhoea, and it had been particularly effective for pain due to cancer. The benoxaprofen group included a much higher proportion of patients with rheumatoid arthritis.

Pattern of events

The duration of use of the various drugs differed widely; consequently so did the period of follow-up after the drug had been stopped. Comparisons between the total number of events and the total number of patients do not, therefore, yield much useful information. Table 4 shows the frequency of events expressed as the number of events per thousand patient-years of treatment. The average period of follow-up after patients had stopped or changed treatment was rather longer than the mean duration of treatment, but where the period of follow-up was lengthy, doctors tended to record rather fewer events, presumably because patients made less frequent visits to the surgery or because the doctor felt that this was less important. For this reason we have compared

Table 3 Distribution of indications for the five NSAIDs (percentages)

Indication	Benoxaprofen (n=12 396)*	Fenbufen (n=4516)	Zomepirac (n=6391)	Piroxicam (n=8435)	Osmosin (n=9927)
Osteoarthritis	47	46	18	46	48
Rheumatoid arthritis	18	10	4	9	10
Unspecified arthritis	12	11	6	10	12
Spondylitis	5	5	4	6	5
Back and neck pain	4	7	6	7	7
Prolapsed disc	-	1	3	1	1
Trauma	1	2	6	2	1
Cancer	-	-	4	-	-
Headache	-	-	3	-	-
Other	13	18	46	19	16

*n = Number of patients for whom the indication was recorded

the distribution of events during and following treatment by expressing each type of event as a proportion of all the events recorded. In Table 5 these proportions are expressed as the number of events of a particular type per thousand events of all kinds. This enables comparisons to be made during ("on") and following ("off") treatment with each of the five drugs.

Tables 4 and 5 list some of the skin, (CNS) cardiovascular and gastrointestinal events separately. Other classes of events are shown only as class totals.

Table 4 Rates of events per 1000 patient-years of exposure to the five NSAIDs

Events	Benoxaprofen	Fenbufen	Zomepirac	Piroxicam	Osmosin
Skin					
Onycholysis, nail change	30	1	1	1	1
Photosensitivity	99	1	1	<1	1
Acute rash	54	46	30	15	23
Other	65	49	48	53	68
All	248	97	80	69	93
CNS, eye and ear					
Anxiety, depression	25	23	26	19	48
Headache	10	10	14	8	94
Other	60	46	72	43	132
All	95	79	112	70	274
Cardiovascular					
Cerebrovascular accidents*	3	4	3	4	2
Myocardial infarction	6	5	2	4	4
Ischaemic heart disease	2	2	1	1	1
Hypertension	9	8	6	12	19
Other	67	64	54	64	98
All	87	83	66	85	124
Gastrointestinal					
Diarrhoea	11	14	20	11	57
Dyspepsia, gastritis	70	54	39	34	145
Nausea, vomiting	26	19	32	13	64
Peptic ulcer with complications	4	3	6	5	7
Other peptic ulcer	3	2	6	3	6
Other	78	56	84	69	168
All	192	148	187	135	447
Respiratory	88	70	112	80	124
Hepatic	6	2	3	3	2
Metabolic and endocrine	13	12	12	12	17
Renal	35	25	26	24	38
Blood	9	8	10	8	13
Cancer	5	6	8	5	8
Other	131	124	163	154	185
OVERALL RATE	909	654	779	645	1325

* Excluding haemorrhage

Table 5 Event rates per 1000 events "on" and "off" treatment for the five NSAIDs

Events	Benoxaprofen		Fenbufen		Zomepirac		Piroxicam		Osmosin	
	"On"	"Off"	"On"	"Off"	"On"	"Off"	"On"	"Off"	"On"	"Off"
Skin										
Onycholysis, nail change	33	3	2	2	1	-	1	1	1	-
Photosensitivity	109	2	1	5	1	0	1	2	1	0
Acute rash	59	25	71	18	38	17	23	16	17	23
Other	72	73	74	65	62	60	82	67	51	57
All	273	103	148	90	102	77	107	86	70	80
CNS, eye and ear										
Anxiety, depression	27	43	36	44	33	42	29	36	36	41
Headache	11	13	15	12	18	15	12	14	71	20
Other	66	61	70	74	93	73	68	68	100	79
All	104	117	121	130	144	130	109	118	207	140
Cardiovascular										
Cerebrovascular accident*	3	11	7	7	3	8	6	9	2	5
Myocardial infarction	7	16	7	10	2	10	7	16	3	10
Ischaemic heart disease	2	5	4	2	1	5	2	4	1	2
Hypertension	10	17	12	19	8	6	19	13	15	15
Other	74	99	97	92	70	72	98	83	73	84
All	96	148	127	130	84	101	132	125	94	116
Gastrointestinal										
Diarrhoea	12	12	21	13	25	13	17	13	43	18
Dyspepsia, gastritis	77	30	83	41	50	22	52	26	110	64
Nausea, vomiting	29	12	30	12	40	18	20	11	49	21
Peptic ulcer with complications	4	4	4	3	7	5	8	5	5	7
Other peptic ulcer	4	6	3	6	4	4	4	3	4	4
Other	85	101	86	98	114	93	108	94	126	103
All	211	165	227	173	240	155	209	152	337	217
Respiratory	97	124	107	142	144	138	124	147	94	153
Hepatic	7	11	3	5	4	6	5	7	2	5
Metabolic and endocrine	14	19	18	19	16	18	18	19	13	14
Renal	38	41	38	41	33	37	37	42	28	38
Blood	9	12	12	12	13	10	13	7	10	14
Cancer	6	23	8	14	11	44	9	17	6	17
Other	145	237	191	244	209	284	237	280	139	206

*excluding haemorrhage

SIDE-EFFECTS OF ANTI-INFLAMMATORY DRUGS

1. Skin events

A total of 909 patients developed photosensitivity while taking benoxaprofen, corresponding to 99 cases per thousand patient-years' use of the drug. Much of the period of observation was in the winter and spring when exposure to sunlight is low. Onycholysis was reported by 164 patients and a further 113 developed "nail changes" which were probably of a similar nature. Sporadic records of photosensitivity were noted in the other four drug groups including 31 cases of photosensitivity where a patient's treatment had been changed to benoxaprofen.

2. CNS events

The frequency of CNS events recorded for Osmosin was higher than with the other drugs, and to a great extent this was due to reports of headache which were seven to eight times more frequent with this product.

3. Cardiovascular events

With both zomepirac and Osmosin there appear to be a marked deficit of reports of myocardial infarction during treatment and, on closer inspection, a similar though less marked trend was noted with the other NSAIDs. A trend is also suggested in the data for thrombotic stroke and ischaemic heart disease.

4. Gastrointestinal events

Gastrointestinal events, mostly of a non-serious nature, were recorded two or three times more frequently with Osmosin than with the other drugs. This effect was best shown for the category "dyspepsia and gastritis". It will be noted in Table 5, however, that the proportion of these complaints after Osmosin had been withdrawn was also greater than the proportion after stopping treatment with the other four drugs.

No noteworthy differences are apparent between the proportion of serious complications of peptic ulcer (haematemesis, melaena and perforation) either between the drugs or between the treatment and follow-up period with any of the five.

5. Other types of events

Some differences in the pattern of respiratory events are likely to be due to seasonal differences and are not considered to be of any significance. Hepatic, metabolic, endocrine, renal and haemopoietic events show no important differences during or following treatment, and the only important difference was the relative excess of events relating to cancer after zomepirac had been withdrawn. This is largely due to the inclusion of patients with terminal cancer who died following withdrawal of the drug.

IV. DISCUSSION

In spite of the fact that two of the five studies (benoxaprofen and fenbufen) were aimed at testing the method of PEM rather than the drugs themselves, and although zomepirac and Osmosin and about half the patients treated with benoxaprofen were studied after the drugs had been withdrawn from the market, these preliminary results show a remarkable consistency. Although a number of problems arose during the course of the studies, including two separate industrial disputes which affected the collection of prescriptions and the distribution of documents briefing general practitioners about the conduct of these studies, approximately half of the green forms were returned with valid information.

Although many green forms were not returned, this would only affect comparisons of the pattern of events associated with various drugs, or estimates of their incidence, if doctors deliberately and selectively withheld evidence of certain types of event. We believe this to be extremely unlikely, especially since the recording of an "event" does not imply an opinion that the event might be causally related to treatment. In some cases doctors returned blank or "void" forms which indicated that the chief reasons for non-response were that many patients had moved to another practice during the two or more years of the study. Many doctors had ceased to practise, for various reasons. Difficulties had also been encountered in the identification or interpretation of the names of patients on handwritten and sometimes scarcely legible prescriptions. In some patients the doctor could not remember or had made no note of a prescription for an NSAID. Although it is impossible to exclude bias linked with the fact that some doctors do not respond, none of these reasons suggest that the patients in whom events were not monitored differ significantly from those for whom green forms were returned.

Because of the publicity following the benoxaprofen affair and the withdrawal of zomepirac and Osmosin, we believe it is very unlikely that any fatalities attributed to, respectively, hepato-renal toxicity, anaphylactic shock or perforation of the small bowel, will have escaped identification, although this possibility cannot be entirely ruled out.

One particular difficulty with the analysis has been related to the advanced age of many of the patients and the fact that many died of old age. In octogenarians, for example, the overall death rate exceeded 12% per annum. It is often impossible to ascertain whether or not patients continued treatment after moving to homes for the elderly or admission to hospital. In such cases the period of observation should be considered to have ended when the patient ceased to be cared for by the general practitioner. A further problem is the very high probability that diagnoses recorded on death certificates are inaccurate, particularly in elderly patients who do not come to autopsy.

If events are not related in any way to treatment we would expect to see no appreciable differences between the incidences of events in populations of patients treated with the various NSAIDs, nor would we expect to see differences in the proportions of events "on" or "off" treatment (i.e. no differences between the rows of figures in Tables 4 and 5). Any substantial differences could be related to changes in the severity of the disease, to differences in the composition of the five populations of patients with regard to factors such as age or diagnosis, or to beneficial or harmful effects of the drugs. Several examples can be seen in Tables 4 and 5 where side-effects such as photosensitivity with benoxaprofen or headache with indomethacin were expected, and they are quite clearly "signalled" in both the between-drug and the treatment and post-treatment comparisons.

It must be appreciated that the period of observation during treatment always precedes the period of observation after stopping or changing treatment. As a result of this there has been a tendency for doctors to under-report the less serious events during the follow-up period, particularly when the treatment period was exceptionally long. Another important difficulty is the fact that with benoxaprofen, zomepirac and Osmosin, all but the minority who died during treatment had a period of follow-up (i.e. "off" treatment) following removal of the drug from the market. With piroxicam and fenbufen, on the other hand, some of the patients were still taking the drug at the time the questionnaire was returned so these patients contributed no follow-up experience. We suspect that some other patients would have continued to be treated with another NSAID after the drug we were studying by PEM had been stopped. For these and other reasons we do not believe it is appropriate to apply formal tests for statistical significance to these data.

In 1983 we supplemented the study of benoxaprofen by sending doctors lists of all the patients who had received prescriptions in addition to the four patients for whom green forms were enclosed. In this way the total number of patients included in the study was increased to some 24,000. Among them were 54 cases with renal failure or jaundice. These have been reported elsewhere[4]. Extensive attempts to follow up these cases revealed information about all but six cases (in whom the relationship must be regarded as "possible" by default). At the end of the investigation we concluded that only one case was due to benoxaprofen overdosage (and that was not fatal) and that the number possibly related to it was 11, of whom five died. The majority of the cases were clearly attributable to other causes such as gallstones or cancer of the pancreas.

PEM has been criticized for its apparent failure to detect a problem with benoxaprofen[5]. Certainly we were unable to estimate an attributable death rate for the very good reason that deaths due to the drug were too rare, but PEM certainly detected a number of treatment-associated deaths, most of which were not caused by the drug.

The Committee on Safety of Medicines (CSM) has not published the scientific evidence for withdrawal of benoxaprofen. If we assume that all the hepato-renal deaths reported to the CSM were causally related to drug, the incidence might be in the order of one per 20,000 to 30,000 patients. Clearly PEM, in populations of less than 30,000 patients, cannot be relied on to measure the incidence of such rare events.

We investigated allergic reactions to zomepirac. There were four cases of anaphylaxis, 16 of urticaria, 74 other rashes and 26 reports of asthma. Two cases of anaphylaxis were probably drug-related and so were 17 of the rashes. A further 26 cases were considered to be possibly related and the remaining 75 were unrelated to the drug. None of the allergic reactions had been fatal.

We investigated one patient with a perforated ileum associated with Osmosin. His treatment had been changed 1 month before the perforation to another form of indomethacin, but the possibility remains that he may have retained some Osmosin tablets and taken one shortly before he perforated and died.

The fact that Osmosin appeared at first sight to be associated with more gastrointestinal disturbances than the other NSAIDs is important in view of its promotion as a drug that should have produced fewer gastrointestinal side-effects. The reason for this paradoxical result is not hard to suggest. Because the drug was believed to be less irritant, it would have been used in patients who were particularly prone to develop dyspepsia. This is borne out by the larger proportion of patients in this group who still had dyspepsia and gastritis after the drug had been withdrawn.

While we would not deny that NSAIDs may occasionally cause serious gastrointestinal complications such as bleeding or perforation, one important result of this study is the observation that the distribution of cases both during and following treatment seemed to be very similar. This leads us to conclude that any differences caused by treatment are likely to have been small. In order to emphasize that this is not an artefact due to the method of analysis we show, in Table 6, the number of deaths and the death rates expressed as the rate per 1000 patients. There were eight deaths from gastrointestinal haemorrhage or perforated peptic ulcer during treatment and 12 following treatment. No important differences are apparent.

While some events were more frequently recorded during treatment than during the follow-up period, the reverse was sometimes the case. There were more events linked with cancer, for example, after withdrawal of zomepirac, and this is easily explained by the deaths of patients who were being treated for terminal cancer. On the other hand the marked deficit of myocardial infarction and other thrombotic diagnoses during treatment ran contrary to the general trend and suggests the possibility of a genuine cardioprotective effect. While we do not claim that some of these NSAIDs are cardioprotective we certainly feel that our hypothesis should be tested by other workers. The overall risks of using NSAIDs are so small that it would, in our opinion, be perfectly justifiable to set up formal experimental studies of certain NSAIDs in the primary and secondary prevention of cardiovascular mortality.

PEM is a major advance in post-marketing surveillance. Unlike spontaneous reporting systems in which both numerator and denominator are usually lacking, PEM enables the incidence of

Table 6 Deaths from upper gastrointestinal haemorrhage or perforation during and after stopping or changing treatment reported in the five studies

	Number of deaths		Death rate per 1000 patients	
	"On"	"Off"	"On"	"Off"
Benoxaprofen	1	2	0.1	0.1
Fenbufen	0	1	0	0.2
Zomepirac	1	2	0.1	0.2
Piroxicam	4	6	0.3	0.5
Osmosin	2	1	0.2	0.1

events to be measured and compared in association with different drugs. "Off" treatment follow-up of events also provides crude estimates of the background incidence of non-drug-related events. PEM cannot, however, identify very rare events, and it can only be applied to new products after they have been on the market for some time. In no sense does PEM compete with the CSM's yellow card scheme, which can be applied to all drugs all the time. The two national schemes are complementary.

V. SUMMARY AND CONCLUSIONS

A study of events recorded in the general practice notes of 55 642 patients who have been identified by means of prescriptions for five non-steroidal anti-inflammatory drugs (NSAIDs) has shown the expected side-effects and a low incidence of serious adverse reactions. With few exceptions the general pattern of events during and following treatment was very similar for benoxaprofen, fenbufen, zomepirac, piroxicam and a slow-release formulation of indomethacin known as Osmosin. The incidence of side-effects that have led to the withdrawal of three of the drugs from the market was extremely low. Benoxaprofen was associated with large numbers of skin events, but there were very few cases of renal or hepatic damage. Zomepirac was responsible for a few allergic reactions, none of which was fatal. It was noted that some drugs which were expected to be less irritant to the gut were associated with relatively more gastrointestinal events. This paradoxical result was probably due to their selective use in patients who were especially prone to them. Complications of peptic ulcer were uncommon, and deaths from this cause extremely rare. No difference was apparent in the incidence of serious gastrointestinal complications during or after stopping treatment or changing to another NSAID. There was a deficit of cases of myocardial infarction during treatment with some of the NSAIDs which might reflect a possible cardioprotective effect.

VI. ACKNOWLEDGEMENTS

We wish to thank the Prescription Pricing Authority for their help in identifying doctors who prescribed the various drugs included in this study, the innumerable general practitioners who enthusiastically supported the investigation, and the staff of the Drug Surveillance Research Unit for processing the prescriptions and questionnaires. The Unit is supported by unconditional grants from nearly 30 pharmaceutical companies and by the office of the Chief Scientist of the Department of Health and Social Security. Our thanks are also due to the Office of Population Censuses and Surveys for their help in establishing the cause of deaths in some patients and many of the 90 Family Practitioner Committees in England who have assisted in our enquiries. Finally, we wish to thank Mr Tom Lucas for his help with the assessment of fatal events.

REFERENCES

1. Inman, WHW (1981). Post-marketing surveillance of adverse drug reactions in general practice. 1: Search for new methods. Br Med J, 282, 1131
2. Inman, WHW (1981). Post-marketing surveillance of adverse drug reactions in general practice. 2: Prescription event monitoring at the University of Southampton. Br Med J, 282, 1216
3. Inman, WHW (1985). Iatrogenic hazards. In: Holland, WW, Detels, R and Knox, G (eds) Oxford Textbook of Public Health, vol 3. (Oxford: Oxford University Press), pp. 334-349
4. Prescription-Event Monitoring News No. 2 (1984). (Southampton: Drug Surveillance Research Unit)
5. Dukes, MNG (1984). The seven pillars of foolishness. Side Effects of Drugs Annual, 8. (Amsterdam: Elsevier)

Discussion

Dr A Calin, UK With your suggestion that there is a relationship between the period after stopping the non-steroidal agent and the cardioprotective effect [of zomepirac], how did you break down the second part of the bar graph [the "off period"], how many of those individuals changed to another non-steroidal, and how many stopped the non-steroidal completely?

Professor Inman This is one of the weaknesses of the method in that we cannot be absolutely sure how many of the patients did change to another non-steroidal. We think that it is probably about 20-30%. But an awful lot of patients go to their doctors and are treated with non-steroidal anti-inflammatory for what are self-limiting conditions.

Dr Calin Do you know how they were more or less likely to have an infarct, whether they stopped or changed, or can you not break your data down any further?

Professor Inman I don't think so. All we can say is that there was a very large difference between the number of events occurring while the patients were taking the drugs we were interested in and what happened after they stopped or in some cases switched. We need to do more work on this [aspect].

Dr A Herxheimer, London You mentioned that relative risk is important and that comparisons are the best antidote to panic, but you didn't actually compare one drug with another drug. Also, the statement that you quoted that Stevens-Johnson Syndrome is not unusual is, in the context, a comparative statement [it] wasn't unusual by comparison with other drugs in the same therapeutic class. So I would like you to say something about comparisons between drugs? Or are the frequencies too low to enable you to do that with any degree of confidence?

Professor Inman I hoped that I made it clear we were comparing those five drugs, one with the other. But we may have picked five which were less likely to cause GI disturbance than another five. We were certainly comparing one drug with another in a group of patients who seemed to be the same with respect to indication, age, sex and so forth.

Dr Herxheimer You drew that negative conclusion but what about benoxaprofen and the skin [side effects]. Did you analyze that any further because the persistence of the skin effects is particularly interesting?

Professor Inman Well a high proportion of the patients were taking benoxaprofen or had recently stopped taking this drug, and the longest period of follow-up was 2 years and we did not detect more than a handful of patients who had reports of photosensitivity in that group. I have serious doubts about whether it causes permanent photosensitivity. Maybe if we did another follow up in 2 or 3 years we would find some cases.

Professor WM O'Brien, Charlottesville, USA I was intrigued that in your data it appears that bad things may happen to patients right after they stop taking non-steroidal. This may I think be important, a thing which has been overlooked. One thing we do know is that when they stop taking a non-steroidal they develop a very intense pruritis. Apparently they may have a rebound and over-produce prostaglandins. One would wonder if other bad things could occur. The other comment I would like to make is your failure to detect Osmin [Osmosin]. Your surveying mainly family practitioners whereas if they had a perforation they would most likely go to hospital. Is it possible that the family practitioner is unaware that the patient had a perforation?

Professor Inman I think it is very unlikely that they would be unaware if a patient had a perforation. I think that the quality of records that general practitioners in this country is vastly better than we give them credit for. When the patient is admitted [to hospital] then they [the general practitioner(s)] will get a letter from the consultant telling them what had happened. If they go to the trouble of sending in a green form then they should know. We have a "long-stop" arrangement to pick up death certificates. I do not believe we have missed many but we may have missed a few.

10
Side-effects of non-steroidal anti-inflammatory drugs in children with juvenile rheumatoid arthritis

TK Kvien*, HM Høyeraal*, B Sandstad**
and E Kåss*
*Oslo Sanitets forening, Rheumatism Hospital, Oslo, Norway
**University of Oslo, Oslo, Norway

CONTENTS

I. INTRODUCTION

Different adverse reactions to non-steroidal anti-inflammatory drugs (NSAIDs) may be seen in children with juvenile rheumatoid arthritis (JRA) and adults with rheumatoid arthritis. For example, liver enzymes are frequently elevated in patients with JRA receiving acetylsalicylic acid (ASA)[1,2], whereas such elevations are rare in adults. Some other types of adverse reactions, e.g. gastrointestinal bleedings and nephrotoxicity, are probably more frequent in adults than in children.

A few controlled studies have investigated the comparative tolerance of various NSAIDs in children. This presentation includes data from a comparative 24-week double-blind study of naproxen (NAP) and ASA in patients with JRA[3]. Tolerance data from other comparative studies and some open studies without control groups will be reviewed and discussed.

Side-effects of Anti-inflammatory Drugs. Rainsford, KD and Velo, GP (eds)
Part 1: Clinical and Epidemiological Aspects. (Lancaster: MTP Press)

II. NAPROXEN/ACETYLSALICYLIC ACID STUDY

A. Methods

Patients were consecutively enrolled according to the following entry criteria; (1) diagnosis of JRA[4,5]; (2) age between 3 and 16 years; (3) pauciarticular or polyarticular present disease type without signs of systemic manifestations; (4) mild or moderate disease activity with indication for therapy with NSAIDs without need for slow-acting antirheumatic drugs, immunoregulatory drugs or corticosteroids; (5) no use of slow-acting antirheumatic drugs, corticosteroids or immunoregulatory drugs during the preceding 6 months prior to the study; and (6) no use of joint surgery or local corticosteroid injections during the preceding 2 months.

The study design was parallel and double-blind, NAP was given b.i.d. 10 mg/kg daily (range 8-12) as 100 mg tablets, and NAP placebo tablets were used midday. Microencapsulated ASA (Glob-entyl) was given t.i.d. 75 mg/kg daily (range 62-82) as 500 mg tablets. All tablets had a similar appearance and were produced especially for this study (manufacturers: Naproxen; Astra AB, Södertälje, Sweden. Glob-entyl; Nyegaard & Co., Oslo, Norway). The dissolution of the NAP and ASA tablets in gastric acid was tested prior to the study. A cross-over study in healthy volunteers confirmed that the relative bioavailability of the NAP 100 mg tablets was similar to the marketed preparation NAP 250 mg tablets (Naprosyn). All drugs were dispensed by the local pharmacy. Medication containers were used and the compliance was assessed by tablet count to be 95%[6]. Concomitant drug therapy was not allowed except for the use of mild analgesics i.e. paracetamol (acetaminophen), codeine. Physiotherapy was preferably to be kept unchanged.

The patients were assessed at the study clinic at baseline, after 12 and 24 weeks in accordance with specified guidelines[7]. Adverse reactions were assessed by spontaneous reporting from the patients/parents and by answers to general questions about side-effects. In order to monitor safety the patients were examined after 2 weeks and then at monthly intervals by their local physician in accordance with written guidelines issued by the study group. The serum salicylic acid level was determined after 2 weeks. One physician received the results of the analyses, and reported name and result of patients with levels exceeding 2.0 mmol/l.

Wilcoxon rank sum test or Kruskall-Wallis test was used for the statistical analysis of quantitative measurements. A chi-square test was used for categorical measurements.

B. Results

Eighty patients with JRA entered the study. Median age was 125 months (range 38-188 months). Female to male ratio was 60:20. Median disease duration was 14 months (3-133 months). The treatment groups were comparable with regard to descriptive data at baseline, previous therapy and baseline values of clinical and disease activity measurements (data not shown, see ref. 3). Two patients in the ASA group were withdrawn from further analyses because of errors in the drug handling.

Table 1 Adverse reactions to naproxen (NAP) (n=40) and acetylsalicylic acid (ASA) (n=38)

Adverse reactions	NAP	ASA
Abdominal pain	4	9
Nausea	0	2
Headache	2	2
Dizziness	2	5
Tinnitus	0	4
Drowsiness	1	7
Irritability	0	2
Rash	2	1
Pruritus	1	3
Bronchial constriction	1	1
Bleeding susceptibility	2	1
Faecal blood loss	1	2
Elevated ALAT/ASAT[a]	0	14
Total	16 (12)[b]	53 (30)[b]

[a] More than twice the upper normal value

[b] Number of different patients with adverse reactions in parentheses

Adverse reactions were observed in 12 NAP-treated and 30 ASA-treated patients during the study (Table 1). More than one type of side-effect was seen in several patients (Table 1). Five NAP-treated and 20 ASA-treated patients were withdrawn from the trial because of adverse reactions ($p<0.01$). As indicated in Table 2, most of the adverse reactions necessitating discontinuation of the therapy occurred during the first weeks of the study. The median daily dose of ASA was 76 mg/kg (range 69-80 mg/kg) in the 20 patients withdrawn because of adverse reactions compared to 71 mg/kg (range 62-82 mg/kg) in the other 18 patients ($p<0.01$).

The thrombocyte count and the values of alanine aminotransferase (ALAT) and aspartate aminotransferase (ASAT) seemed to increase in the ASA group compared to the NAP group during the study (changes in values week 12 minus week 0, NAP/ASA (median values): thrombocyte count (10^9/l) -5/25 ($p=0.05$), ALAT (U/l) 0/3 ($p<0.01$) ASAT (U/l) 0/7 ($p<0.01$); week 24 minus week 0: thrombocyte count 3/34.5 ($p=0.03$), ALAT 1/4 ($p=0.05$), ASAT 1/3 ($p=0.20$)). Group differences were not seen for other laboratory measurements (haemoglobin, haematocrit, erythrocyte count, leukocyte count, creatinine, urea, immunoglobulins).

Table 2 Number of patients withdrawn because of adverse reactions in the naproxen (NAP) and acetylsalicylic acid (ASA) groups

Weeks of treatment	Withdrawals NAP (n=40)	Withdrawals ASA (n=38)	Reasons[a] Gastrointestinal NAP	Gastrointestinal ASA	CNS[b] NAP	CNS[b] ASA	Cutaneous NAP	Cutaneous ASA	Bronchial constriction NAP	Bronchial constriction ASA
1-4	3	9	1	4	2	7	0	0	0	0
5-8	0	6	0	5	0	3	0	0	0	1
9-12	1	2	0	1	0	1	1	1	0	0
13-16	0	1	0	1	0	1	0	0	0	0
17-20	1	1	0	0	0	0	1	1	0	0
21-24	0	1	0	0	0	0	0	1	0	0
Total	5	20	1[c]	11[d]	2	12	2	3	0	1

[a] More than one adverse reaction were observed in some patients
[b] Central nervous system (headache, tinnitus, dizziness, drowsiness, irritability)
[c] Radiographic examination revealed gastritis and duodenal ulcer in this patient
[d] Of these 11 patients, eight had elevated ALAT/ASAT (more than twice the upper normal value)

III. OTHER CLINICAL STUDIES

Two controlled comparative studies with more than a few weeks duration have been performed by the Pediatric Rheumatology Collaborative Study Group. Both studies were designed as 12-week, parallel double-blind studies comparing one of the newer NSAIDs with ASA[8,9]. In the tolmetin sodium versus ASA study 107 patients were enrolled[8]. The initial daily dose of tolmetin sodium was 15 mg/kg and of ASA 50 mg/kg. The dose was increased at weekly intervals until efficacy was noted, adverse reactions appeared or maximum allowable daily dose was reached (30 mg/kg or 1800 mg for tolmetin sodium, 100 mg/kg or 5900 mg for ASA). The number of adverse reactions observed was 106 in 37 tolmetin sodium-treated patients, 98 in 34 ASA-treated patients. The types of side-effects were similar in the two groups. One patient in the tolmetin sodium group, compared to six in the ASA group, discontinued the trial drug because of limiting side-effects (Table 3).

Ninety-nine patients were enrolled in the fenoprofen versus ASA trial[9]. Fenoprofen was given 900 mg/m^2 daily increased during 4 weeks to 1800 mg/m^2 daily, ASA 1500 mg/m^2 daily increased to 3000 mg/m^2 daily. No fenoprofen treated, and seven ASA-treated patients were withdrawn because of limiting side-effects (hepatotoxicity in four, nausea and vomiting in two, hyperventilation in one). The total number of adverse reactions was 78 in the fenoprofen group (28 patients) and 90 in the ASA group (40 patients) (Table 3).

Trial drugs have been given for shorter periods of time in other comparative studies of NSAIDs in children, including trials of NAP versus ASA[10,11], ibuprofen versus ASA[12], diclofenac sodium versus ASA versus placebo[13], and ketoprofen versus indomethacin[14] (Table 3). The data from these studies seem to be consistent with the data from the studies with treatment for longer periods of time[3,8,9], indicating that ASA is not as well tolerated as some of the newer NSAIDs.

Knowledge about children's tolerance to NSAIDs has also been obtained from some open retrospective and prospective studies. A retrospective survey of 101 patients with JRA having previously received more than one NSAID showed that 79 of these patients had to discontinue the treatment because of toxicity, and 22 stopped the NSAID because of insufficient therapeutic response[15]. Fifteen of the 40 patients with toxicity to more than one NSAID experienced different toxicity to the subsequent NSAID. Toxicity from the gastrointestinal and the central nervous systems seemed to be most frequently observed. Clinical significant elevation of serum transaminases was seen in 22 of 147 ASA trials (15%), in 3 of 53 NAP trials (5.7%), but in none of the 90 tolmetin sodium trials, 46 fenoprofen trials or 33 ibuprofen trials[15].

Mäkelä et al[16] found that toxicity occurred in about 40% of the JRA patients receiving ASA therapy. The toxicity appeared early after start of treatment and seemed to be closely related to the serum salicylic acid level[16]. In a North American study toxicity was found in 16% of the ASA-treated patients[17].

Table 3 Tolerance data from comparative studies of non-steroidal anti-inflammatory drugs in patients with juvenile rheumatoid arthritis

Reference	Number of patients	Design	Duration of therapy (weeks)	Drugs compared	Daily dose	Number of patients with adverse reactions	Number of patients discontinuing the trial drug because of adverse reactions
3	80	Double-blind parallel	24	Naproxen	10 mg/kg	12	5
				Acetylsalicylic acid	75 mg/kg	30	20
8	107	Double-blind parallel	12	Tolmetin sodium	15-30 mg/kg	37	1
				Acetylsalicylic acid	50-100 mg/kg	34	6
9	99	Double-blind parallel	12	Fenoprofen	900-1800 mg/m^2	28	0
				Acetylsalicylic acid	1500-3000 mg/m^2	40	7
10	18	Double-blind cross-over	8	Naproxen	160 mg	0	0
				Acetylsalicylic acid	1500 mg	0	0
11	23	Double-blind cross-over	4	Naproxen	10 mg/kg	1	1
				Acetylsalicylic acid	80 mg/kg	6	3
12	20	Double-blind cross-over	2	Ibuprofen	200-800 mg	1 (?)[b]	?[b]
				Acetylsalicylic acid	--[a]	4 (?)[b]	?[b]
13	45	Double-blind parallel	2	Diclofenac sodium	2-3 mg/kg	0	0
				Acetylsalicylic acid	50-100 mg/kg	4	4
				Placebo		2	0
14	30	Double-blind cross-over	2	Indomethacin	50-100 mg	9	0
				Ketoprofen	50-100 mg	9	0

[a] Modified to give salicylate level 25 mg%
[b] Data are insufficiently stated in the report cited

Table 4 Tolerance data from some open studies of non-steroidal anti-inflammatory drugs in patients with juvenile rheumatoid arthritis

Reference	Number of patients	Therapy (weeks)	Drug studied	Daily dose	Number of patients with adverse reactions	Number of patients discontinuing the trial drug because of adverse reactions
18	81	46 (mean)	Indomethacin	0.7-6.6 mg/kg	41	25
19	35	36 (mean)	Indomethacin	1.5-3.0 mg/kg	15	14
20	10	2	Piroxicam	5-20 mg	?[a]	1
21	25	4	Ketoprofen	100-200 mg/m^2	20	1
22	39	4	Sodium meclofenamate	3-7.5 mg/kg	25	7
23	33	4	Proquazone	400-800 mg/m^2	24	1
24	32	4	Pirprofen	300-600 mg/m^2	19	0

[a] Data are insufficiently stated in the report cited

Some of the newer NSAIDs have not been tested in comparative trials with ASA as a reference substance. Table 4 summarizes the results of open studies without control groups of some of these drugs, including indomethacin[18,19], piroxicam[20], ketoprofen[21], sodium meclofenamate[22], proquazone[23] and pirprofen[24]. Adverse reactions seem to be frequently occurring during treatment with indomethacin (Table 4)[18,19], and fatal toxic reactions to this drug have been reported in children[25,26]. A high proportion of patients experienced adverse reactions in the sodium meclofenamate study and 18% of the patients were withdrawn due to such reactions (Table 4). In addition, nearly half of the patients experienced a fall in haematocrit of 4% or more during the 4-week study period[22].

IV. DISCUSSION

It is difficult to draw definite conclusions from the investigations reviewed in this presentation because the studies are not directly comparable. However, the present data indicate that ASA is less favourable than some of the newer NSAIDs with regard to tolerance (Table 3).

The highest withdrawal rate in ASA-treated patients was found in the NAP versus ASA trial[3] and in the study performed by Mäkelä et al.[16]. The different results with regard to proportion of patients withdrawn during ASA therapy may be related to such factors as dose[16] or compliance[3]. Small dose increments of ASA above the therapeutic dose may be followed by major increments of the serum salicylic acid level[27,28]. A small alteration in compliance may have a similar effect. A three-dose regimen of ASA was used in the studies where the highest withdrawal rate was found[3,16]. It is not likely that differences in number of doses in itself leads to different occurrence of adverse reactions. Recent investigations have indicated that stable serum salicylic acid levels are achieved after 6 days[16] and that stable concentrations during the day also may be obtained with a two-dose regimen of ASA[29]. It seems advisable to start with a moderate dose of ASA in patients with JRA (for example 60 mg/kg daily). The ASA dose should then be adjusted in accordance with the serum level of salicylic acid[30,31] accounting for the great inter-individual variations in serum levels obtained by identical doses of ASA in different patients[29,32].

Different tolerance to NSAIDs in the various types of JRA (systemic, pauciarticular, polyarticular) have not been observed. However, in the tolmetin sodium versus ASA and the fenoprofen versus ASA studies[8,9] only a few patients with systemic disease type were studied. The NAP versus ASA study was limited to patients with pauciarticular and polyarticular disease[3]. Further studies of NSAIDs in patients with the systemic type of JRA are needed.

The comparative studies of NSAIDs in patients with JRA have not revealed any definite difference in efficacy between the drugs studied. The tolerance data available indicate that ASA may be replaced as the first drug among NSAIDs in patients with pauciarticular and polyarticular JRA. Further studies should be performed to investigate the comparative long-term tolerance between the various NSAIDs in children, and especially focus on differences in tolerance between various age and disease type subsets of patients.

ACKNOWLEDGEMENTS

This work was supported by Norsk Hydro Research Foundation for Rheumatology, and Norma and Leon Hess' Foundation for Support of Rheumatological Research at Oslo Sanitetsforening Rheumatism Hospital.

REFERENCES

1. Athreya, BH, Moser, G, Cecil, HS and Myers, AR (1975). Aspirin-induced hepatotoxicity in juvenile rheumatoid arthritis. Arthritis Rheum, 18, 347
2. Miller, JJ and Weissman, DB (1976). Correlations between transaminase concentrations and serum salicylate concentration in juvenile rheumatoid arthritis. Arthritis Rheum, 19, 115
3. Kvien, TK, Høyeraal, HM and Sandstad, B (1984). Naproxen and acetylsalicylic acid in the treatment of pauciarticular and polyarticular juvenile rheumatoid arthritis. Assessment of tolerance and efficacy in a single-centre 24-week double-blind parallel study. Scand J Rheumatol, 13, 342
4. Brewer, EJ, Bass, J, Baum, J, Cassidy, JT, Fink, C, Jacobs, J, Hanson, V, Levinson, JE, Schaller, J and Stillman, JS (1977). Current proposed revision of JRA criteria. Arthritis Rheum, 20 (suppl.), 195
5. Kvien, TK, Høyeraal, HM and Kåss, E (1982). Diagnostic criteria of rheumatoid arthritis in children. Proposed criteria for controlled clinical studies. Scand J Rheumatol, 11, 187
6. Kvien, TK and Reimers, S (1983). Drug handling and patient compliance in an outpatient paediatric trial. J Clin Hosp Pharm, 8, 251
7. Kvien, TK, Høyeraal, HM and Sandstad, B (1982). Assessment methods of disease activity in juvenile rheumatoid arthritis - evaluated in a prednisolone/placebo double-blind study. J Rheumatol, 9, 696
8. Levinson, JE, Baum, J, Brewer, E, Fink, C, Hanson, V and Schaller, J (1977). Comparison of tolmetin sodium and aspirin in the treatment of juvenile rheumatoid arthritis. J Pediatr, 91, 799
9. Brewer, EJ, Giannini, EH, Baum, J, Bernstein, B, Fink, CW, Emery, HM and Schaller, JG (1982). Aspirin and fenoprofen (Nalfon) in the treatment of juvenile rheumatoid arthritis. Results of the double blind trial. A segment II study. J Rheumatol, 9, 123
10. Mäkelä, A-L (1977). Naproxen in the treatment of juvenile rheumatoid arthritis. Scand J Rheumatol, 6, 193
11. Moran, H, Hanna, DB, Ansell, BM, Hall, M and Engler, C (1979). Naproxen in juvenile chronic polyarthritis. Ann Rheum Dis, 38, 152
12. Menon, ND, Whelton, JJ, Ansell, BM and Goldberg, AAJ (1974). A comparative study of ibuprofen and aspirin in Still's disease (juvenile chronic polyarthritis). Curr Med Res Opin (suppl.), 17
13. Haapasaari, J, Wuolijoki, E and Ylijoki, H (1983). Treatment of juvenile rheumatoid arthritis with diclofenac sodium. Scand J Rheumatol, 12, 325
14. Bhettay, E and Thomson, AJG (1978). Double-blind study of ketoprofen and indomethacin in juvenile chronic arthritis. S Afr Med J, 54, 276

15. Barron, KS, Person, DA and Brewer, EJ (1982). The toxicity of nonsteroidal anti-inflammatory drugs in juvenile rheumatoid arthritis. J Rheumatol, 9, 149

16. Mäkelä, A-L, Yrjänä, T and Mattila, M (1979). Dosage of salicylates for children with juvenile rheumatoid arthritis. A prospective clinical trial with three different preparations of acetylsalicylic acid. Acta Paediatr Scand, 68, 423

17. Doughty, RA, Giesecke, L and Athreya, B (1980). Salicylate therapy in juvenile rheumatoid arthritis. Dose, serum level, and toxicity. Am J Dis Child, 134, 461

18. Sänger, L, Stoeber, E and Kölle, G (1967). Langzeittherapie mit Indometacin bei der juvenilen rheumatoiden Arthritis und beim Morbus Still. Arzneimittelforsch, 17, 1414

19. Brewer, EJ (1977). Nonsteroidal anti-inflammatory agents. Arthritis Rheum, 20 (suppl.), 513

20. De Vere-Tyndall, AG and Ansell, BM (1980). Piroxicam in juvenile chronic arthritis: a pilot study. In: Dessain, P (ed.), Proc Int Symp Rheumatology in the 80's. (Princeton, NJ: Excerpta Medica), p. 45

21. Brewer, EJ, Giannini, EH, Baum, J, Bernstein, B, Fink, CW, Schaller, JG and Knee, CM (1982). Ketoprofen (Orudis) in the treatment of juvenile rheumatoid arthritis. A segment I study. J Rheumatol, 9, 144

22. Brewer, EJ, Giannini, EH, Baum, J, Cassidy, JT, Fink, CW, Hanson, V, Levinson, JE and Schaller, JG (1982). Sodium meclofenamate (Meclomen) in the treatment of juvenile rheumatoid arthritis. A segment I study. J Rheumatol, 9, 129

23. Brewer, EJ, Giannini, EH, Baum, J, Fink, CW, Hanson, V, Jacobs, JC and Schaller, JG (1982). Proquazone (Biarsan) in the treatment of juvenile rheumatoid arthritis. A segment I study. J Rheumatol, 9, 135

24. Bass, JC, Giannini, EH, Brewer, EJ, Athreya, BH, Brandstrup, NE, Goldsmith, DP, Miller, JJ and Pachman, LM (1982). Pirprofen (Rengasil) in the treatment of juvenile rheumatoid arthritis. A segment I study. J Rheumatol, 9, 140

25. Kelsey, WM and Scharyj, M (1967). Fatal hepatitis probably due to indomethacin. J Am Med Assoc, 199, 154

26. Jacobs, JC (1967). Sudden death in arthritic children receiving large doses of indomethacin. J Am Med Assoc, 199, 182

27. Paulus, HE, Siegel, M, Mongan, E, Okun, R and Calabro, JJ (1971). Variations of serum concentrations and half-life of salicylate in patients with rheumatoid arthritis. Arthritis Rheum, 14, 527

28. Levy, G and Tsuchiya, T (1972). Salicylate accumulation kinetics in man. N Engl J Med, 287, 430

29. Kvien, TK, Olsson, B and Høyeraal, HM (1985). Acetylsalicylic acid and juvenile rheumatoid arthritis. Effect of dosage interval on the serum salicylic acid level. Acta Paediatr Scand, 74, 755

30. Pachman, LM, Olufs, R, Procknal, JA and Levy, G (1979). Pharmacokinetic monitoring of salicylate therapy in children with juvenile rheumatoid arthritis. Arthritis Rheum, 22, 826

31. Bardare, M, Cislaghi, GU, Mandelli, M and Sereni, F (1978). Value of monitoring plasma salicylate levels in treating juvenile rheumatoid arthritis. Observations in 42 cases. Arch Dis Child, 53, 381

32. Brewer, EJ (1966). Acetylsalicylic acid and juvenile rheumatoid arthritis. In: Lamont-Havers, RW and Wagner, BM (eds), Proc. of the Conference of Effects of Chronic Salicylate Administration. (New York: US Department of Health, Education and Welfare), p. 26

Discussion

Dr KD Rainsford, UK: You must have a very large patient group from your two childrens centres as well as a registry in Oslo, is that correct?

Dr Kvien: In Norway most of the patients with juvenile rheumatoid arthritis go to Oslo and are treated in our special unit there, so we see about 70 new cases there each year.

Dr Rainsford: Regarding the ad lib allowance of paracetamol which you regard as a weak analgesic, but paracetamol is none-the-less about equianalgesic with aspirin. Just how much paracetamol have your patients taken in the different groups and is this intake appreciably different in these groups?

Dr Kvien: Only a few patients, less than 10, received paracetamol at all. As you know the juvenile patients experience little pain, but we allowed the possibility in the protocol for them to receive a paracetamol, but that was not necessary in most of the patients.

Dr Rainsford: What was the quantity of the drug involved?

Dr Kvien: It was only a very small quantity so it can't make any difference.

Dr Rainsford: It seemed in your tolmetin study that the aspirin dosage was high and the tolmetin dosage a little low. Is that right?

Dr Kvien: Yes, I think so. The aspirin dose is higher in the studies performed in the US than in Scandinavia. We used lower doses. That's a problem to explain why we have much more adverse reactions with acetyl salicylic acid in Finland and Norway than they have in the US in spite of them using more higher doses of aspirin in the US than in Scandinavia, so I have no explanation. We have talked about compliance as a possible explanation.

Dr SG Mann, UK: I was interested to see the high number of hepatoxic reactions you had in your acetyl salicylic acid group. Adult SLE patients are known to have an increased incidence of hepatoxic effects on aspirin and I wondered if you had looked to see if there was any correlation between the hepatoxic effects in the children that you studied and whether they had antinuclear antibodies.

Dr Kvien: We have not been especially interested in that but I think that there is no indication from other studies that there is any correlation between antinuclear antibodies and hepatoxicity.

11
Non-steroidal anti-inflammatories: outpatient audit of patient preferences and side-effects in different diseases

NL Cox* and SM Doherty**
*Royal Hants County Hospital, Winchester, UK
**Hull Royal Infirmary, Humberside, UK

CONTENTS

I. INTRODUCTION

Can patients detect any difference between anti-inflammatory agents which clinical trials have shown to be equipotent (or more accurately not to be statistically different from one another)? Does it matter which drug is chosen for a specific disease? To answer these questions we have asked patients attending routine rheumatology outpatient clinics to try quartets of NSAIDs. So far 1200 patients have been recruited into eight quartets. This paper

Side-effects of Anti-inflammatory Drugs. Rainsford, KD and Velo, GP (eds)
Part 1: Clinical and Epidemiological Aspects. (Lancaster: MTP Press)

reports the preliminary results of patient preferences in six groups as shown:

Group A
Piroxicam 30 mg nocte
Naproxen 500 mg b.d.
Indomethacin-R 75 mg b.d.
Fenbufen 300 mg a.m. 600 mg p.m.

Group B
Fenoprofen 600 mg t.d.s.
Diclofenac 500 mg t.d.s.
Ibuprofen 400 mg q.i.d.
Azapropazone 600 mg b.d.

Group C
Flurbiprofen 100 mg t.d.s.
Feprazone 200 mg t.d.s.
Benorylate 10 ml b.d.
Sulindac 200 mg b.d.

Group D
Ketoprofen 100 mg t.d.s.
Tiaprofenic acid 200 mg t.d.s.
Fenclofenac 600 mg b.d.
Aloxiprin 1200 mg q.i.d.

Group E
Ketoprofen C-R 200 mg b.d. (Oruvail)
Naproxen 500 mg b.d.
Indomethacin S-R 105 mg b.d. (Osmosin)
Indoprofen 400 mg b.d.

Group G
Piroxicam 30 mg nocte.
Ketoprofen C-R 200 mg b.d. (Oruvail)
Fenoprofen 600 mg t.d.s.
Flurbiprofen 100 mg t.d.s.

Nomenclature

Where two different formulations of a drug have been used we have used the pharmacological name for the original preparation and the trade name for the newer preparation to avoid confusion e.g. indomethacin-R & Osmosin, and ketoprofen & Oruvail. S-R = Sustained release, C-R = Controlled release, R = Regular formulations, respectively.

II. METHODS

Anybody seen in outpatients who needed an anti-inflammatory agent (either de novo or because their present one was not ideal) was eligible for inclusion into the study. Patients were only excluded from a quartet if they had previously been exposured to one of the agents in that quartet. Patients were given a simple instruction sheet outlining the reasons for the study. They were requested to take each of the four NSAIDs in the order indicated on the bottles for 3 weeks, and to record the order of their preference, if any, and any side-effects experienced. Where an adverse reaction occurred the drug was stopped for 48 hours and then restarted at a lower dose which was then gradually increased. If the patient was further upset the drug was stopped and the next in the sequence started. All medication was provided by prescription from the hospital pharmacy or retail chemist. Concurrent analgesia was permitted but only one NSAID was allowed to be taken at any one time. A "latin square" sequence of drugs was used with all 24 possible order permutations of four drugs to eliminate any bias from order effect.

Patients were asked wherever possible to rank drugs in an order of preference from 1 to 4, but were allowed to rank drugs equally if really unable to distinguish between them. The mean rank for a drug was derived:

$$\textbf{Mean rank} = \frac{\text{Aggregate of patient choices for a given drug}}{\text{Number of patients who took that drug}}$$

If all four drugs were equally preferred the mean rank of each would be 2.5. If a drug is preferred more often than the others the average score is lower, i.e. the lower the mean rank the better the drug performance. The results so obtained may be expressed as shown in Table 1.

Table 1 Group B osteoarthritis (N = 22)

	Rank							Total score	Mean rank
	1	1.5	2	2.5	3	3.5	4		
Fenoprofen	12	-	2	2	4	-	2	41.0	1.86
Diclofenac	7	-	5	3	3	1	3	49.0	2.23
Ibuprofen	2	-	2	4	10	1	3	61.5	2.80
Azapropazone	1	-	4	1	7	1	9	68.5	3.11

Any discrepancy between the average ranking and side-effect profile may suggest a relatively ineffective or more effective agent, e.g. in Group A fenbufen, though upsetting fewer patients, was ranked significantly below indomethacin, suggesting that indomethacin is more effective than fenbufen quite independently of the side-effects.

Alternatively if the cumulative mean rank taken every 10 completed patients is graphed for the group as a whole a picture emerges of the relative preference for each drug. The significance of any differences was calculated using Friedmann's rank test. (For non-statisticians: ranking differences of 1.0 are significant at 5% with 20 patients corresponding to a considerable difference in clinical terms. Similarly differences of 0.5, 0.25 and 0.20 require 50, 160 and 200 patients respectively to be significant at 5%). Quite large numbers are needed, and we hope to recruit 60 patients into each diagnostic group of interest. We hope this system will uncover any differences which may exist between NSAIDs rather than have a built-in bias towards equivalence as most comparative studies on NSAIDs do.

Additional information recorded included patients' age, sex, weight, cigarette consumption, serum albumen, and the number of different agents being taken. Side-effects were elicited by the question "Has the drug upset you in any way?" without any leading question.

Numbers in groups C (feprazone), D (fenclofenac), E (Osmosin & indoprofen) are curtailed due to withdrawal of some drugs. It is hoped to recruit further numbers into the remaining groups.

III. PATIENT PREFERENCES

Overall preferences to date are shown in Figures 1-6.

Group A

Overall piroxicam and naproxen were preferred more often than indomethacin-R and fenbufen ($p<0.05$). In rheumatoid arthritis (RA) both naproxen and piroxicam were better than fenbufen ($p<0.05$). In psoriatic arthritis piroxicam was more often preferred than fenbufen ($p<0.05$). In osteoarthritis (OA) both piroxicam and naproxen were more often preferred than indomethacin-R and fenbufen ($p<0.05$). When analysed by age naproxen and piroxicam were significantly more often preferred than indomethacin-R and fenbufen in the age group 51-70 ($p<0.05$). In the 71-90 age group naproxen was the most often preferred but numbers were too small to yield a result significant at 5%.

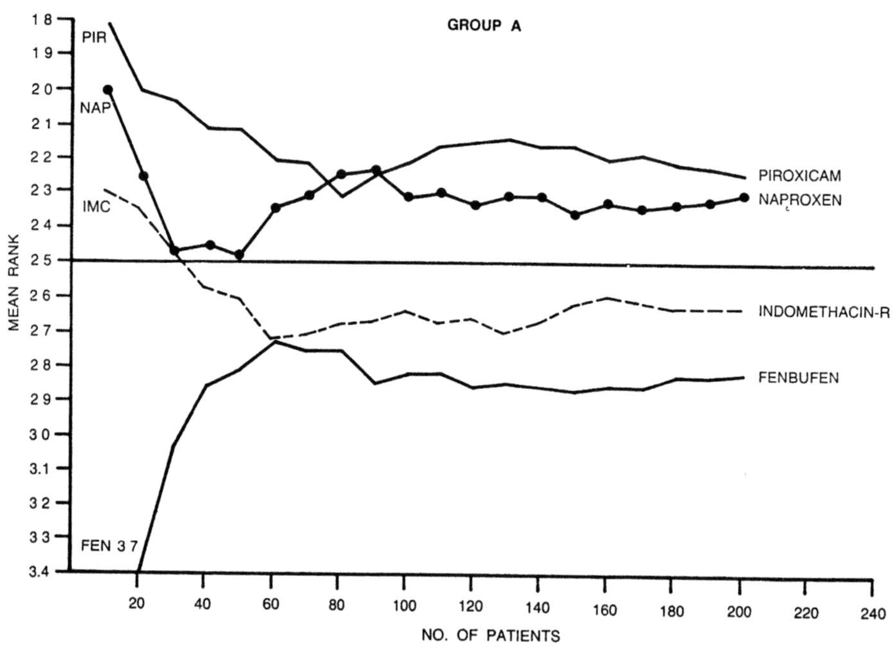

Figure 1 Cumulative mean rank of patients on NSAIDs: Group A (piroxicam, naproxen, indomethacin S-R (Indocid-S), fenbufen).

Group B
In group B fenoprofen was ranked above ibuprofen and azapropazone both overall and in OA ($p<0.05$). In the 71-90 age group ibuprofen was highest ranked and was significantly so compared with azapropazone ($p<0.05$) despite relatively low numbers.

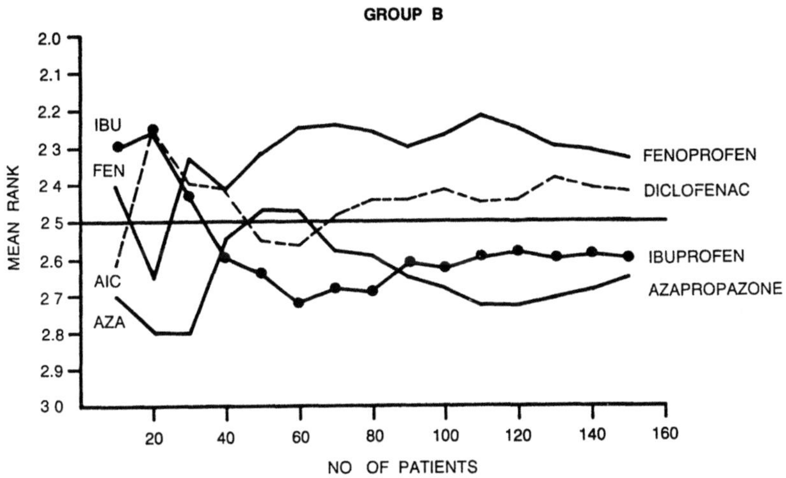

Figure 2 Cumulative mean rank of patients on NSAIDs: Group B (fenoprofen, diclofenac, ibuprofen, azapropazone).

Group C
Group C was curtailed by the withdrawal of feprazone from the market, and numbers are inadequate. Froben (flurbiprofen) was the most often preferred drug ($p<0.05$) overall and was notably so in males where it was ranked significantly above benorylate and sulindac.

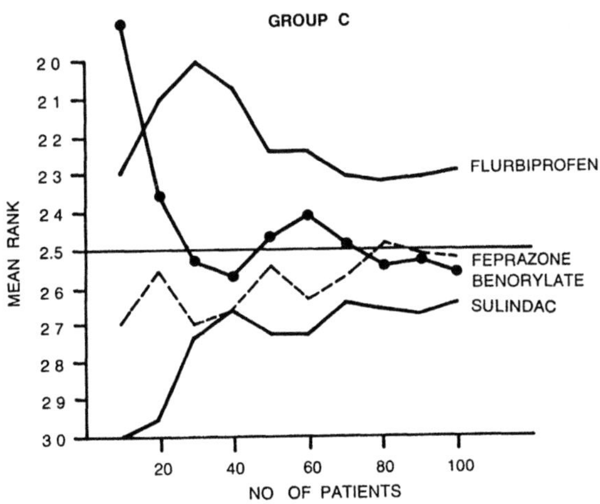

Figure 3 Cumulative mean rank of patients on NSAIDs: Group C (flurbiprofen, feprazone, benorylate, sulindac).

Group D

Group D died when fenclofenac was withdrawn; overall both ketoprofen and tiaprofenic acid were significantly better ranked than Aloxiprin ($p<0.05$). In RA both ketoprofen and tiaprofenic acid were better ranked than Aloxiprin ($p<0.05$). Aloxiprin is an aluminium oxide formulation complex with aspirin.

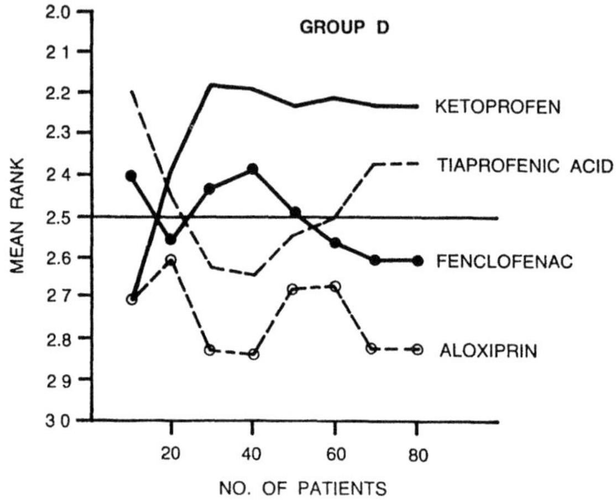

Figure 4 Cumulative mean rank of patients on NSAIDs: Group D (ketoprofen, tiaprofenic acid, fenclofenac, aloxiprin).

Group E

Group E stopped when Osmosin was withdrawn. Overall Oruvail, naproxen and Osmosin were all significantly ranked higher than indoprofen ($p<0.05$). In psoriatic arthritis Oruvail was preferred more often than Osmosin and indoprofen ($p<0.05$). Numbers are insufficient to determine a final relative placing of Oruvail, naproxen and Osmosin.

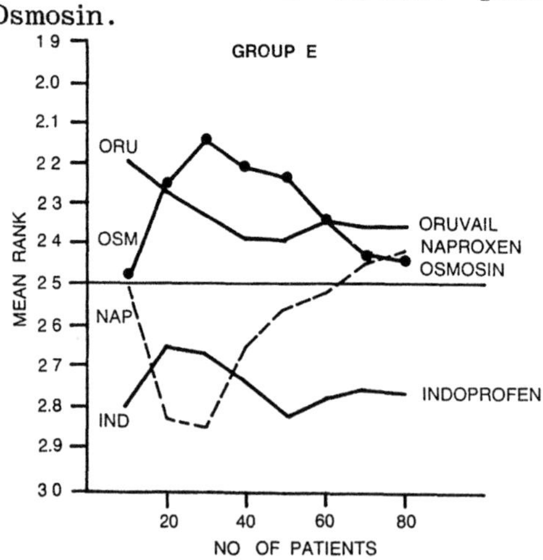

Figure 5 Cumulative mean rank of patients on NSAIDs: Group E (ketoprofen C-R (Oruvail), naproxen, indomethacin S-R (Osmosin), indoprofen).

Group G

Group G represents the winners of Groups A, B, C, and E and so can be regarded as a more final heat. Overall piroxicam was better ranked than Oruvail, fluribiprofen and fenoprofen ($p<0.05$). In RA the difference between piroxicam and the other three agents was significant at 5%, and in seronegative arthritis Oruvail was ranked better than fenoprofen.

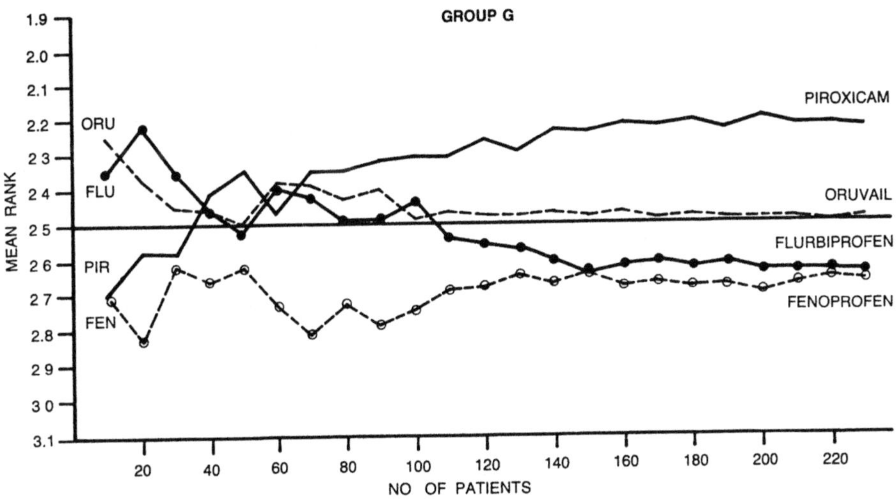

Figure 6 Cumulative mean rank of patients on NSAIDs: Group G (piroxicam, ketoprofen C-R (Oruvail), flurbiprofen, fenoprofen).

IV. SIDE-EFFECTS

Side-effects were common and occurred 35.9% (1331/3711) of patient drug exposures. Viewed overall there was no significant difference between groups (range 33.8% in Group D to 38.3% in Group C).

A. Gastrointestinal side-effects

These were most common and were present in 15.9% (590/3711) of all patient drug exposures. They are listed in Table 2.

Unfortunately, we have not graded side-effects for severity. Benorylate has a relatively poor showing due to the nausea induced at least in part by its taste. One patient died after perforating a duodenal ulcer on Osmosin; another died from faecal peritonitis after perforating a colonic diverticulum on indoprofen (? not drug-related). One patient required an emergency gastrectomy for a haematemesis on indoprofen. One patient perforated a duodenal ulcer on piroxicam but had had abdominal pain for the last 2 weeks of the preceding drug (naproxen). In all groups women had more gastrointestinal side-effects than men.

Table 2 Gastrointestinal side-effects

No.		%	No.		%
306	Naproxen	12.1	180	Azapropazone	15.6
477	Piroxicam	12.4	179	Diclofenac	17.3
220	Fenbufen	12.7	79	Fenclofenac	17.7
180	Ibuprofen	14.4	366	Flurbiprofen	18.3
109	Feprazone	14.7	109	Benorylate	19.2
435	Fenoprofen	14.9	78	Aloxiprin	20.5
80	Osmosin	15.0	111	Sulindac	21.6
223	Indomethacin-R	15.2	83	Indoprofen	22.9
339	Oruvail	15.3	79	Ketoprofen	24.1
78	Tiaprofenic acid	15.4			
	TOTAL 3711	15.9			

B. Lower gastrointestinal side-effects

These occurred in 3.5% (129/3711) of all patient drug exposures but were only infrequently a clinical problem. Diarrhoea was relatively more common with Osmosin (6%) and flurbiprofen (5%). Aloxiprin caused constipation in 7.7%.

V. CNS SIDE-EFFECTS

These were quite common and occurred in 9.8% (364/3711) of patient drug exposures. Interpreting such "soft data" without placebo controls is difficult. Indomethacin as indomethacin-R 150 mg a day caused side-effects in 40% of women compared with 18% of men, and as Osmosin 210 mg a day upset 21% of women compared with 8% of men. In group E Osmosin caused side-effects in 26.1% of rheumatoid patients (12/46) compared to 5.7% (2/35) of non-rheumatoid patients. In group A indomethacin-R upset 37% of RA patients compared to 26% of non-RA patients. When side-effects are plotted against weight they appear to be directly dose-related in men but less so in women, suggesting a genuine difference in susceptibility independent of weight (Figure 7); see also Table 3.

CNS side-effects in patients taking drugs other than indomethacin were a small but significant problem. Headaches, dizziness, and drowsiness were the commonest complaints but a few complained of severe confusion, and some volunteered that they did not think they were safe to drive.

In all groups women complained of more CNS side-effects than men. Cigarette smokers were less likely to develop side-effects on indomethacin than were non-smokers.

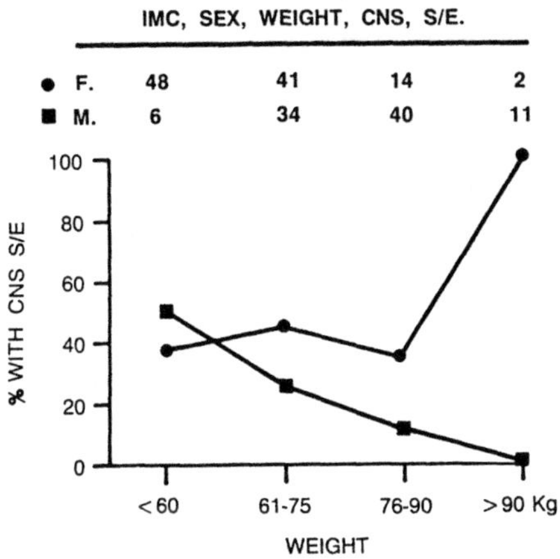

Figure 7

Table 3 Central nervous system side-effects

No.		%	No.		%
220	Indomethacin R	30.0	106	Benorylate	8.5
78	Aloxiprin	20.5	180	Azapropazone	8.3
80	Osmosin	18.1	220	Fenbufen	8.2
179	Diclofenac	11.7	180	Ibuprofen	7.8
108	Sulindac	10.2	79	Fenclofenac	7.6
435	Fenoprofen	9.0	303	Naproxen	6.9
78	Ketoprofen	8.9	479	Piroxicam	6.7
78	Tiaprofenic acid	8.9	83	Indoprofen	6.0
362	Flurbiprofen	8.8	339	Oruvail	5.0
106	Feprazone	8.5			

VI. MUCOCUTANEOUS SIDE-EFFECTS

These occurred in 4.1% (153/3711) of patients. Only in azapropazone (9.4%), fenbufen (10.9%), feprazone (11.0%) and fenclofenac (11.4%) were these a clinical nuisance. None of the rashes was severe. In most groups women developed more mucocutaneous side-effects than men. The overall incidence of side-effects is shown in Table 4.

Table 4 Mucocutaneous side-effects

No.		%	No.		%
79	Fenclofenac	11.4	111	Sulindac	2.7
109	Feprazone	11.0	366	Flurbiprofen	2.7
220	Fenbufen	10.9	78	Aloxiprin	2.6
180	Azapropazone	9.4	79	Tiaprofenic acid	2.6
83	Indoprofen	4.8	79	Ketoprofen	2.5
339	Oruvail	3.8	179	Diclofenac	2.2
109	Benorylate	3.7	306	Naproxen	1.9
180	Ibuprofen	3.3	223	Indomethacin R	1.3
435	Fenoprofen	3.2	80	Osmosin	1.2
477	Piroxicam	2.9			
	Total 3711				4.1%

VII. MISCELLANEOUS SIDE-EFFECTS

A miscellany of side-effects were present in 3.6% (135/3711) of patients. Fluid retention occurred in 5/479 patients on piroxicam and was also seen in flurbiprofen(3), fenoprofen(3), Oruvail(2).

VIII. DISCUSSION

We have described a simple method of ranking NSAIDs which can be applied in routine outpatient clinics. The study is based on the assumptions that (1) NSAIDs do differ in efficacy, and (2) patients can detect such differences, even if small. Unless a non-steroidal shows some evidence that it may modify inflammatory joint disease patient preference will be the largest factor determining prescription in drugs which aim to give symptomatic relief. Advantages of the system are that it is part of normal outpatient practice and therefore any placebo reaction will be less than in a more formal trial, it is simple and so large numbers can be recruited, and it is more likely to detect differences than most NSAID comparative studies. Limitations of the study include the absence of any placebo control data, or washout period between drugs, the initial fixed dose regime and minimal laboratory data. Greater numbers are needed to detect rare side-effects. Only symptomatic side-effects are picked up, and 3 weeks is a very short period for a chronic NSAID taker. Longer-term side-effects, particularly gastrointestinal, are likely to be under-reported.

Patients can usually make a choice between the drugs, and rankings are obtained in 85% of patients. About 3% default, and the remainder are unable to choose between agents (usually when none have helped much) or fail to complete the quartet. About 75% of patients are satisfied with one of the drugs offered, but some have to rotate through two or three quartets before finding an anti-inflammatory which suits them. Even drugs which perform poorly have a few staunch supporters.

Given adequate numbers significant differences do emerge between agents, both overall and in different diagnoses. Results at both centres correspond, as shown in Table 5.

Table 5

	MEAN RANKING		
	Winchester	Hull	Both
Group A	(N=134)	(N=71)	(N=205)
Piroxicam	2.25	2.25	2.25
Naproxen	2.33	2.27	2.31
Indomethacin R	2.57	2.72	2.62
Fenbufen	2.85	2.77	2.82
Group G	(N=188)	(N=51)	(N=239)
Piroxicam	2.32	1.88	2.23
Oruvail	2.49	2.46	2.48
Flurbiprofen	2.59	2.90	2.66
Fenoprofen	2.60	2.73	2.64

This system may demonstrate small differences in patient preference which some would not regard as clinically significant. We would suggest that differences which emerge with 50 patients and are significant at the 5% level will be intuitively recognizable by most clinicians, and that any significant difference emerging with only 20 patients represents a large difference in efficacy (or incidence of side-effects). With greater numbers small but real differences may be demonstrated which may allow a broader evaluation of the drugs against each other, and may provide a basis for a strategy of drug choice likely to suit a given type of patient best. For example, try men with indomethacin or flurbiprofen earlier than women, and OA patients with piroxicam. If the above database is further expanded an overall picture may emerge enabling prescription of the most appropriate NSAID for a given patient. Such a system may also provide a sensible basis for choosing which drugs should be included in a hospital or district formulary, and provide a system for fairly swift evaluation in a routine clinical setting of any new agent against those currently in wide use.

IX. CONCLUSIONS

1. A simple method for ranking patient preference in anti-inflammatory treatment is described.
2. Patients do prefer some agents significantly more than

others, and there may be preferred NSAIDs for different conditions, age groups and sexes.

3. Women get side-effects more often than men.
4. No clear differences in susceptibility to side-effects in different diseases has so far emerged.
5. 9.8% of all patients put on NSAIDs develop CNS side-effects, which are occasionally severe.

Discussion

Dr A Herxheimer, UK: I wonder what the effect of the dose is of the drugs used. It sounded from your presentation as if you were using the recommended dose for each one and that introduces the luck of the draw in the manufacturers' decision on what dose to recommend, and it makes the comparison confounded by the dose factor so you're comparing one dose of each of the drug with that of others?

Dr Cox: The fixed dose regime is a limitation, yes, they're all hospital cases, they're hospital referants, so I've used the upper end of the recommended dose. I accept that's a limitation of the study and the doses were not related to weight.

Dr Herxheimer: Have you titrated the dose?

Dr Cox: Patients in fact had the option. If they were upset they were told to stop the drug for 48 hours, and to start again at a small dose and to titrate up till they got symptomatic relief or if they didn't get relief but they got side effects, they were told to stop it and go onto the next.

Professor A Bennett, UK: Another problem with your study is that you've done so many comparisons, and of course you can't avoid it, but if you do enough comparisons some of them are likely to arise by chance. What have you done to avoid this bias?

Dr Cox: All I can do is to continue with the study and get the numbers up to a point until you get higher degrees of significance, but that is built in if you do lots of studies and you accept a 5% probability, 1 in 20 is goint to be by chance.

Professor Bennett: You might do better not to just add the numbers but to take a separate cohort of patients and see whether in that separate cohort you get the same results because once you've swung the results one way or the other adding numbers to them may make that much difference. So what I'm saying, you've done that study, do another one on a completely different set of data which you could analyse separately.

Dr Cox: My target was that the patients went into each quartet depending upon which one we were recruiting for at the time and it was mainly historical order. Having got quite a large number in I have then selectively added psoriatic and spondyloarthritics into group A because I had 30 and I counted to get the number up to 60 in each diagnostic bracket which should give a difference if there's a real one.

Professor Bennett: No but you see the problem is if you have already had 10 patients preferring one and one preferring another and then you randomly added and it tended to come out 6 preferred as opposed to 15. In other words there was no difference in the second group, when you still analyzed the combined data you'll still have a significant difference, even though if you had analyzed the second lot separately you would have shown no difference. Do you understand that point?

Dr Cox: Not entirely, but all I can say is that if you compare the mean rankings between the Winchester and the Gall patients they correspond very closely, these two populations.

Dr KD Rainsford, UK: I would like to take up a point you made about the differences in the GI susceptibility of the drugs in the sexes. As I understood it you said that with all the drugs you looked at the females appeared to have greater susceptibility than the males, but your data showed that the proportion was about equal in the 2 sexes. Is that so?

Dr Cox: That was so, yes, but overall nevertheless there is a preponderance. Looking at the body weights though we find that those who are very light are more likely to get gastro-intestinal side effects. People with a moderate weight have a low incidence. Then as the weight of the patients increased though they were'nt complaining of acid reflux the incidence went up quite so fat women and men got more side effects than people of the appropriate weight.

Dr Walker: My question is an extension of the first one. I would like your comments on the frequency of dosage, not the total daily dose. Some patients were taking one unit at night and others were taking it 2 or 3 times a day. From my experience there is a very strong patient preference for taking a drug once or twice a day and after that their preference tails off very rapidly.

Dr Cox: In the various groups, piroxicam did well. Fenoprofen is taken 3 times a day and Ibuprofen is taken 4 times a day. My impression has been that given equal efficacy patients don't mind taking it more often or according to their choice. If there is greater efficacy they'll take a drug more often but they're equal they'll go for the more convenient one.

Professor PF D'Arcy, UK: I was very interested in this variation that you've got in the adverse events. Could it have been that the women were taking other analgesics during the period you were examining?

Dr Cox: They were only allowed one back up analgesia or asked to take one analgesia and no other anti-inflammatories were taken. Certainly across the group as a whole women took a greater number of drugs than men. We've also recorded the number of drugs they take, their cigarette consumption, albumin levels and weight, and women consistently take more drugs in virtually all diagnostic groups and age groups so it may be related to that.

12
Non-steroidal anti-inflammatories in the elderly

PP Lamy
Centre for the Study of Pharmacy and Therapeutics for the Elderly, School of Pharmacy, and Department of Epidemiology and Preventive Medicine, University of Maryland at Baltimore, Baltimore, MD 21201, USA

CONTENTS

I. INTRODUCTION

The population at risk to serious side-effects of the NSAIDs is rapidly expanding by the aging of the population. Eighty-five percent of randomly selected patients attending an outpatient-arthritis department in a British city were women, one-half were over 64. Elderly patients often presented with multiple problems and lived alone[1]. In Britain, 23% of all visits to primary care

Side-effects of Anti-inflammatory Drugs. Rainsford, KD and Velo, GP (eds)
Part 1: Clinical and Epidemiological Aspects. (Lancaster: MTP Press)

physicians are for rheumatic complaints and in the US, patients with rheumatic arthritis (RA) average 7 physician visits annually[2]. One-half of all people with RA are 50 years and older[3]. By retirement, 80% of people in the US complain about some rheumatic problem. After age 75, almost 24% of women and 14% of men have RA[4]. Of 3097 elderly studied, 24% of females and 18% of males reported low back pain[5]. Overall, possibly 12 million elderly in the US suffer from some type of joint and musculoskeletal disease. Non-steroidals are often used to treat all of these complaints, osteoarthritis (for analgesia), acute attacks of gout and pseudogout, and polymyalgia rheumatica in the absence of giant cell arthritis. Consequently, use of non-steroidals is high (Table 1). In the UK, the number of prescriptions for non-steroidals has doubled to 20 million in the last decade, and more than 75% of these are written for the elderly[6]. The number of prescriptions for NSAIDs rises with age, but the incidence of all side-effects rises disproportionally with age[7].

Table 1 Use of systemic anti-arthritics correlated with age

Age (yrs)	Number of R_x/ 1000 patients/yr
0-44	113
45-54	419
55-64	590
65-74	747
75 +	785

Source: FDA Drug Analysis Branch. Washington DC 1984

The NSAIDs have an exceptionally high incidence of side-effects (Tables 2 and 3)[8], and non-steroidals should be used with caution in the elderly[9], but some relatively recent publications do not even speak to the effect of these drugs in the elderly[10]. Much of current knowledge regarding the elderly and NSAIDs is based on data gathered on phenylbutazone and highly toxic drugs such as benaxoprofen[11]. In general, non-steroidals have not been comparatively studied in most rheumatic disorders, especially in the older population[12]. Some data are available. Phenylbutazone, for example, causes agranulocytosis in elderly 30 times as often than in younger people. Flurbiprofen is more toxic to elderly than younger patients[13].

II. THE NSAIDs

All non-steroidals are weakly acidic and highly protein bound. Those with a higher pKa usually have a longer duration of action.

Non-steroidals have been causatively linked to acute liver and renal failure, and acute autoimmune haemolytic anaemia[14]. They can interfere with the cellular respiratory chain, but multisystem failures have not often been reported. Gastritis and peptic ulceration, perhaps most often caused by piroxicam, occur relatively often. Occurring less often but serious in nature are hypersensitivity reactions, such as blood dyscrasias (aplastic anaemia, thrombocytopenia, agranulocytosis, haemolytic anaemia), erythema

Table 2 Non-fatal NSAID-induced ADRs/million R_x - 1984

Drug	ADRs/Mill. R_x
Diflunisal	95.31
Piroxicam	91.16
Tolmetin	59.09
Meclofenamate	47.72
Sulindac	46.61
Indomethacin	25.39
Phenylbutazone	25.29
Fenoprofen	24.85
Naproxen	20.75
Ibuprofen	10.22

Source: FDA Arthritis Advisory Committee, 1985 (ref. 8)

Table 3 Fatal NSAID-induced ADRs/million R_x - 1984

Drug	ADRs/mill. R_x
Phenylbutazone	4.99
Diflunisal	4.00
Piroxicam	2.66
Sulindac	2.01
Fenoprofen	1.84
Indomethacin	1.66
Tolmetin	1.55
Meclofenamate	1.11
Naproxen	0.67
Ibuprofen	0.44

Source: FDA Arthritis Advisory Committee, 1985 (ref. 8)

multiforme, and hepatitis. Blood dyscrasias, while rare, are among the main causes of death attributed to NSAIDS. Agranulocytosis can occur with indomethacin, ibuprofen, fenoprofen, naproxen, tolmetin and piroxicam. Some non-steroidals interact with oral anticoagulants with the potential for displacing warfarin from its protein binding sites and inhibiting hepatic metabolism, the synthesis of clotting factors, and platelet aggregation. Those highly protein bound may displace oral hypoglycaemics and phenytoin from their binding sites[15-19].

III. THE ELDERLY: AT HEIGHTENED RISK?

Most reports of NSAID-related renal effects have involved patients over 60 years of age[20]. Anecdotal evidence seems to indicate that reversible acute renal failure (ARF) is more frequently seen in hospitalized elderly patients than ever before, but the question whether or not advancing age, itself, predisposes a patient to an increased risk has not yet been answered. One factor involved may be a greater prevalence of NSAID exposure in older patients. Other factors involved may be primary age changes (physiological changes) such as reduction in kidney and liver function, alteration in protein metabolism, or an altered thirst mechanism[21-24]. These changes can lead to altered pharmacokinetic and pharmacodynamic profiles of drugs and a greater incidence of drug toxicity. Other primary age changes may not yet have been recognized. For example, senescent cells appear to have a diminished capacity to convert fatty acids to prostaglandins[25]. Secondary age changes (pathophysiological changes) also could alter drug action. Multiple pathology is not unusual in elderly patients, including hypertension, cardiovascular disease, arteriosclerosis, diabetes mellitus and others. Moreover, the drugs used to manage these chronic diseases may account for undesirable interactions with NSAIDs[26].

For some non-steroidals, alterations in pharmacokinetics have been documented. Naproxen kinetics are altered with impaired renal[27] or hepatic function and with changes in plasma protein[28]. The fraction of naproxen unbound to plasma protein is doubled in elderly both at peak and trough concentrations[28]. These effects may be age related, an effect of undernutrition, widely perceived in the elderly population[29], or disease-related. In one case, the effect was age-related, since only healthy elderly were studied[28]. Alteration in half-life of piroxicam has been reported[30]. The half-life of piroxicam, which is much longer than that of most other non-steroidals (Table 4), was prolonged to 61.7 hrs, leading to a body clearance approximately 33% lower in elderly than in younger women. The latter observation is of extreme importance, since women outnumber men at a ratio of 3 : 1 (in nursing homes) and 2 : 1 among community-living elderly and women, in general, are more sensitive to adverse drug reactions than are men[23].

Alteration in drug action and heightened risk to toxicity could, in these cases, be related to patient age, drug dose and duration of treatment. By contrast, certain drugs, i.e. fenoprofen, can cause an interstitial nephritis that seems to be unrelated to the prostaglandin-synthesis-inhibiting effect of the drug, its dose, or duration of use[10] and correlation with age is difficult to achieve. Perhaps, a risk assessment process is needed[31], involving a three-step process. First would be hazard identification, the process of gathering and validating data on the hazard of a drug, i.e. its ability to potentially cause harm and to ascertain whether a hazard exists. The second step, hazard evaluation, seeks to determine characteristics of the hazard and the expression of the hazard in terms of human health effects. Finally, step three, risk evaluation, determines whether and to what extent the potential hazard of the drug is realized. Actual exposure levels, frequencies, and identification of those most exposed will aid in the assessment of risk and the acceptability of the degree of risk.

Table 4 Half-life of some non-steroidals

Drug	Half-life (hrs)
Tolmetin	1-3
Ibuprofen	2
Indomethacin	2-3
Ketoprofen	3
Fenoprofen	3
Mefenamic acid	3-4
Flurbiprofen	4
Diflunisal	8-12
Flufenamic acid	9
Naproxen	12-15
Sulindac	18
Piroxicam	45

IV. THE EXISTING DATA BASE

Preclinical and clinical trials cannot provide a full description of all adverse drug reactions (ADRs). Formal phase IV data will probably not be too helpful, either[32]. Observations by individual physicians would be most helpful, but in the case of the elderly, kidney changes and mental status changes, for example, may be overlooked, ascribed to old age, or may be too difficult to separate from the effect of other drugs in the presence of multiple pathology, multiple drug regimens, and poor self-reporting. Furthermore, it is difficult to separate an increase in reported side-effects from an increase in sales. Sometimes, individual reporting is very successful as was the case with tolmetin-induced anaphylactoid reactions[33].

The FDA relies on voluntary reporting[8]. The system may reflect biases. Incidence data cannot be obtained. It is also difficult to accurately estimate reporting rates. Key information is sometimes not reported in as many as one-half of the reports. Other useful data show a "high level of nonreporting", including age and sex of patient. Finally, the system cannot be used to validate that a drug may cause a particular side-effect in particular patients. It must be kept in mind, too, that the rate of reporting usually increases toward the end of the second year and then declines, despite an increasing rate of prescribing. Even though, useful comparisons can be made between fractions consisting of the number of adverse reactions as the numerator and the number of prescriptions as the denominator[34].

In the case of the elderly, one needs to approach these data with particular caution. Some time ago, the FDA Drug Analysis Branch reported that 25% of all prescriptions written for elderly are not filled. In 1981, the non-compliance with non-steroidals was found to vary between 30% and 40% among the elderly[35], perhaps because they could not open the containers[36]. In 1985, non-compliance with non-steroidals was called "rampant", since 44% of patients treated for arthritis and chronic pain did not take the NSAID as prescribed, mainly because of gastrointestinal side-effects[37]. Thus, the denominator in the fraction used to estimate side-effects may well be incorrect. Some recent developments may make it even more difficult to define the risk of NSAIDs to elderly. First is the availability of ibuprofen as a non-prescription product[38]. In itself probably a giant step backward in containing NSAID-induced ADRs in the elderly, it also probably enhances the chances of elderly for using more than one analgesic at a time. Elderly, traditionally, have used either acetaminophen or aspirin to enhance the analgesic properties of a NSAID, and may well now add a NSAID to their regimen without realizing that it is, indeed, a non-steroidal. In view of the recent NIH conclusion that long-term use of analgesic/antipyretic combinations can enhance patient risk to kidney disease and chronic renal failure[38], it would appear that elderly are now more at risk than ever, a risk that will almost certainly not be identified by the current FDA reporting system. Finally, a major shift in health care delivery in the US finds more and more seriously ill elderly being cared for at home. It is questionable how well ADRs due to non-steroidals will be recognized and reported and, indeed, lack of supervision of chronic care drugs has been cited as one of the major reasons for a high incidence of ADRs among the elderly[39].

V. IDENTIFYING AND EVALUATING THE HAZARD

A. Drug-induced asthma

Aspirin-sensitive patients are more sensitive to urticaria, bronchospasm, and proctocolitis[19]. Patients with aspirin intolerance often have similar allergic responses to non-steroidals[40]. Asthmatic attacks may be precipitated in 5% to 10% of adult asthmatic patients[41] but sensitivity increases with age and occurs more often in females[42]. Younger adults seem to be less likely to have polyps, one part of the predisposing triad, than older adults[43]. It has been proposed that an imbalance between the "bronchodilator" prostaglandin E and the "bronchoconstrictor" F2 alpha occurs, leading to bronchospasm[44] and, in older people, bronchospasm may be caused by increased leukotriene synthesis[45]. Drug-induced asthma may be particularly dangerous in the elderly. At the recent meeting of the American Thoracic Society, rises in asthma death rates were documented for Oregon (87%), California (56%) and Washington (41%). Increased mortality was seen only in older age groups, particularly those 75 years and older[46]. Identifying the old patient with drug-induced asthma may be difficult. Elderly may present only with cough and exertional dyspnoea. Finally, it should be noted that with increasing age, the incidence of kerato-conjunctivitis sicca in association with RA (Sjoegren's syndrome) increases and patients presenting with this syndrome are more likely than others to show evidence of hypersensitivity to drug effects[7]. It is clear that the cumulative prevalence of aspirin intolerance increases steadily with age and that aging and disease factors are involved. Among drugs absolutely contraindicated in patients with aspirin-induced asthma are indomethacin, mefenamic acid, flufenamic acid, meclofenamic acid, ibuprofen, fenoprofen, ketoprofen, naproxen, diclofenac, and phenylbutazone[41].

B. Haematological disorders

The elderly seem to be at particular risk of abnormalities of haematological indices. Perhaps a significant number of elderly have this abnormality but are not reported. Platelet dysfunction is well-recognized as a side-effect of NSAIDs[47] and thrombocytopenia, leukopenia, and agranulocytosis have been reported for some non-steroidals, including sulindac[48-50] and piroxicam[51]. A number of elderly patients, treated with sulindac, often for only two weeks, developed aplastic anaemia[52-54]. Five cases of mefenamic acid-induced leukopenia in elderly (78 to 89 years) have been reported over one specific six month period[55]. Obviously, elderly are at risk to haematological problems which can be fatal, but it is not clear whether these are causally linked only to advancing age. In any case, regular haematological review is mandatory for elderly, particularly the very old, receiving non-steroidals.

C. CNS effects

Some non-steroidals, particularly indomethacin, are associated with a high incidence of CNS effects. In general, CNS effects are associated with headaches and dizziness. However, primary age changes in brain sensitivity and the blood-brain barrier, as well as use of many drugs that may cause psychiatric side-effects in the elderly[56,57] would suggest that other, more serious CNS effects are likely to occur. Recognition of cognitive dysfunction in the elderly is particularly difficult. Often, complaints may be ascribed to old age "symptomatology". Complaints are often subjective and can only be elicited by specific questioning of patient or family, neither of whom are likely to ascribe CNS effects to drug therapy. Indeed, it has been suggested that memory loss, inability to concentrate, confusion, and personality changes are frequent toxicities of the newer non-steroidals in the elderly[58], albeit still mainly unrecognized or unreported. The risk is high, since loss of mental acuity is often associated with "senility" and subsequent institutionalization.

D. Cutaneous reactions

The NSAIDs frequently induce cutaneous reactions. Reactions to piroxicam have been most often reported[59]. Piroxicam-induced phototoxicity seems to be due to a metabolite preferentially formed in affected patients[60]. There are no data to indicate whether the elderly would be at heightened risk. However, of 135 dermatological reactions reported over 30 months, two resulted in fatalities, both patients over 80 years of age[59].

E. Activation and masking of infections

The non-steroidals have antipyretic action and evaluation of general health problems in the elderly can be complicated by NSAID-masked fever. NSAIDs may activate, spread, and mask infections. Scattered reports document a statistically significant relation between reactivation of tuberculosis and use of NSAIDs in elderly patients[61,62]. Since tuberculosis is on the rise among the elderly, this would present a hazard, even though it may not be purely age-related.

Table 5 NSAID-induced hepatic reactions per million R_x - 1984

Drug	ADRs/mill. R_x
Phenylbutazone	4.99
Sulindac	4.39
Piroxicam	4.25
Diflunisal	2.40
Meclofenamate	1.66
Fenoprofen	0.92
Naproxen	0.76
Indomethacin	0.44
Tolmetin	0.39
Ibuprofen	0.29

Source: FDA Arthritis Advsiory Committee, 1985 (ref. 8)

F. Hepatic toxicity

The incidence of NSAID-induced hepatic toxicity is probably underestimated[7], but the FDA Arthritis Advisory Committee has now agreed that liver injury should be considered a class characteristic of NSAIDs[63]. Non-fatal hepatic toxicity is reported fairly often (Table 5). Liver disease in RA may range between 25% to 50% of patients not receiving drug therapy, serum phosphatase levels decreasing with improvement of the disease[64]. Hepatocellular necrosis or degeneration can occur with phenylbutazone, sulindac, ibuprofen, indomethacin and naproxen[65,66]. It has a potential case fatality of 10% or more. Since females predominate in older age groups, it is of note that phenylbutazone and sulindac hepatotoxicity occur often in females[64,67]. Hepatic toxicity may be particularly difficult to see in elderly, since anorexia, fatigue and nausea are symptoms of clinical presentation, which may often be overlooked. Elderly may be more at risk, then, because of gender and a certain non-recognition factor, but also because they may be taking several drugs with the potential to cause hepatic injury (Table 6). Aminotransferase levels three or more times the upper limit mandate prompt withdrawal of the NSAID.

Table 6 Some drugs known to cause liver injury which are frequently used by elderly

Acetaminophen	Isoniazid
Antidepressants	Manganese*
Antipsychotics	Methyldopa
Chlorothiazide	Phenytoin
Chlorpropamide	Propylthiouracil
Chlorthalidone	Quinidine
Copper*	Selenium*
Erythromycin	Sulphonamides
Iron*	Tolbutamide

* Elderly likely to obtain as non-prescription items in health food stores, often in megadoses

G. Renal effects

In patients with even mild impairment of renal function, renal blood flow (RBF) and glomerular filtration rate (GFR) depend critically on prostaglandin E production[68]. NSAIDs can abolish renal blood flow autoregulation (Figure 1). Thus, because there is a progressive decline in GFR with age, associated with a high incidence of superimposed conditions impacting on renal action, elderly patients are at risk for renal complications when treated with NSAIDs (Table 7). These drugs can decrease RBF and GFR by 33%[69] and ibuprofen (1.2 g/day) has reduced creatinine clearance by as much as 19%[68]. A clear consensus labels advanced age as a risk factor to NSAID-induced renal effects.

A predisposing factor is dehydration[70], relatively common among elderly, who exhibit a diminished thirst mechanism. Patients with poor appetites or inability to feed themselves, such

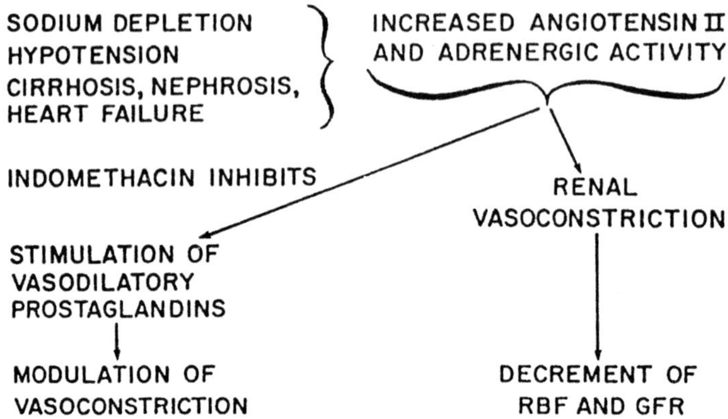

Figure 1 Suppressed prostaglandin counterregulations.

as chair- or bed-bound patients, are at heightened risk[24]. Other risk factors, associated with age-related pathophysiological changes, abound. Common to all these is a need for increased renal synthesis of vasodilator prostaglandins.

Table 7 The aging kidney

Change	Consequences
Primary aging	
Reduced cardiac output	Less perfusion
Decline in GFR	Kidney depends critically on endogenous prostaglandins
Decreased thirst mechanism	Dehydration
Secondary aging	
Intercurrent diseases (hypertension, diabetes CHF)	Increased risk to ADRs of NSAIDs
Concomittant drugs	Nephrotoxicity, volume depletion

Hyporeninaemic hypoaldosteronism with hyperkalemia usually involves elderly patients with congestive heart failure (CHF), diabetes mellitus, chronic renal insufficiency, hypertension, infection, and gout. Acute illness or stress are apparently not predisposing factors, but use of potassium-sparing diuretics and potassium supplements is important[71,72]. The use of potassium-sparing diuretics is increasing. A potassium-sparing diuretic ranks sixth among the most frequently used drugs for those 85 years and older[73]. Prescribed potasssium supplements rank fifth, and the FDA has estimated that about 25% of the elderly purchase potassium supplements in health food stores. Elevated potassium levels may be exacerbated by hyponatraemia, hypocalcaemia and acidosis. Fatal cardiac arrhythmias may result. In patients with suppressed prostaglandin counterregulatory mechanism, reduction in RBF will augment salt and water retention. Patients with underlying CHF are at risk for both severe hyponatraemia and oedema[74]. NSAID interference with fluid and electrolyte homeostatis, therefore, is a major hazard to the elderly. Acute renal failure is one of the major effects of prostaglandin inhibition. It is most often noted in females over 50[16,75]. Common to all instances is a reduction in cardiac output caused by CHF or myocardial infarction and reduced plasma volume, resulting in sodium retention and reduced urine output. Volume depletion may be caused by haemorrhage, gastrointestinal losses via diarrhoea or vomiting, urinary losses due to diuretics, salt wasting, a decreased "effective" volume as in cirrhosis, and peripheral vasodilation due to sepsis or drugs. Urethral obstruction, prostatic hypertrophy and bladder infections contribute, as do tubular lesions often caused by nephrotoxic drugs. Respiratory tract infection is a frequent complication and elderly over 60 are less likely to recover completely[76,77]. Obviously, older patients have a higher mortality rate than younger patients.

Patients at risk to haemodynamic or functional ARF are generally female, of advanced age, being treated with diuretics, with underlying intrinsic renal disease with or without obvious renal insufficiency, with volume contraction (CHF, liver disease), hypertension, diabetes mellitus or atherosclerotic cardiovascular disease. Advanced age and atherosclerosis may be associated with fixed renal microvascular disease (long-standing hypertension) and glomerulosclerosis[78-80]. Diuretic-induced gouty arthritis is fairly common in these patients. If ARF develops, it will happen within 24 hrs of initiation of drug therapy or an increase in dose. Elderly may be at particular risk because use of digitalis for this population is high. Digitalis ranks second among drugs most frequently used for those 85 and older[73]. Toxicity due to reduced clearance of digoxin and also aminoglycosides, secondary to decreased creatinine clearance, may occur.

NSAID-induced interstitial nephritis, leading to renal failure, is idiosyncratic, and has been reported with tolmetin, fenoprofen, mefenamic acid, phenylbutazone and naproxen. Risk factors have not yet been identified. It is usually accompanied by glomerular lesions and proteinuria, and possibly by the nephrotic syndrome. Patients developing this type of renal failure are usually older and female, suffering from RA, osteoarthritis, non-specific arthritis, bursitis, tendinitis and low back pain. Underlying renal lesions are usually absent. Severity of renal failure is usually greater than in haemodynamic ARF. Patients developing this type of renal failure are probably at greater risk than patients with haemodynamic ARF. The former type develops slowly, often in patients on chronic therapy who are not hospitalized. Thus, considering the developing home care sector, observation and recognition may be difficult.

Table 8 Renal failure and NSAIDs

Drug	Renal failure (any sign/million R_x)
Diflunisal	6.41
Fenoprofen	5.52
Piroxicam	4.12
Meclofenamate	2.77
Sulindac	2.74
Phenylbutazone	1.78
Naproxen	1.35
Indomethacin	1.33
Tolmetin	0.78
Ibuprofen	0.54

Source: FDA Arthritis Advisory Committee, 1985 (ref. 8)

FDA-reported cases of renal failure indicate a fairly high number (Table 8), and the incidence of NSAID-associated renal insufficiency may reach 20% in the elderly[79,82]. It is likely that all non-steroidals decrease renal clearance, particularly in patients 60 years old and older[83]. The major risk factors are advanced age, atherosclerotic cardiovascular disease, and concurrent diuretic therapy.

Table 9 NSAID-induced upper GI adverse effects of reported cases in people over 50*

Drug	Percent
Overall	62.1
Piroxicam	91.6
Sulindac	83.8
Indomethacin	81.6
Meclofenamate	75.0
Diflunisal	67.5
Phenylbutazone	67.2
Tolmetin	60.0
Ibuprofen	57.0
Naproxen	52.8
Fenoprofen	47.1

Source: FDA Arthritis Advisory Committee, 1985 (ref. 8)
* Percent of ADR cases reported

H. GI effects

The undesirable effects of NSAIDs most often involve the GI tract. Patients on anti-inflammatory drugs have a high incidence of gastric lesions (Table 9). GI complaints centre around dyspepsia, nausea, diarrhoea, constipation, abdominal pain and stomatitis. Diffuse gastritis may occur, with a slow but steady loss of small volumes of blood, leading to chronic iron deficiency anaemia[84], a condition worsened by alcohol and coffee intake, as well as by hypovitaminosis C. Gastrointestinal microbleeding occurs even in healthy normal males[85]. The gastric mucosa is affected even by pro-drugs (sulindac, fenbufen) since their prostaglandin-inhibiting effect is systemic and not local. Large ulcers can occur. One-third of ulcers in treated RA patients are gastric versus only 5% in the general population. Clearly, non-steroidals are a significant cause of gastric lesions[86]. Haemorrhage can occur, which can be life-threatening. The danger is most acute when the NSAIDs antiplatelet effects are combined with pre-existing coagulation defects and a high frequency of erosive gastritis[87]. There may also be an association between complicated lower bowel disease and NSAIDs[88,89] and unmasking of idiopathic inflammatory bowel disease[90,91] which is fairly frequent among elderly[92]. Gastric injury is particularly dangerous in the elderly as there is often no relation between subjective symptoms and endoscopic findings[93]. Clearly, there is a significant association between UGI pathology and NSAID ingestion[94], the NSAIDs causing gastric lesions in more than 20% of patients on a single drug[95], an incidence that rises sharply when two analgesics are given concomittantly[16]. Moreover, the elderly are at increased risk to these side-effects[96,97]. NSAID consumption by old patients places them at considerable risk of upper GI bleeding in which old age is an important adverse prognostic factor.

Table 10 The aging stomach

Change	Consequences
Primary aging	
Decreased mucosal thickness mucosal blood flow	Devitalization of mucosa, atrophic gastritis, greater risk for ulcers
Delayed gastric emptying	Longer residence time for erosive agents
Reduced gastric secretion	Increased incidence of ulcers Less rapidly repaired Less resistance to injury
Secondary aging	
Intercurrent diseases and drug use	Greater risk to injury
Behavioural changes	Increased incidence of GI complaints

Vulnerability to GI problems increases with age. Devitalization of the gastric mucosa and less resiliency increase the risk of GI injury and prolong healing time. Increased vulnerability is due to morphological and secretory changes with age, increased GI pathology with age and multiple drug therapy (Table 10). After age 50, about 80% of stomachs show muscular atrophy, thinning of gastric mucosa, and infiltration of the submucosa with elastic fibres[98]. In addition to this age-related factor, atrophy and dedifferentiation result from cumulation of the effects of repeated superficial injury and repair. There is an elevation of both cell destruction and renewal, but, histologically, atrophy will result[99]. Intestinal blood flow may be reduced by as much as 50% by age 65, further diminished by stress, CHF, hypoxia and hypovolaemia[21]. This can result in ischaemia and subsequent arterial occlusion. Blood flow in the gastric mucosa is also reduced by inhibitors of prostaglandin synthesis, and damage can occur in relatively ischaemic areas[100,101]. Perhaps that is the reason why bioflavonoids, such as mecladanol, protect against GI bleeding, since they maintain vascular integrity and protect gastric mucosal blood flow[102,103]. With advancing age, there is a decrease in gastric cell function and an elevation of gastric pH[104], the secretory volume declining by as much as 50%[105]. Age-associated diseases such as diabetes mellitus, untreated hyperthyroidism and hypothyroidism may further decrease gastric secretion[106]. Age-associated decrease in gastric emptying[107] which is further depressed by diseases and drugs, as well as nutritional changes, mandates longer residency time of these drugs, and therefore, higher risk.

Importantly, 31% of the GI complaints of the elderly are behaviourally-induced[92], by stress due to fear of death and disease, anxiety, depressive illness and worry, all of which influence stomach motility and secretory function. Thus, Rainsford's work in stressed rats and proposed experimental ulcerogenic index has important relevance in predicting ulcerogenic activity of NSAIDs in the elderly (Table 11)[108-110].

Table 11 An experimental ulcerogenic index for non-steroidals: anti-inflammatory vs ulcerogenic activity$^+$

Drug	AI dose (mg/kg)	Ulcerogenic dose (mg/kg)	u.I.*
Sulindac	5.6	70.5	0.08
Fenbufen	50	165	0.30
Indomethacin	2.8	2.7	1.03
Naproxen	4.5	1.6	2.81
Piroxicam	4.5	0.10	45

$^+$ Source: Rainsford, KD: Br J Pharmacol 1981; 73, 226P-7P

* Ulcer index = AI dose/ulcerogenic dose. The smaller the number, the safer the drug

The cumulative effects of all of these changes are associated with an increased incidence of gastritis and gastric ulcers[111]. Symptoms may be either absent or non-specific. About one-third of duodenal ulcer patients are 60 years and older and up to 20% of those 70 to 79 years suffer from chronic peptic ulcer[112]. Ulcer disease is more virulent in the elderly and has a higher mortality rate than in the young[113]. Bleeding is a fairly common complication of ulcers in the elderly. Fifteen to 20% of GI bleeding in the elderly is caused by acute ulcers or erosions[114]. Complications rise from 31% for those 60 to 64 to 76% for those 70 to 79 years old. Re-bleeding may occur in up to 40% of patients. Mortality reaches 25% in those 80 years and older[92].

Table 12 Drugs that can cause gastric erosion

Alcohol	Chemotherapeutics
Anticoagulants	Corticosteroids
Antimalarials	Non-steroidals
Antimetabolites	Potassium suppl.
Aspirin	Reserpine
Ascorbic acid	

Table 13 Adverse UGI reports and NSAIDs

Drug	Perforation/bleeding/ulcer per million R_x Non-fatal	Fatal
Piroxicam	20.60	0.90
Diflunisal	8.62	0.96
Phenylbutazone	5.34	0.53
Sulindac	3.77	0.17
Indomethacin	3.58	0.23
Meclofenamate	2.61	0.15
Naproxen	2.10	0.14
Tolmetin	1.36	0.08
Fenoprofen	1.29	0.05
Ibuprofen	0.85	0.06

Source: FDA Arthritis Advisory Committee 1985 (ref. 8)

All non-steroidals can cause gastritis for which the elderly, taking a host of drugs with erosive capabilities (Table 12) are at great risk. Gastric haemorrhage from superficial lesions is the most life-threatening ADR of the non-steroidals, but peptic ulceration and perforation also occur[93]. The majority of NSAID-induced ulcers occur in elderly women, in whom it is a significant problem. Those on concurrent diuretic therapy are most likely to develop a giant ulcer and need a blood transfusion[115]. Non-steroidals account for about one-third of all ADRs reported to the UK Committee on Safety of Medicines[116]. It is important to realize that the ulcerogenic activity of the non-steroidals in the elderly varies greatly (Table 13). Apparently, piroxicam is the most gastrotoxic drug, a problem recognized by several reports[117-120].

The evidence is strong that the elderly are at great risk to NSAID-induced GI problems because of advanced age, secondary age changes, and concomittant drug therapy.

VI. CONCLUSIONS

Hazard identification

NSAIDs pose a hazard to elderly patients by causing bronchospasm in aspirin-sensitive patients, by inducing haematological, CNS, and cutaneous disorders, by activation and masking of infections, by their hepatotoxicity, and via their renal and GI effects. All of these have been validated, affecting patients of all ages.

Hazard evaluation

Some hazards have been identified as potentially fatal: asthma, haematological disorders, cutaneous reactions, renal effect, GI effects. CNS effects can be devastating in terms of quality of life and independent living.

Risk evaluation

Elderly are at heightened risk to these hazards of NSAIDS:

All hazards: Increased level of exposure, often for problems where NSAID is not indicated.

Bronchospasm: Aspirin sensitivity increases with age. Mortality among elderly asthmatics is increasing sharply.

Haematological disorders: Elderly seem to be at particular risk. Although not proven, haematological review for elderly receiving an NSAID is mandatory.

CNS effects: Memory loss, inability to concentrate, confusion, and personality changes may be frequent, but unrecognized. May be due to primary age changes, multiple pathology and polymedicine.

Cutaneous reaction: Increased risk to elderly not demonstrated, although two fatalities reported were elderly.

Activation and masking of infection: Elderly are at risk, but not due to primary age changes.

Hepatotoxicity: Elderly may be at risk because of gender factor, a certain non-recognition factor, intake of other hepatotoxic drugs.

Renal effects: Elderly at definitely heightened risk because of primary and secondary age changes, multiple drug use, possible drug interactions. Home care patients at heightened risk.

GI effects: Elderly at a definite increased risk, due to primary and secondary age changes, gender factor, multiple drug use.

REFERENCES

1. Chamberlain, MA, Buchanan, JM and Hanks, H (1979). The arthritic in an urban environment. Ann Rheum Dis, 38, 51-6
2. Kraag, GR (1985). Rare toxicity with nonsteroidal anti-inflammatory drugs. J Rheumatol, 12, 1-3
3. Ehrlich, GE (1982). Diagnosis and management of rheumatic diseases in older patients. J Am Geriatr Soc, 30, 45-51
4. Meenan, RF, Goldenberg, DL, Murrman, MK and Cohen, AS (1982). An evaluation strategy for rheumatology education. Arthritis Rheum, 25, 92-7
5. Lavsky-Shulan, M, Wallace, RB and Kohout, FJ et al. (1985). Prevalence and functional correlates of low back pain in the elderly: the Iowa 65+ Rural Health Study. J Am Geriatr Soc, 33, 23-8
6. Nuki, G and Burley, L (1984). Nonsteroidal analgesic anti-inflammatory drugs in the elderly. In: Butler, RN and Bearn, AG (eds), The Aging Process: Therapeutic Implications, pp. 207-26. (New York: Raven Press)
7. Mowat, AG (1979). Drug treatment of arthritis in the elderly. Age Ageing, 8 (Suppl.), 14-25
8. Hersey, DF and Weisman, MH (1985). Minutes (19th Meeting) FDA Arthritis Advisory Committee, Washington DC. Food and Drug Administration (June), 1-22
9. Gall, EP (1982). Analgesic and anti-inflammatory agents. In: Conrad, KA and Bressler, R (eds), Drug Therapy for the Elderly, 225-54. (St. Louis: CV Mosby)
10. Dick, WC and De Ceulaer, K (1981). Nonsteroidal antirheumatic drugs. In: Kelley, WN, Harris, ED Jr, Ruddy, S and Sledge, CB (eds), Textbook of Rheumatology, 768-84. (Philadelphia: WB Saunders)
11. Calin, A (1984). Clinical and pharmacological considerations in the use of nonsteroidal anti-inflammatory drugs in the elderly. Geriatr Med Today, 3 (7), 77-84
12. Ziminski, CM (1985). Treating joint inflammation in the elderly: an update. Geriatrics, 40 (1), 73-88
13. Innes, EH (1977). Efficacy and tolerance of flurbiprofen in the elderly using liquid and tablet formulations. Curr Med Res Opin, 5, 122-6
14. Patmas, MA, Wilborn, SL and Shankel, SW (1984). Acute multisystem toxicity associated with the use of nonsteroidal anti-inflammatory drugs. Arch Intern Med, 144, 519-20
15. Svihovec, J (1980). Anti-inflammatory analgesics and drugs used in gout. In: Dukes, MNG (ed.), Meyler's Side Effects of Drugs, 141-61. (Amsterdam: Excerpta Medica)
16. Del Favero, A (1981). Anti-inflammatory analgesics and drugs used in rheumatism and gout. In: Dukes, MNG, and Elis, J (eds), Side Effects of Drugs Annual 5, 88-117. (Princeton: Excerpta Medica)
17. Anon (1983). Toxicity of nonsteroidal anti-inflammatory drugs. Med Letter, 25, 15-6
18. Nuki, G (1983). Non-steroidal analgesics and anti-inflammatory agents. Br Med J, 287, 39-43

19. O'Brien, WM and Bagby, GF (1985). Rare adverse reactions to non-steroidal anti-inflammatory drugs. J Rheumatol, 12 (1), 13-20

20. Clive, DM and Stoff, JS (1985). Nonsteroidal anti-inflammatory drugs and the kidney. Resident Staff Phys, 31 (5), 5PC-10PC

21. Lamy, PP (1980). Prescribing for the Elderly, 249-92. (Littleton MA: John Wright-PSG)

22. Lamy, PP (1983). Drug prescribing for the elderly. In: Reichel, W (ed.), Clinical Aspects of Aging, 21-71. (Baltimore MD: Williams & Wilkins)

23. Lamy, PP (1981). Drug prescribing for the elderly. Bull NY Acad Med, 57 (8), 718-30

24. Lamy, PP (1984). Modifying drug dosage in elderly patients. In: Covington, TR and Walker, JI (eds), Current Geriatric Therapy, 35-72. (Philadelphia: WB Saunders)

25. Polgar, P and Taylor, L (1980). Alterations in prostaglandin synthesis during senescence of human lung fibroblasts. Mech Ageing Dev, 12, 305-10

26. Miehlke, K (1979). Symptomatic antirheumatic problems with the older patient: drug interactions. Rheumatol Rehab, 18 (Suppl. 1), 104-8

27. Antilla, M, Haataja, M and Kasanan, A (1980). Pharmacokinetics of naproxen in subjects with normal and impaired renal function. Eur J Clin Pharm, 18, 263-8

28. Upton, RA, Williams, RL, Kelly, J and Jones, RM (1984). Naproxen pharmacokinetics in the elderly. Br J Clin Pharm, 18, 207-14

29. Lamy, PP (1983). The elderly, undernutrition, and pharmacokinetics. J Am Geriatr Soc, 31, 560-2

30. Richardson, CJ, Blocka, KLN, Ross, SG and Verbeek, RK (1985). Effects of age and sex on piroxicam disposition. Clin Pharmacol Ther, 37, 13-18

31. Deisler, PF Jnr (1983). Science, regulations and the safe handling of chemicals. Reg Toxicol Pharmacol, 3, 60-70

32. Lasagna, L (1985). Techniques for ADR reporting. RS 8583. (Boston: Tufts University)

33. Rossi, AC and Knapp, DE (1982). Tolmetin-induced anaphylactoid reactions. New Engl J Med, 307, 499-500

34. Weber, JCP (1984). Epidemiology of adverse reactions to non-steroidal antiinflammatory drugs. In: Rainsford, KD and Velo, GP (eds), Advances in Inflammation Research, 1-7. (New York: Raven Press)

35. Deyo, RA, Inui, TS and Sullivan, B (1981). Non-compliance with arthritis drugs: magnitude, correlates, and clinical implications. J Rheumatol, 8, 931-6

36. Lisberg, RB, Higham, C and Jayson, MI (1983). Problems for rheumatic patients in opening dispensed drug containers. Br J Rheumatol, 22, 95-8

37. Anon (1985). Noncompliance with NSAID therapy is rampant. Drug Topics, 129 (10), 74-5

38. Lamy, PP (1984). OTC Ibuprofen and the elderly. Maryland Pharm, 60 (8), 22-3

39. Anon (1984). Medication for the elderly. A report of the Royal College of Physicians. J R Coll Physicians (London), 18 (1), 7-17

40. Fisherman, EW and Cohen, GN (1978). Hypersensitivity to five non-steroidal antiinflammatory agents: ibuprofen, fenoprofen, indomethacin, naproxen and tolmetin. Ann Allergy, 41, 75-7

41. Szczeklik, A (1983). Anti-cyclo-oxygenase agents and asthma. J Asthma, 20 (S-1), 23-9

42. Falliers, CJ (1983). Acetaminophen and aspirin challenges in sub-groups of asthmatics. J Asthma, 20 (S-1), 39-49

43. Settipane, GA and Chafee, FH (1977). Nasal polyps in asthma and rhinitis.

J Allergy Clin Immunol, 59, 17-22

44. Szczeklik, A, Gryglewski, RJ and Czerniawska-Mysik, G (1975). Relationship of inhibition of prostaglandin biosynthesis by analgesics to asthma attacks in aspirin-sensitive patients. Br Med J, 1, 67-9
45. Bardana, EJ Jr and Andrash, RH (1983). Reviewing bronchial astham and its pharmacotherapy. Geriatrics, 38, 73-95
46. Anon (1985). US asthma mortality rising. Med World News, 26 (11), 68
47. Guthbert, MD (1974). Adverse reactions to nonsteroidal anti-rheumatic drugs. Curr Med Res Opin, 2, 600-10
48. Romeril, KR, Duke, DS and Hollings, PE (1981). Sulindac-induced agranulocytosis on bone marrow culture. Lancet, 2, 523
49. Rosenbaum, JT and O'Connor, M (1981). Thrombocytopenia associated with sulindac. Arthritis Rheum, 753-4
50. Stambaugh, JE, Bordon, RL and Geller, R (1980). Leucopenia and thrombocytopenia secondary to clinoril therapy. Lancet, 2, 594
51. Lee, SH, Fawcett, V and Preece, JM (1982). Aplastic anaemia associated with piroxicam. Lancet, 1, 1186
52. Miller, JL (1980). Marrow aplasia and sulindac. Ann Intern Med, 92, 129
53. Bennett, L, Schlossman, R and Rosenthal, J et al. (1980). Aplastic anemia and sulindac. Ann Intern Med, 92-874
54. Morris, EL, Hochberg, MC and Dorsch, CA (1981). Agranulocytosis and sulindac. Arthritis Rheum, 24, 752-3
55. Burns, A and Young, RE (1984). Mefenamic acid induced leucopenia in the elderly. Lancet, 2, 46
56. Lipowski, ZJ (1983). Transient cognitive disorders (delirium, acute confusional states) in the elderly. Am J Psychiatry, 14, 1426-36
57. Erman, MK and Guggenheim, FG (1981). Psychiatric side effects of commonly used drugs. Drug Ther, 11, 117-9, 123-6
58. Goodwin, JS and Regan, M (1982). Cognitive dysfunction associated with naproxen and ibuprofen in the elderly. Arthritis Rheum, 25, 1013-5
59. Stern, RS and Bigby, M (1984). An expanded profile of cutaneous reactions to nonsteroidal anti-inflammatory drugs. J Am Med Assoc, 252, 1433-7
60. Kochevar, IE, Lamm, JK and McAuliffe, DJ et al. (1985). Antiphlogistics: mechanism of piroxicam-induced photosensitivity. Clin Res, 33, 656A
61. Brennan, M (1980). Activation of latent tuberculosis by non-steroidal anti-inflammatory agents. Can Med Assoc J, 122, 400-1
62. Tomasson, HO, Brennan, M and Bass, MJ (1984). Tuberculosis and non-steroidal anti-inflammatory drugs. Can Med Assoc J, 120, 275-8
63. Lewis, JH (1984). Hepatic toxicity of nonsteroidal anti-inflammatory drugs. Clin Pharm, 3, 128-38
64. Weinblatt, ME, Tesser, JRP and Gilliam, JH III (1982). The liver in rheumatic diseases. Sem Arthrit Rheum, 11, 399-405
65. Mills, PR and Sturrock, RD (1982). Clinical associations between arthritis and liver disease. Ann Rheumatic Dis, 41, 292-307
66. Zimmerman, HJ (1984). Drug-induced liver disease. In: Bayless, TM (ed.), Current Therapy in Gastroenterology and Liver Disease, 424-30. (Philadelphia: BC Decker)
67. Babany, G and Pessayre, D (1984). Hepatites dues aux nouveaux anti-inflammatoires non steroidens. Gastroenterol Clin Biol, 8, 523-9
68. Ciabattoni, GC, Cinotti, GA and Pierucci, A et al. (1984). Effects of sulindac and ibuprofen in patients with chronic glomerular disease. New Engl J Med, 310, 279-83
69. Dunn, MJ, Scharschmidt, L and Zambraski, E (1984). Mechanism of nephrotoxicity of non-steroidal anti-inflammatory drugs.

Arch Toxicol, (Suppl. 7), 328-37

70. Cove-Smith, JR (1981). Analgesic nephropathy in the United Kingdom: incidence, clinical features and pathogenesis. J Clin Pathol, 1255-60
71. Torres, VE (1982). Present and future of nonsteroidal anti-inflammatory drugs in nephrology. Mayo Clin Proc, 57, 389-93
72. Meier, DE, Myers, WM, Swenson, R and Bennet, WM (1983). Indomethacin-associated hyperkalemia in the elderly. J Am Geriatr Soc, 31, 371-3
73. Lamy, PP (1984). Patterns of prescribing and drug use. In: Butler, RN and Bearns, AG (eds), The Aging Process: Therapeutic Implications, 53-82. (New York: Raven Press)
74. Clive, DM and Stoff, JS (1984). Renal syndromes associated with nonsteroidal antiinflammatory drugs. New Engl J Med, 310, 563-72
75. Robertson, CE, Ford, MJ and Van Someren, V et al. (1980). Mefenamic acid nephropathy. Lancet, 2, 232-3
76. Harter, HR and Martin, KJ (1982). Acute renal failure. 1. Classification, evaluation and clinical consequences. Postgrad Med, 72 (6), 47-53
77. Harter, HR and Martin, KJ (1982). Acute renal failure. 2. Pathophysiology, prevention, management and prognosis. Postgrad Med, 72 (6), 54-62
78. Garella, S and Matarese, RA (1984). Renal effects of prostaglandins and clinical adverse effects of nonsteroidal anti-inflammatory agents. Medicine, 63 (3), 165-81
79. Stillman, MT, Napier, J and Blackshear, JL (1984). Adverse effects of nonsteroidal anti-inflammatory drugs on the kidneys. Med Clin North Am, 68, 371-85
80. Dunn, MF and Zambraski, EJ (1980). Renal effects of drugs that inhibit prostaglandin synthesis. Kidney Int, 18, 609-22
81. Ward, JR (1984). Update on ibuprofen for rheumatoid arthritis. Am J Med, 77, (1A), 3-9
82. Blackshear, JL, Davidman, M and Stillman, MT (1983). Identification of risk for renal insufficiency from non-steroidal anti-inflammatory drugs. Arch Intern Med, 43, 1130-4
83. Stewart, RB, Hale, WE and Marks, RS (1982). Effects of nonsteroidal anti-inflammatory drugs on renal function in the elderly. South Med J, 75, 824-6
84. O'Brien, WM (1983). Pharmacology on nonsteroidal anti-inflammatory drugs. Am J Med, 76, 32-9
85. Salom, IL, Jacob, G and Jallad, N et al. (1984). Gastrointestinal microbleeding associated with the use of etodolac, ibuprofen, indomethacin, and naproxen in normal males. J Clin Pharmacol, 24, 240-6
86. Sun, DC, Roth, SH and Mitchell, CS (1974). Upper gastrointestinal disease in rheumatoid arthritis. Am J Dig Dis, 19, 405-10
87. O'Reilly, RA (1980). Anticoagulant, antithrombotic, and thrombolytic drugs. In: Gilman, AG, Goodman, LS and Gilman, A (eds), The Pharmacologic Basis of Therapeutics VI, 1347-66. (New York: Macmillan)
88. Langman, MJS, Morgan, L and Worral, A (1985). Use of anti-inflammatory drugs by patients admitted with a small or large bowel perforation and haemorrhage. Br Med J, 290, 347-9
89. Schwartz, HA (1981). Lower gastrointestinal side effects of non-steroidal anti-inflammatory drugs. J Rheumatol, 8, 952-4
90. Hall, RI, Petty, AH, Cobden, I and Lendrum, R (1984). Enteritis and colitis associated with mefenamic acid. Br Med J, 287-1182
91. Rampton, DS and Sladen, GE (1981). Relapse of ulcerative proctocolitis during treatment with non-steroidal anti-inflammatory drugs. Postgrad Med, 57, 297-9
92. Sklar, M (1983). Gastrointestinal diseases in the elderly. In: Reichel, W

(ed.), Clinical Aspects of Aging, 205-17. (Baltimore MD: Williams & Wilkins)

93. Lanza, FL (1984). Endoscopic studies of gastric and duodenal injury after the use of ibuprofen, aspirin, and other non-steroidal anti-inflammatory agents. Am J Med, 77 (1A), 19-24

94. Clinch, D, Banerjee, AK, Ostick, G and Levy, DW (1983). Nonsteroidal anti-inflammatory drugs and gastro-intestinal adverse effects. J R Coll Phys, 17, 228-30

95. Caruso, I and Bianchi, PG (1980). Gastroscopic evaluation of anti-inflammatory agents. Br J Med, 1, 75-8

96. Antler, AS, Pitchumoni, CS and Thomas, E et al. (1981). Gastrointestinal bleeding in the elderly. Am J Surg, 142, 271-3

97. Caradoc-Davies, TH (1984). Nonsteroidal anti-inflammatory drugs, arthritis, and gastrointestinal bleeding in elderly patients. Age Ageing, 13, 295-8

98. Schuster, MM (1978). Disorders of the ageing GI system. In: Reichel, W (ed.), The Geriatric Patient, 73-81. (New York: HP Publ Co)

99. Almy, TP (1981). Factors leading to digestive disorders in the elderly, 57, Bull NY Acad Med, 57, 709-17

100. Simon, LS and Mills, JA (1980). Nonsteroidal antiinflammatory drugs. Part I. New Engl J Med, 302, 1179-85

101. Simon, LS and Mills, JA (1980). Nonsteroidal antiinflammatory drugs. Part II. New Engl J Med, 302, 1237-43

102. Konturek, SJ, Kitler, ME, Kwiecien, N, Obtulowicz, B, Olesky, J and Kopp, B (1984). Effect of meciadanol on gastric secretion and aspirin-induced gastric mucosal injury in humans. Scand J Gastroenterol, 19, 1099-1103

103. Jayaraj, AP, Kitler, ME and Tovey, FI et al. (1984). The protective effect of a new histidine decarboxylase inhibitor (meciadanol, Zy 15029) on experimental ulceration and on mast cell degranulation in several rat models. Internatl Congr Gastroenterology. Lisbon, Portugal, Abstract 587

104. Geokas, MD and Haverback, BJ (1969). The aging gastrointestinal tract. Am J Surg, 117, 881-92

105. Krentz, K and Jablonowski, H (1984). Functional and histological gastric changes with age. In: Hellemans, J and Vantrappen, G (eds), Gastrointestinal Tract Disorders in the Elderly, 62-9. (New York: Churchill Livingstone)

106. Holt, PR (1985). Age related changes in the gut. Geriatr Med Today, 4 (2), 44-53

107. Evans, MH, Triggs, EJ and Cheons, M et al. (1981). Gastric emptying in the elderly: implications for drug therapy. J Am Geriatr Soc, 29, 201-5

108. Rainsford, KD (1977). Aspirin and gastric ulceration: light and electron microscopic observations in a model of aspirin plus stress-induced ulceration. Br J Exp Pathol, 58, 215-9

109. Rainsford, KD (1978). The role of aspirin in gastric ulceration: some factors involved in the development of gastric mucosal damage induced in rats exposed to various stress conditions. Dig Dis, 23, 521-30

110. Rainsford, KD (1981). Comparison of the gastric ulcerogenic activity of new non-steroid anti-inflammatory drugs in stressed rats. Br J Pharmacol, 73, 226P-7P

111. Baron, JH (1970). The clinical use of gastric function tests. Scand J Gastroenterol, 6 (Suppl.), 9-46

112. Permutt, KP and Cello, JP (1982). Duodenal ulcer disease in the hospitalized elderly patient. Dig Dis Sci, 27 (1), 1-6

113. Narayanan, M and Steinheber, FU (1976). The changing face of peptic ulcer in the elderly. Med Clin North Am, 69, 1159-72

114. Schiller, KF, Truelove, SC and Williams, DG (1970). Haematemesis and melaena with special reference to factors influencing the outcome. Br Med J, 2, 7-14
115. Cooke, P and Thompson, MR (1981). Old ladies, drugs, and gastric ulceration. Gut, 22, A430
116. Rogers, JD (1983). Biopharmaceutical evaluation of "Osmosin". Curr Med Res Opin, 8 (Suppl 2.), 38-54
117. Emery, P and Grahame, R (1982). Gastrointestinal blood loss and piroxicam. Lancet, 11, 1302-3
118. Pisko, EJ, Rahman, MA, Turner, RA and Agudelo, CA (1980). Long-term efficacy and safety of piroxicam in the treatment of rheumatoid arthritis. Curr Ther Res, 27, 852-9
119. Semble, E, Metcalf, D and Turner, R (1980). Genetic predictors of patient response and side effects in the treatment of rheumatoid arthritis. Curr Ther Res, 27, 852-9
120. Ward, K and Weir, DG (1982). Piroxicam and upper gastrointestinal hemorrhage. Ir Med J, 75, 10-11

Discussion

Dr SM Doherty, UK: Could you expand a little on the association of non-steroidals with non-skin tuberculosis. In what organs was this evident and how?

Professor Lamy: This was published in Canada where they have seen patients in which old TB was reactivated. It was not normal TB. It was old TB that was reactivated by the use of NSAIDs, and I think they have 5 or 6 patients by now.

Dr Doherty: Are you not able to quote the drugs involved?

Professor Lamy: No I can't, but I will tell you afterwards from my papers which I have here.

13
Ibuprofen overdose - the first year following over-the-counter release*

S Perry, P Streete and GN Volans
Poisons Unit,
New Cross Hospital,
London SE14,
UK

CONTENTS

I. MONITORING OF IBUPROFEN OVERDOSE

The National Poisons Information Service (NPIS) has been monitoring overdose with NSAIDs since 1980. On the basis of the results to date it has been reported that most of these drugs appear safer in overdose than do aspirin or paracetamol[1]. Ibuprofen, however, is the only member of the group where sufficient data have been collected to substantiate this claim.

The results of this study support the decision to grant a licence for over-the-counter (OTC) sales of ibuprofen, but since analgesic poisoning largely involves OTC products[2], a marked increase in the incidence of ibuprofen overdose was expected once that drug became available without prescription.

*This is an summary of a poster presentation

Side-effects of Anti-inflammatory Drugs. Rainsford, KD and Velo, GP (eds)
Part 1: Clinical and Epidemiological Aspects. (Lancaster: MTP Press)

II. METHODS

Details are collected of all telephone enquiries related to suspected buprofen overdose, and outcome assessment is made by sending out a specially designed questionnaire for each case. Blood and urine samples are requested at the time of the telephone enquiry. At the point where OTC sales began, the follow-up questionnaire was modified to facilitate computer input of data and to determine certain additional features about the products ingested and their sources. The covering letter was also changed to draw attention to the OTC release of the drug and the importance of continued monitoring.

III. RESULTS

During the 12-month period immediately following the launch of OTC ibuprofen at the end of August 1983, the NPIS saw a dramatic rise in enquiries about the drug. This amounted to a 169% increase on the figure for the period August 1982 to September 1983. The rise was not entirely due to the easier availability of the drug, and it is thought that other possible factors were increased interest in the problem, and also an increased overall number of enquiries.

So far the increased incidence of overdose has not been associated with any increase in severity of poisoning. Many patients remained asymptomatic (64%) even after quite substantial overdoses. Symptomatic patients typically exhibited mild gastrointestinal and CNS disturbances. More severe problems were rare, and usually occurred when the case had been complicated by the ingestion of other drugs.

IV. CONCLUSIONS

Although these results show an encouraging trend towards lower toxicity from analgesic overdoses, continued monitoring is necessary. This project is planned to continue for several years and up-to-date results will be presented here.

REFERENCES

1. Court, H and Volans, GN (1984). Drug React. Ac. Pois. Rev. 3, 1
2. The National Poisons Information Service Monitoring Group (1981). Human Toxicol, 1, 7

Discussion

Anonymous: What is the dose of Brufen taken in poisonings with the over counter preparations as opposed to those prescribed?

Dr Perry: I don't think it's really possible to tell. I think generally we don't see very large overdoses of ibuprofen in reports from either the over the counter product or from prescriptions only.

Dr A Herxheimer, UK: How near can you get? Can we have some semi-quantitative answer

Dr Perry: Well I can give you an estimate, and I would say that with the over the counter products the packaging does tend to mean there are fewer tablets, but I don't honestly think there is that much difference.

Prof. PF D'Arcy, UK: The whole object of over the counter medicines is to sell them in much smaller packs and I think in the normal pack of Brufen in Britain there are 25. Now if you say the average number is 36 it means they are buying more than one packet at a time and this is probably intentional and not accidental if they would take 36. Is that right?

Dr Perry: We don't really go into circumstances behind the overdose because we don't really have the facilities to be able to do that.

Prof. D'Arcy: If that is so, it would be rather going against the ideal of selling packs of 25. If people are going to buy multiple packs of 25 that's doing away with the safeguard of selling small packs.

Dr Rainsford: Going back to the point made by Dr Herxheimer, you actually state in your abstract that you have obtained blood and urine samples. You should be able to do some drug assays and estimate of toxic levels of the drug and from nomograms estimate the amount which was ingested.

Dr Perry: Yes, I don't think at this point in time we actually have enough samples available to do that and hopefully in the future we will be able to do so. But at the moment we do experience difficulty in getting samples, because I think a large number of patients who come into hospital with ibuprofen overdoses don't really become particularly ill and are quite often discharged from casualty. So doctors just don't bother to take the samples whereas if the patients were more severly ill they might, and also we have problems with accurate timing of collection of the samples. This is another factor.

Dr M Geldman, UK: Judging by your average overdose number that would be quite an expensive overdose to take over the counter, if you look at the pricing policy. You are probably talking about £UK 10 in an overdose. I think probably people would stick to something cheaper like paracetamol or alcohol.

SECTION II

DRUG INTERACTIONS AND DRUG METABOLISM

14
Drug interactions between the anti-inflammatory drugs and with other agents

PF D'Arcy and JC McElnay
Department of Pharmacy,
The Queen's University of Belfast,
Northern Ireland,
UK

CONTENTS

I. INTRODUCTION

Although drug interactions have often been over-estimated and over-stated there still remains a spectrum of clinically relevant interactions involving drugs that are in common use. The anti-inflammatory analgesic drugs are no exception to such occurrence. This is not unexpected because of the wide use of these drugs in the community. For example, latest figures available in Great

Side-effects of Anti-inflammatory Drugs. Rainsford, KD and Velo, GP (eds)
Part 1: Clinical and Epidemiological Aspects. (Lancaster: MTP Press)

Britain[1] show that some 19 million prescriptions for anti-inflammatory agents are issued each year by family practitioners. These represent some 5% of all drugs prescribed, and over the past 10 years they have consistently ranked between 7 and 9 in the list of most frequently prescribed groups of preparations.

The problem of drug interactions arises because many patients, particularly the elderly, receive more than one drug at the same time. This, however, is often necessary in treatment since a patient may suffer from more than one disease or have different symptoms of a single disease which require separate and different treatments.

Interactions involving non-steroidal anti-inflammatory drugs (NSAIDs) can take place by different mechanisms, and an understanding of these interactions can best be approached by considering the mechanisms and the sites at which the interactions take place.

II. SITES AND MECHANISMS OF DRUG INTERACTIONS

All drug interactions can be divided into three major categories:

(a) pharmacokinetic interactions in which one drug changes the pharmacokinetic profile of another drug;

(b) pharmacodynamic interactions in which two drugs interact giving summation, potentiation or antagonism of their pharmacological (and toxicological) effects;

(c) miscellaneous drug interactions that do not fit well into either of the former two categories (e.g. drugs causing interference with diagnostic laboratory tests).

III. PHARMACOKINETIC INTERACTIONS

There are four types and sites of drug interactions that relate to the majority of interactions involving NSAIDs:

A. Drug absorption interactions

Drug interactions in the gastrointestinal tract can occur for a variety of reasons. Changes in gastric pH will lead to changes both the rate of drug dissolution and the rate of drug absorption. The effects of pH and pK_a (dissociation constant) have been discussed elsewhere by McElnay and D'Arcy[2].

Antacids influence both gastrointestinal pH and its motility, and by doing so can influence the effects of co-administered drugs. For example, an aluminium/magnesium mixture decreases the bioavailability of indomethacin[3], while magnesium trisilicate and kaolin decrease the bioavailability of chloroquine when it is used in an anti-inflammatory role[4] (Figure 1)

Foodstuffs also sometimes enter into interactions with drugs, and they commonly decrease gastric emptying rate. This can result in a reduced rate of drug absorption. This type of interaction, however, has little relevance in the use of NSAIDs which, because of their gastrointestinal irritant effects, are best taken after food.

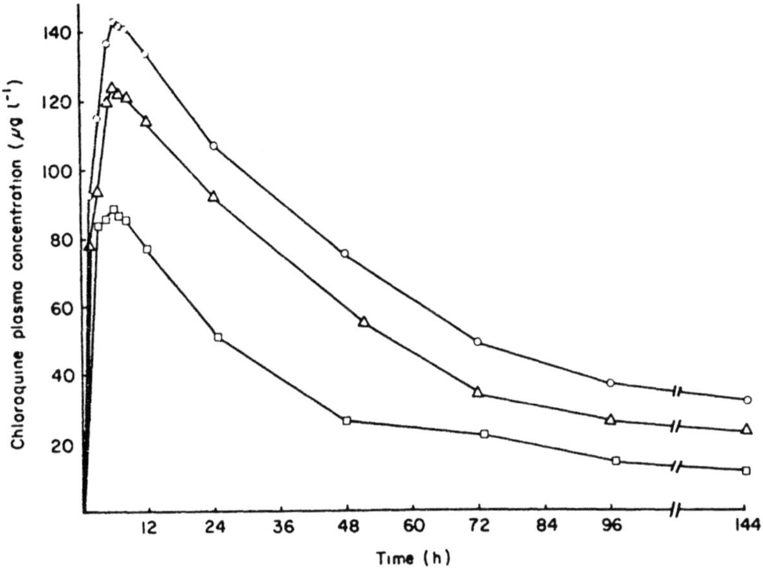

Figure 1 The effect of magnesium trisilicate (triangles) and kaolin (squares) on the absorption of chloroquine in a single dose study (600 mg chloroquine base, by mouth) compared with the control period (circles) (chloroquine alone) in one healthy volunteer (From McElnay et al.[4]).

B. Interactions at plasma and tissue protein binding sites

The binding of drugs to protein is an important pharmacokinetic parameter. Although much emphasis has been placed on the binding of drugs in the plasma, binding also takes place in the tissues[5,6]. The distribution of drugs between plasma and tissues can be represented diagrammatically (Figure 2). Once distribution of a drug is complete, the drug concentration throughout the extracellular water will equal that of the serum water (i.e. free concentration in the serum). Only free drug is therapeutically active, and the therapeutic response will depend on the percentage of drug unbound. Many of the NSAIDs are highly bound to plasma (e.g. phenylbutazone is 90-98% bound). At higher plasma concentrations of drug the protein binding declines because of saturation of binding sites[7]. Drugs often compete for plasma binding sites (a type of molecular "musical chairs"), thus altering the ratios of free and bound drugs in the plasma; in this respect the most important displacing agents at plasma albumin binding sites are acidic compounds[8].

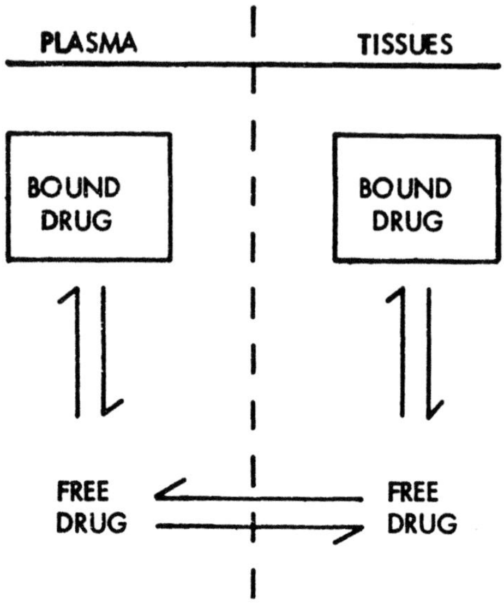

Figure 2 Distribution of drug between plasma and tissue compartments. Free drug alone can diffuse out of the plasma, and free drug in plasma and tissues is of equal concentration. Bound drug concentration, however, will depend on the amount of binding materials present in both plasma and tissues, and the affinity of the drug for the binding sites on these materials (redrawn from Tillement et al.[9]).

When a displacing agent is added to a primary drug regimen there is an increase in the free concentration of the displaced drug in the plasma. It is often falsely assumed, however, that the free drug concentrations will remain raised; this is not so. What in fact occurs is that the increased free drug in the plasma quickly distributes throughout the body and may localize in tissues[9] (see Figure 2). When equilibrium is again reached, assuming the volume into which the drug distributes is large, the free concentration in the plasma will be the same as, or near to, its pre-interaction level. After this redistribution, however, the percentage of free drug in the plasma will increase, as also will the free fraction of drug in the plasma and the drug's apparent volume of distribution. All these increased values are due to the decreased "total" drug concentration in the plasma after the new equilibrium is reached. Any increased pharmacological effect seen after displacement is therefore usually of a transient nature and, in most cases, is clinically unimportant. Elevated free drug concentrations will also cause increased amounts of free drug to be presented at sites of drug metabolism and excretion; this will minimize the potential augmented therapeutic (or toxic) effect of the displaced drug[6]. In most cases for which drug displacement in the plasma has been implicated as the cause of increased therapeutic effect, it is clear that a second interaction mechanism is also involved. For example, work in volunteer studies showed that azapropazone displaced phenytoin from its protein binding sites. It was also demonstrated, however, that a secondary interaction mechanism was involved in which azapropazone decreased phenytoin clearance due to competitive inhibition of the para-hydroxylation of phenytoin[10,11].

The interaction between phenylbutazone and warfarin is another good example of a double interaction mechanism. In the past this interaction was generally attributed to plasma binding displacement; it is now clear, however, that phenylbutazone inhibits the metabolism of the more potent S-isomer of warfarin[12].

These latter two examples serve to emphasize a point concerning the involvement of anti-inflammatory drugs in protein binding displacement. It is this: NSAIDs usually have a high therapeutic plasma concentration, and because of this they become involved in interactions as displacing agents. The drugs which they displace are often compounds with a narrow therapeutic concentration range, for example warfarin, phenytoin and sodium valproate. Warfarin is perhaps the drug most commonly involved in interactions with NSAIDs (see Table 2). This is due primarily to the anti-platelet effects of the prostaglandin synthetase inhibition of the NSAIDs and also to their toxicity in the gastrointestinal tract, although protein binding displacement is often reported to be involved. In vitro studies have shown that azapropazone and phenylbutazone are potent displacers of warfarin from plasma binding sites while naproxen, indomethacin, mefenamic acid, ketoprofen, and ibuprofen have a very much smaller effect[13] (Table 1).

Table 1 Decreased protein binding (human serum albumin) of warfarin as measured by fluorescence quenching methodology (from McElnay and D'Arcy[13])

Drug	Typical therapeutic plasma concentration ($\mu g\ ml^{-1}$)	Fluorescence quenching* (%)
Azapropazone	90	85.37
Phenylbutazone	75	74.22
Naproxen	50	14.89
Indomethacin	2	11.11
Mefenamic acid	5	10.76
Ketoprofen	6	6.47
Ibuprofen	35	-5.69

*Increased fluorescence quenching reflects decreased protein binding. Displacing agents (NSAIDs) were examined at concentrations in the same ratios as typical therapeutic plasma concentrations shown in the table.

Clinical findings so far published agree well with this experimental assessment. For example the two potent displacers azapropazone and phenylbutazone are known to cause clinically significant increases in warfarin anticoagulation [14,15]. The other agents appear to be relatively free from interaction. Penner and Abbrecht[16] found no interaction between ibuprofen and warfarin, and Jain et al[17] showed that naproxen had little effect on warfarin anticoagulation. Although Self et al.[18] described one case of warfarin potentiation by indomethacin, they commented that the interaction had low incidence. The lack of case reports would also suggest that ketoprofen and mefenamic acid do not enter into clinically important interactions with warfarin by this mechanism.

Table 2 Clinically relevant interactions involving NSAIDs

Interacting combination	Sequel and management	References
NSAID/oral anticoagulant	Over-anticoagulation (bruising, haemorrhage) due to changed warfarin metabolism and/or coumarin displacement from plasma protein binding sites. NSAID may exert antiplatelet effect or intestinal toxicity. Avoid or monitor carefully.	Aspirin[39-41] Azapropazone[14,42] Diflunisal[43] Flurbiprofen[44] Indomethacin[13,18] Phenylbutazone[12] Sulindac[45-47]
NSAID/oral hypoglycaemic	Hypoglycaemia potentiated; possibly multiple mechanisms involved including displacement of hypoglycaemic drug from protein binding sites, inhibition of its metabolism or changed urinary excretion. Avoid or monitor blood sugar levels closely.	Aspirin[48,49] Azapropazone[50] Fenclofenac[51] Phenylbutazone[52]
NSAID/lithium salts	Increased steady-state plasma lithium concentrations; possible lithium intoxication. Monitor lithium concentrations and anticipate reduction in lithium dosage.	Diclofenac[25] Indomethacin[26,53] Ibuprofen[53]
NSAID/phenytoin sodium	Phenytoin toxicity due to decreased phenytoin binding to plasma proteins and/or competition for hepatic hydroxylation systems giving rise to decreased phenytoin clearance. Avoid combined use of NSAIDs with stabilized phenytoin treatment if possible; if not, anticipate reduction in phenytoin dosage.	Aspirin[6,54,55] Azapropazone[10,11,56]

Table 2 continued

Interacting combination	Sequel and management	References
NSAID/frusemide	Reduced diuretic effect; the natriuretic response is mediated by prostaglandins which are inhibited by NSAIDs. Avoid combination when possible	Flurbiprofen[57] Indomethacin[58]
NSAID/digoxin	Increased serum digoxin concentrations due to changed digoxin clearance and displacement from tissue binding sites. Reduce digoxin dosage and monitor serum levels during concomitant treatments.	Aspirin[59] Chloroquine[60] Indomethacin[59] Ibuprofen[59,61]
NSAID/oxprenolol	Reduced anti-hypertensive effect; prostaglandins play a role in hypotensive action of oxprenolol and NSAIDs are prostaglandin synthetase inhibitors. Avoid combination if possible but if essential monitor blood pressure and anticipate increasing oxprenolol dosage	Indomethacin[27]
NSAID/phenylpropanolamine	Hypertensive episode; NSAID caused enhanced sympathomimetic action of phenylpropanolamine due to its inhibitory action on prostaglandin synthesis. Avoid sympathomimetic formulations (especially non-prescription OTC products) when taking NSAIDs.	Indomethacin[28]
NSAID/antacid	Generalizations cannot be made; for example Mg-Al-hydroxide gels do not alter the absorption of aspirin, fenoprofen, tolmetin, or piroxicam, but they do delay the time to achieve peak serum levels of indomethacin.	General[2-4,62]

Table 2 continued

Interacting combination	Sequel and management	References
	Absorption of naproxen is reduced by Al-hydroxide gel alone but not by Mg-Al-hydroxide gel. Effect of antacids on gastric and urinary pH may be significant in altering drug absorption, and reabsorption at renal sites, respectively. If antacids are indicated to control NSAID-induced gastrointestinal irritation then combination Mg-Al products are recommended since they are less likely to affect the NSAID kinetics.	
NSAID/NSAID	Apart from interactions involving aspirin and other NSAIDs (see text for details), few relevant data are available on interactions between the NSAIDs themselves. However, the general concensus is that their combined use presents little clinical advantage. Indeed there is some evidence that multiple use of these drugs may be hazardous (e.g. enhanced toxicity, gastric irritation and reduced blood level of one component).	Aspirin[31-37] General[30]

C. Metabolic drug interactions

Drug metabolism takes place primarily in the liver, although other tissues (e.g. lungs and gut) also contain enzymes capable of drug metabolism. There are two categories of interaction depending on whether the interaction is due to enzyme induction or enzyme inhibition.

1. Enzyme induction. Many drugs are inducers of microsomal enzyme systems, particularly the cytochrome-P450 system. A consequence of this type of interaction is a shortening not only of the plasma half-life of the inducing agent, but also

that of other drugs taken concomitantly that are metabolized by the same pathway. Enzyme induction is more commonly seen with drugs that are relatively lipid-soluble and which are themselves slowly metabolized. Drugs that enter into clinically significant induction interactions include: barbiturates, chloral hydrate, glutethimide, griseofulvin, phenazone, phenylbutazone, phenytoin, rifampicin, and commonly alcohol, which may not always be recognized as an interaction component. Apart from phenylbutazone, NSAIDs do not normally activate this type of interaction; they more commonly inhibit liver enzyme activity (see review by Griffin and D'Arcy[19]).

2. Enzyme inhibition. A range of drugs inhibit the metabolic degradation of other drugs and thus cause an increase in both their duration and intensity of their pharmacological and therapeutic action. Drugs causing enzyme inhibition include: allopurinol, aspirin (high dosage), chloramphenicol, cimetidine, dicoumarol, disulfiram, influenza vaccine, isoniazid, morphine, oral contraceptives (combined type), para-aminosalicylic acid, pethidine, phenylbutazone and other NSAIDs (see Table 2), sulphaphenazole and also some psychotropic drugs, notably the phenothiazines and the MAOI-antidepressants, e.g. iproniazid, nialamide, etc.) (see review by Griffin and D'Arcy[19]).

An example of a NSAID which is involved in both enzyme induction and enzyme inhibition is phenylbutazone; it has been shown to decrease the plasma clearance of the S-isomer of warfarin while increasing the metabolism of the R-isomer[12]. The rate of clearance of racemic warfarin is unaffected by phenylbutazone as the depression of the clearance of the S-isomer masks the stimulation of the clearance of the R-isomer. S-warfarin has been shown to be some five to six times more potent that the R-isomer[20], and therefore the reduced clearance of the more potent S-isomer predominates in this interaction and results in augumented anticoagulation.

D. Interactions during drug elimination in the kidney

Most drugs are eliminated via a renal mechanism either as unchanged drug or as its metabolite. Many factors can influence this type of drug elimination; for example, reabsorption of a drug depends on its state of ionization which in turn depends on the pK_a of the drug and the pH of the glomerular filtrate (see McElnay and D'Arcy[21]). Active secretion and reabsorption mechanisms in the kidney are often troublesome when drug interactions are concerned. The retention or loss of drugs which are actively secreted or reabsorbed can be influenced by other drugs when they compete for the same transport systems.

An important drug interaction at the renal site involving NSAIDs is their interaction with lithium ions (see Table 2). Renal prostaglandins are important mediators of renal electrolyte excretion for chloride, sodium and potassium ions[22-24] and this action has led to an examination of the effects of NSAIDs (prostaglandin synthetase inhibitors) on lithium ion excretion. For example, Reimann and Frölich[25] showed that diclofenac decreased the renal clearance of lithium by 23% and increased lithium plasma concentration by 26%. Earlier work by the same group had demonstrated a similar interaction between lithium and indomethacin[26].

General inhibition of prostaglandin synthetase by indomethacin has also been indicated as a possible mechanism for the reduced anti-hypertensive activity of oxprenolol[27] and enhanced sympathomimetic action of phenylpropanolamine leading to a hypertensive episode[28]. It has also been suggested that the reversible acute renal failure that occurred in four healthy subjects during concomitant dosage with indomethacin and triamterene was due to prostaglandin inhibition unmasking the nephrotoxic potention of the diuretic[29].

IV. PHARMACODYNAMIC DRUG INTERACTIONS

Drugs which give summation or synergism of pharmacological effect are said to interact by a pharmacodynamic mechanism. On occasion, interactions of this type can be used to clinical advantage. Drug combinations may give an enhanced therapeutic profile at an individual dosage that is less than when the components of the mixture are used alone. This sparing effect on individual drug dosage may reduce the resultant toxicity of the treatment.

The ready availability of a large number of NSAIDs has made it tempting to suggest that combinations of them might be more effective than single agents, and that a sparing of individual dosage might reduce the incidence of gastric intolerance that is common to them all. Experience has, however, shown otherwise and Miller[30], who reviewed the combinations of NSAIDs, reached the conclusions that there were no good clinical data to suggest that combined use of NSAIDs was beneficial. Furthermore, he suggested that the use of aspirin with other NSAIDs should be discouraged since aspirin reduced the blood levels of many of the combinant drugs. He stressed that NSAIDs should be used one at a time, and that supplementary analgesics should only be added on a "when required" (prn.) basis. The appropriateness of this advice is well illustrated by some of the interactions summarized in Table 2. In particular it should be noted that aspirin decreases the gastrointestinal absorption (and thus the serum concentration) of diclofenac[31], flurbiprofen[32], and indomethacin[33-36]; it also increases the elimination of fenoprofen[37].

V. CONCLUSIONS

Clinically relevant interactions involving NSAIDs occur mainly with oral anticoagulants (coumarins), oral hypoglycaemics, lithium salts, phenytoin sodium, frusemide, digoxin, oxprenolol, phenylpropanolamine and antacids. The mechanisms of interaction involved are mainly metabolic inhibition of the concomitant drug by the NSAID, or an interference with renal elimination due to the prostaglandin synthetase inhibition of the NSAIDs. Drug absorption interactions expecially involving antacids can be relevant, but those involving plasma and tissue binding sites are transient and have little relevance with continuing dosage. Interactions between the NSAIDs themselves are generally disadvantageous and combinations are not recommended. Brief details of these interactions are shown in Table 2. A more detailed account of interactions involving NSAIDs has already been presented by D'Arcy and McElnay[38].

REFERENCES

1. OHE Compendium of Health Statistics (1984). 5th edition, pp. 56-58 (London: Office of Health Economics)
2. McElnay, JC and D'Arcy, PF (1980). Sites and mechanisms of drug interactions I. In vitro, intestinal and metabolic interactions. Int J Pharmaceutics, 5, 167
3. Galeazzi, RL (1977) The effect of an antacid on the bioavailability of indomethacin. Eur J Clin Pharmacol, 12, 65
4. McElnay, JC, Mukhtar, HA, D'Arcy, PF, Temple, DJ and Collier, PS (1982). The effect of magnesium trisilicate and kaolin on the in vivo absorption of chloroquine. J Trop Med Hyg, 85, 159
5. D'Arcy, PF and McElnay, JC (1982). Drug interactions involving the displacement of drugs from plasma protein and tissue binding sites. Pharmac Ther, 17, 211
6. McElnay, JC and D'Arcy, PF (1983). Protein binding displacement interactions and their clinical importance. Drugs, 25, 495
7. Mafouz M, Abdel-Maguid, R and El Dakhakhny, M (1970). Potentiation of hypoglycaemic action of tolbutamide by different drugs. Arzneim Forsch, 20, 120
8. Sellers, EM and Koch-Weser, J (1971). Kinetics and clinical importance of displacement of warfarin from albumin by acidic drugs. Ann. NY Acad Sci, 179, 213
9. Tillement, J-P, Albengres, E and Urien, S (1980). Plasma binding of drugs. Pharmacy Int,1,64
10. Geaney, DP, Carver, JG, Aronson, JK and Warlow, CP (1982). Interaction of azapropazone with phenytoin. Br Med J, 284, 1373
11. Geaney, DP, Carver, JG, Davies, CL and Aronson, JK (1983). Pharmacokinetic investigation of the interaction of azapropazone with phenytoin. Br J Clin Pharmac,15 727
12. Lewis, RJ, Trager, WF, Chan, KK, Breckenridge, A, Orme, M, Rowland, M and Schary, W (1974). Warfarin: stereochemical aspects of its metabolism and interaction with phenylbutazone. J Clin Invest, 53, 1607
13. McElnay, JC and D'Arcy, PF (1980). Displacement of albumin-bound warfarin by anti-inflammatory agents in vitro. J Pharm Pharmacol, 32,709
14. Powell-Jackson, PR (1977). Interaction between azapropazone and warfarin. Br Med J, 1, 1193
15. Aggeler, PM, O'Reilly, RA, Leong, L and Kowitz, PE (1967). Potentiation of anticoagulant effect of warfarin by phenylbutazone. N Engl J Med, 276, 496
16. Penner, JA and Abbrecht, PH (1975). Lack of interaction between ibuprofen and warfarin. Curr Ther Res, 18, 862
17. Jain, A, McMahan, G, Slattery, JT and Levy, G (1979). Effect of naproxen on the steady state serum concentrations and anticoagulant activity of

warfarin. Clin Pharmacol Ther, 25, 61

18. Self, TF, Soloway, MS and Vaughn, D (1978). Possible interaction of indomethacin and warfarin, Drug Intell Clin Pharm, 12, 580
19. Griffin, JP, and D'Arcy, PF (1984). A Manual of Adverse Drug Interactions, 3rd edn, (Bristol:Wright), 25, 29, 222
20. O'Reilly, RA (1971). Interaction of several coumarin compounds with human and canine serum albumin. Mol Pharmacol, 7, 209
21. McElnay, JC and D'Arcy, PF (1980). Sites and mechanisms of drug interactions.II. Protein binding, renal excretion and pharmacodynamic interactions. Int J Pharmaceutics, 6, 205
22. Fulgraff, G and Brandenbusch, G (1974). Comparison of the effects of prostaglandins A_2,E_2, and $F_{2\alpha}$ on kidney function in dogs. Pflugers Arch, 349, 9
23. Tannenbaum, J, Splawinski, JA, Oates, JA and Nies, AS (1975). Enhanced renal prostaglandin production in the dog. I. Effects on renal function. Circ Res, 36, 197
24. Stokes, JB (1979). Effects of prostaglandin E_2 on chloride transport across the rabbit thick ascending limb of Henle-selective inhibition of the medullary portion. J Clin Invest, 64, 495
25. Reimann, IW and Frölich, JC (1981). Effects of diclofenac on lithium kinetics. Clin Pharmacol Ther, 30, 348
26. Frölich, JC, Leftwich, R, Ragheb, M, Oates, JA, Reimann, I and Buchanan, D (1979). Indomethacin increases plasma lithium. Br Med J, 1, 1115
27. Salvetti, A, Arzilli, F, Pedrinelli, R, Beggi, P and Motolese, M (1982). Interaction between oxprenolol and indomethacin on blood pressure in essential hypertensive patients. Eur J Clin Pharmacol, 22, 197
28. Horowitz, JD, Howes, LG, Christophidis, N, Lang, WJ, Fennessy, MR, Rand, MJ and Louis, WJ (1980). Hypertensive responses induced by phenylpropanolamine in anorectic and decongestant preparations. Lancet, 1, 60
29. Favre, L, Glasson, P and Vallotton, MB (1982). Reversible acute renal failure from combined triamterene and indomethacin. Ann Intern Med, 96, 317
30. Miller, DR (1981). Combination use of non-steroidal anti-inflammatory drugs. Drug Intell Clin Pharm, 15, 3
31. Müller, PO, Hundt, HKL and Müller, DG (1977). Pharmacokinetic and pharmacodynamic implications of long-term administration on non-steroidal anti-inflammatory agents. Int J Clin Pharmacol, 15, 397
32. Brooks, PM and Khong, TK (1977). Flurbiprofen-aspirin interaction: a double blind crossover study. Curr Med Res Opin, 5, 53
33. Jeremy, R and Towson, J (1970). Interaction between aspirin and indomethacin in the treatment of rheumatoid arthritis. Med J Aust, 2, 127
34. Yessair, DW, Remington, L, Callahan, M and Kensler, CJ (1970). Comparative effects of salicylic acid, phenylbutazone, probenecid and other anions on the metabolism, distribution and excretion of indomethacin by rats. Biochem Pharmacol, 19, 1591
35. Champion, GD, Paulus, HE, Mongan, E, Okun, R, Pearson, CM and Sarkissian, E (1972). The effect of aspirin on serum indomethacin. Clin Pharmacol Ther, 13, 239
36. Kwan, KC, Breault, GO, Davis, RL, Lei, BW, Czerwinski, AW, Bresselaar, GH and Duggan, DE (1978). Effect of concomitant aspirin administration on the pharmacokinetics of indomethacin in man. J.Pharmacokinet Biopharm, 6, 451
37. Rubin, A, Rodda BE, Warrick, P, Gruber, CM and Ridolfo, AS (1973). Interaction of aspirin with nonsteroidal anti-inflammatory drugs in man. Arthritis Rheum, 16, 635
38. D'Arcy, PF and McElnay, JC (1986). Drug interactions involving anti-rheumatic and anti-inflammatory drugs. In: Rainsford KD (ed)

Antirheumatic and Anti-inflammatory Drugs, vol III. (Boca Raton, Florida, USA: CRC Press) p. 213

39. Udall, JA (1970). Drug interference with warfarin therapy. Clin Med, 77, 20
40. Koch-Weser, J and Sellers, EM (1971). Drug interactions with coumarin anticoagulants, N Engl J Med, 285, 487
41. Anon (1972). The choice of an oral anticoagulant. Drug Therapeutics Bull, 10, 25
42. McElnay, JC and D'Arcy, PF (1978). Interaction between azapropazone and warfarin. Experientia, 34, 1320
43. Serlin, MJ, Mossmann, S, Sibeon, RG and Breckenridge, AM (1980). The effect of diflunisal on the steady state pharmacodynamics and pharmacokinetics of warfarin. Br J Clin Pharmacol, 9, 287
44. Stricker, BHCh and Delhez, JL (1982). Interaction between flurbiprofen and coumarins. Br Med J, 285, 812
45. Carter, SA (1979). Potential effects of sulindac on response of prothrombin time to oral anticoagulants. Lancet, 2, 698
46. Ross, JRY and Beeley, L (1979). Sulindac, prothrombin time and anticoagulants. Lancet, 2, 1075
47. Loftin, JP and Vesell, ES (1979). Interaction between sulindac and warfarin: different results in normal subjects and in an unusual patient with a potassium-losing renal tubular defect. J Clin Pharmacol, 19, 733
48. Cherner, R, Groppe, CW and Rupp, JJ (1963). Prolonged tolbutamide-induced hypoglycemia. J Am Med Assoc, 185, 883
49. Peaston, MJ and Finnegan, P (1968). A case of combined poisoning with chlorpropamide, acetylsalicylic acid and paracetamol. Br J Clin Pract, 22, 30
50. Andreasen, PB, Simonsen, K, Brocks, K, Dimo, B and Bouchelouche, P (1981). Hypoglycaemia induced by azapropazone-tolbutamide interaction. Br J Clin Pharmacol, 12, 581
51. Allen, PA and Taylor, RT (1980). Fenclofenac and thyroid function tests. Br Med J, 281, 1642
52. Szita, M, Gachalyi, B, Tornyossy, M and Kaldor, A (1980). Interaction of phenylbutazone and tolbutamide in man. Int J Clin Pharmacol Ther Toxicol, 18, 378
53. Ragheb, M, Ban, TA, Buchanan, D and Frölich, JC (1980). Interaction of indomethacin and ibuprofen with lithium in manic patients under a steady state lithium level. J Clin Psychiatry, 41, 397
54. Olanow, CW, Finn, AL and Prussak, C (1981). The effects of salicylate on the pharmacokinetics of phenytoin. Neurology, 31, 341
55. Inoue, F and Walsh, RJ (1983). Folate supplements and phenytoin-salicylate interaction. Neurology, 33, 115
56. Roberts, CJC, MacFarlane, D, Daneshmend, TK and Dieppe, PA (1981). Anticonvulsant intoxication precipitated by azapropanone. Postgrad Med J, 57, 191
57. Rawles, JM (1982). Antagonism between non-steroidal anti-inflammatory drugs and diuretics. Scot Med J, 27, 37
58. Chennavasin, P, Seiwell, R and Brater, DC (1980). Pharmacokinetic-dynamic analysis of the indomethacin-furosemide interaction in man. J Pharmacol Exp Ther, 215, 77
59. Wilkerson, RD, Mockridge, PB and Massing, GK (1980). Effects of selected drugs on serum digoxin concentrations in dogs. Am J Cardiol, 45, 1202
60. D'Arcy, PF, McElnay, JC and Sidahmed, AM (1984). Chloroquine digoxin interaction. Br J Pharmacol, 81, 8P
61. Quattrocchi, FP, Robinson, JD, Curry, RW, Grieco, ML and Schulman, SG (1983). The effect of ibuprofen on serum digoxin concentrations. Drug

Intell Clin Pharm, 17, 286
62. Day, RO, Graham, GG, Champion, GD and Lee, E (1984). Anti-rheumatic drug interactions. Clin Rheum Dis, 10, 251

Discussion

Professor A Bennett, UK: The British National Formulary actually says that indomethacin will act against antihypotensives in general and it doesn't actually specify how. The way I thought about this is that prostaglandins in general helped maintain vasomototone and that anything that reduced that will therefore tend to increase the blood pressure as indomethacin does on its own. Any of these class of drugs will therefore be antihypotensive and therefore will also increase the blood pressure effect with agents like phenylpropyl amine.

Professor D'Arcy: I think that's very possible. What I did when we went through the literature was to select out those clinical reports which I was satisfied would give the right indication. The trouble is, as you well know in the history of interactions between drugs, so many animal studies or anecdotal studies have been extrapolated to fact, so I tried to confine myself to those cases that had been reported, but I appreciated what you have said. Yes that could be a possibility.

Dr Cox: I can add that in a study of fenclofenac against gold we ran all patients in on their standard anti-inflammatory and then added gold or fenclofenac and then at month one the fenclofenac group were very much better and I assumed this was an enhanced anti-inflammatory effect.

Professor D'Arcy: Could be, yes. Thank you.

Dr Crowshaw, UK: I thought I would just like to mention one other interaction that you didn't mention which has been shown in animals, and this is the one whereby, if you pretreat rats with sodium salicylate, and then dose them with anti-inflammatory drugs, a whole range of them, you then minimise and decrease markedly the pro-ulcer effect of those anti-inflammatory agents. Now I don't know if this has been repeated in patients, I have a vague memory that it has, but this is one example of a beneficial drug interaction which might be possible to use?

Professor D'Arcy: Thank you very much, that's very useful to know. I did avoid, I must admit, any animal studies apart from our own on chloroquine and digoxin.

Anonymous: Is there any indication of the mechanism of that interaction?

Professor D'Arcy: I've read recently that the thought is that there are binding sites in the stomach which sodium salicylate shares with the anti-inflammatory agents. They may not be the same, they may be adjacent, and then by occupying one of the sites you then prevent the anti-inflammatory agent siting on the adjacent side and therefore producing its pro-ulcer effect.

Dr KD Rainsford, UK: In fact that study with sodium salicylate in combination with indomethacin has in fact been performed in man in Hungary and is the subject of commercial development by a Hungarian company (Gideon Richter) at the moment. The other thing of course is that the suggested interaction of salicylate with indomethacin or aspirin on binding sites of cyclooxygenase in fact has also been shown by Ham and co-workers with diflunisal. While talking of diflunisal there is an interesting study that was performed in man showing a very complex interaction between the type of antacid which is co-administered with this drug and fasting state. It depends on whether you were using magnesium or aluminium hydroxide. This is a very complicated one, and I wondered whether you knew about it and could unravel its mechanism?

Professor D'Arcy: Well actually we are starting in October with a student to look at these particular interactions, because I've thought that the role of antacids need sorting out. There's a lot of evidence in the literature I think which is conflicting.

Professor C Patrono, Italy: To add to the comment of Dr Crowshaw I would like to add a final comment to the last item of your very complete and interesting list that is related to interactions between different non-steroidals and which has bearing to the question of these drugs interacting with 2 different binding sites of the cyclooxygenase. There is the fact that most used NSAIDs can interfere with aspirin's irreversible binding to the enzyme which is necessary for its long-lasting effect on platelet thromboxane production. So whenever aspirin is used as an anti-platelet agent the concomitant use of non-steroidal anti-inflammatory agents can prevent its long lasting anti-platelet effect.

Professor D'Arcy: I'm glad you raised that point because it's so often when you look at a drug interaction you think of how one component is altered and of course both components of the drug mixture are usually altered.

15
Interaction between non-steroidal anti-inflammatory drugs and angiotensin-converting enzyme inhibitors in man

GP Velo, P Minuz, E Arosio*, MG Capuzzo*, G Covi* and A Lechi*
Istituto de Farmacologia
*Clinica Medica, University of Verona, Verona, Italy

CONTENTS

I. INTRODUCTION

Angiotensin-converting enzyme (ACE) inhibitors reduce blood pressure (BP) by two possible mechanisms: reducing the formation of angiotensin II and aldosterone, and increasing the production of kinins (angiotensin-converting enzyme is also a kininase II) (Figure 1). This leads to a decreased vasoconstriction of the kinin and to a potentiation vasodepressor system with vasodilatory and antihypertensive effects[1]. A rise in kinin levels stimulates an increased synthesis of vasodepressor prostaglandins (PGs), especially prostacyclin (PGI_2)[2]. Moreover, some authors have shown an increase in PG production after captopril administration[3-5]. Therefore the prostaglandin system could be involved in the mechanism of action of ACE inhibitors and prostaglandin synthetase inhibitors could reduce their antihypertensive activity. In man a reduction of the antihypertensive activity of ACE inhibitors was observed when non-steroidal anti-inflammatory drugs (NSAIDs) were administered[6,7].

Side-effects of Anti-inflammatory Drugs. Rainsford, KD and Velo, GP (eds)
Part 1: Clinical and Epidemiological Aspects. (Lancaster: MTP Press)

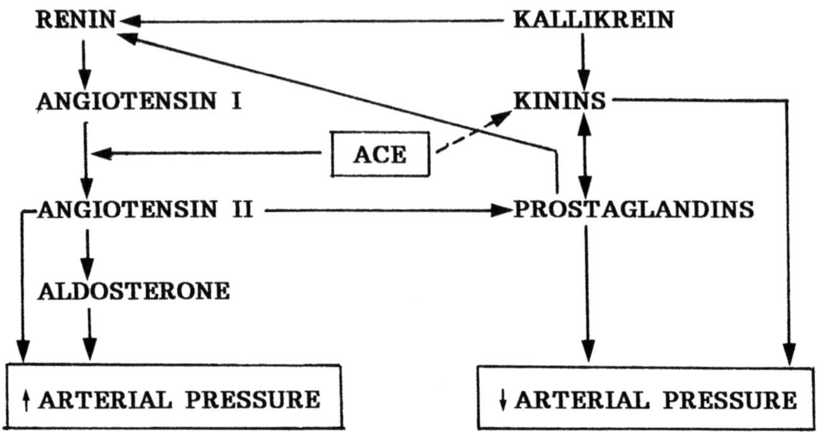

Figure 1 Interrelations between renin-angiotensin-aldosterone and kallikrein-kinin systems, and prostaglandins.

II. CLINICAL STUDIES

The aim was to study the effect of the inhibition of prostaglandin synthesis by NSAIDs on blood pressure and urinary excretion of the prostacyclin metabolite, 6-keto-$PGF_{1\alpha}$, in hypertensive patients treated with ACE inhibitors. 6-Keto-$PGF_{1\alpha}$ excretion, an index of renal PGI_2 formation, was measured by radioimmunoassay (RIA) after purification with high-pressure liquid chromatography (HPLC)[8,9]. A first study was carried out on eight patients with mild or moderate essential hypertension (1 or 2 by WHO criteria); no patients had received antihypertensive therapy for at least 2 weeks before the study. They were treated with captopril (50 mg t.i.d.) for 7 days. After 4 days of treatment the patients received also indomethacin (50 mg t.i.d.) for 3 days. Blood pressure, plasma renin activity (PRA) and plasma aldosterone, in supine and upright positions, were assessed before treatment, after the 4-day period of captopril administration and after the 3-day period of captopril + indomethacin administration. 24-hour urine collections were made at the same time, and urinary 6-keto-$PGF_{1\alpha}$ and kallikrein excretions were measured.

Mean arterial pressure was significantly reduced after 4 days of captopril, but its antihypertensive effect was inhibited by indomethacin (Figure 2). Urinary 6-keto-$PGF_{1\alpha}$ was unchanged after captopril and markedly reduced after combined captopril and indomethacin treatment: the decrease was of 42.8% and was statistically significant ($p \leq 0.05$). In the upright position an increase in plasma renin activity was most noticeable after captopril, and returned to basal values after indomethacin, whereas in the supine position the basal values were much lower and did not increase after ACE inhibitor.

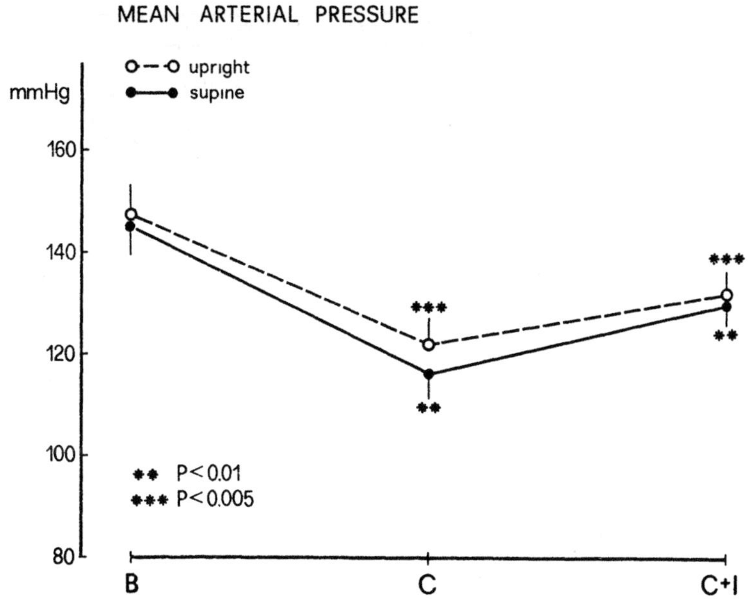

Figure 2 Modification of mean arterial pressure after treatment with captopril and captopril + indomethacin. Values are expressed as mean ± standard deviation. B = basal; C = after captopril; C+I = after captopril + indomethacin; ** and *** = significance of difference between C and B or C + I and C, respectively.

A second study was carried out on 16 hypertensive patients (stage 1 or 2 by WHO criteria). Starting from 3 days before and during the whole time of the treatment eight patients received a low Na^+ diet (40 mEq/day) and the other eight a high Na^+ diet (190 mEq/day). The patients were treated with enalapril (20 mg) for 4 days and the last 2 days also with ibuprofen (400 mg t.i.d.) (Figure 3). Ibuprofen was used in place of indomethacin since the latter also has a direct vasoconstrictory action with effects on renal and peripheral vascular resistances.

Enalapril showed an anti-hypertensive effect lasting 24 hours or more, which was maximum during the first 4 hours of treatment. The effect was more noticeable in the subjects with low sodium diet, and this could be dependent on reduction of their extracellular fluid, and was not modified after the treatment with ibuprofen (Figure 4).

A reduction of ACE levels and a rise of plasma renin activity were also evident, particularly in the group of patients on low sodium diet. The PRA increase could be explained by the loss of the negative feedback control of renin secretion by angiotensin II.

After 3 days of diet and before enalapril treatment the urinary excretions of 6-keto-$PGF_{1\alpha}$ were similar in both groups of patients. An increase in 6-keto-$PGF_{1\alpha}$ excretion was evident after enalapril only in low sodium diet group and after ibuprofen there was a weak inhibition. No modifications were observed in high sodium diet group.

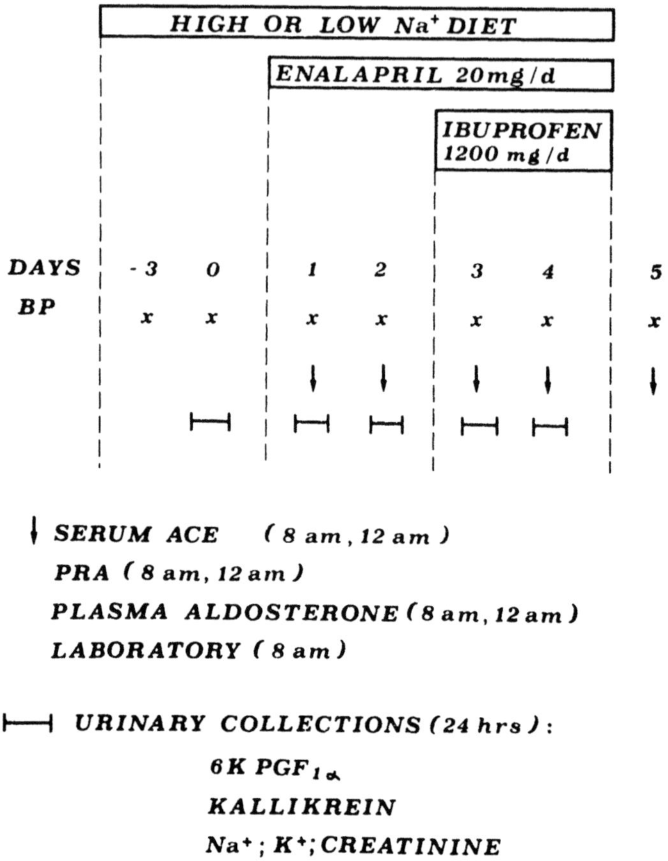

Figure 3 Scheme of treatment with enalapril and ibuprofen. Serum and urinary determinations. BP = blood pressure determinations.

III. DISCUSSION

The role of vasodilator systems (kinins and PGs) in the antihypertensive mechanisms of ACE inhibitors is not yet fully understood.

As far as renal PGI_2 is concerned, the measurements of urinary 6-keto-$PGF_{1\alpha}$ did not provide unequivocal results in patients treated with both captopril and enalapril. Moreover, conflicting results have been also obtained by different authors: captopril and enalapril have been reported to increase[3,10-12], decrease[13], or have no effect on prostaglandin synthesis[14-16]. These discrepancies could depend on the different conditions of renal blood flow and on the activity of the renin-angiotensin system, both conditions known to affect the renal PG synthesis[17].

The effect of NSAIDs on blood pressure and 6-keto-$PGF_{1\alpha}$ excretion during ACE inhibition is also different. Indomethacin significantly reduces the anti-hypertensive effect of captopril, whereas in a short time study (2 days) ibuprofen does not reduce the action of enalapril on both blood pressure decrease and PRA increase. Similarly, a 2-day treatment with ibuprofen does not cause any appreciable change in 6-keto-$PGF_{1\alpha}$ urinary excretion, and this could be due to the short time of ibuprofen administration.

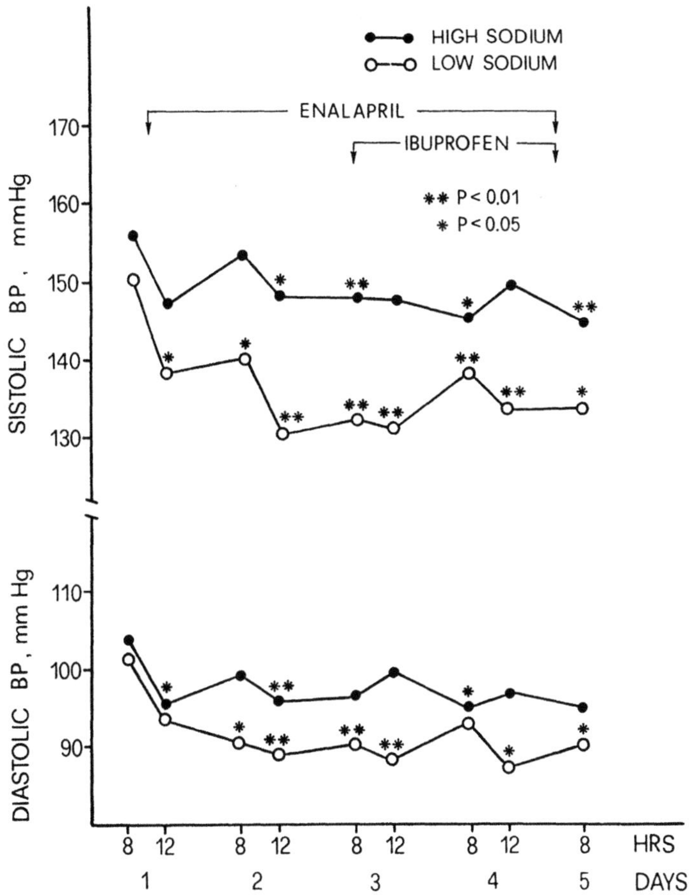

Figure 4 Arterial pressure variations after treatment with enalapril and enalapril + ibuprofen.

In a long-term study Oparil et al.[12] did not demonstrate an attenuation of the anti-hypertensive effects of enalapril when indomethacin or sulindac were also administered in a group of patients with mild to moderate low-renin essential hypertension. However in other studies indomethacin has been reported to show a different behaviour in comparison to other NSAIDs, and this could be due to a direct vasoconstrictory action on renal and systemic vasculature induced by this drug[18].

The varying effects of NSAIDs on blood pressure during their administration with ACE inhibitors could be partially due to variations in the inhibition of renal PGI_2 synthesis, but it could also depend on other mechanisms, such as sodium balance. In sodium-depleted subjects, where the renin-angiotensin system is activated, ACE inhibition causes an increase in renal blood flow, and this could lead to a rise[17] in the synthesis of vascular renal PGI_2. For these reasons the patients treated with ACE inhibitors and on low sodium diet might be more susceptible to NSAIDs[18].

REFERENCES

1. Swartz, SL, Williams, GH, Hollenberg, NK, Moore, TJ and Dluhy, RG (1979) Converting enzyme inhibition in essential hypertension: the hypotensive response does not reflect only reduced angiotensin II formation. Hypertension, 1, 106
2. Mullane, KM and Moncada, S (1980) Prostacyclin release and the modulation of some vasoactive hormones. Prostaglandins, 20, 25
3. Moore, TJ, Crantz, FR, Hollenberg, NK, Koletsky, RJ, Leboff, MS, Swartz, SL, Levine, L, Podolsky, S, Dluhy, RG and Williams, GH (1981) Contribution of prostaglandins to the anti-hypertensive action of captopril in essential hypertension. Hypertension, 3, 168
4. Mullane, KM and Moncada, S (1980) Prostacyclin mediates the potentiated hypotensive effect of bradykinin following catopril treatment. Eur J Pharmacol, 66, 355
5. Zusman, RM (1981) Captopril stimulates prostaglandins E_2 synthesis in vitro: possible mechanism of anti-hypertensive action. Clin Res, 29, 362A
6. Goldstone, R, Martin, K, Zipser, R and Horton, R (1981) Evidence for a dual action of converting enzyme inhibitor on blood pressure in normal man. Prostaglandins, 22, 587
7. Covi, G, Minuz, P, Capuzzo, G, Lechi, C, Delva, P and Lechi, A (1984) Reduction of the anti-hypertensive effects of captopril induced by prostaglandin synthetase inhibition. Int J Clin Pharmacol Res, 4, 47
8. Minuz, P, Capuzzo, G, Degan, M, Lechi, G, Covi, G, Velo, GP, Lechi, A (1985) The effect of 9α-fluorohydrocortisone on the urinary excretion of 6-keto-$PGF_{1\alpha}$ in man. In: Samuelsson, B et al (eds) Drugs Affecting Leukotrienes and other Eicosanoid Pathways, (New York: Plenum Press) p. 211
9. Minuz, P, Capuzzo, MG, Degan, M, Lechi, A and Velo, GP (1986) Determinazione HPLC-RIA della prostaglandina 6-keto-$F_{1\alpha}$ urinaria nell'uomo. Quaderni di Ligand Quarterly, 4, 263
10. Abe, K, Itoh, T, Imai, Y, Sato, M, Goto, T, Otsuka, Y, Yoshinaga, K (1980) Indomethacin inhibits the antihypertensive effect of captopril, SQ 14225, in low renin hypertensive. Tohoku J Exp Med, 132, 117
11. Swartz, SL, Williams, GH, Hollenberg, NK, Grautz, FR, Levine, L, Moore, TJ and Dluhy, RG (1980) Increase in prostaglandins during converting enzyme inhibition. Clin Sci, 59, Suppl 6, 133s
12. Oparil, S, Horton, R, Floyd, Z, Wilkins, L, Irvin, J, Hammett, D and Dustan, H (1983) Increased urinary 6-keto-prostaglandin $F_{1\alpha}$ excretion in patients with low renin essential hypertension treated with enalapril. Clin Res, 31, 876A
13. Lijnen, P, Fagard, R, Staessen, J, Verschueren, LJ and Amery, A (1980) Dose response in captopril therapy on hypertension. Clin Pharmacol Ther, 28, 310

14. Bravo, EL and Tarazi, RC (1979) Converting enzyme inhibition with an orally active compound in hypertensive man. Hypertension, 1, 39
15. Abe, K, Itoh, T, Sato, M, Haruyama, T, Sato, K, Omata, K, Hiwatari, M, Sakurai, Y, Imai, Y and Yoshinga, K (1980) Role of prostaglandin in the antihypertensive mechanism of captopril in low renin hypertension. Clin Sci, 59, Suppl 6, 141s
16. Fitz, A, Lawton, W, Reimer, J and Nelson, G (1982) The effect of enalapril, a non-thiol converting enzyme inhibitor, on vasoactive factors in hypertension. Clin Res, 30, 775A
17. Dunn, MJ (1983) Renal prostaglandins, In: Dunn, MJ (ed) Renal Endocrinology (Baltimore: Williams & Wilkins) p. 1
18. Dunn, MJ and Zambraski, EJ (1980) Renal effects of drugs that inhibit prostaglandin synthesis. Kidney Int, 18, 609

Discussion

Dr AJ Lewis, USA: Have you looked at the effect of indomethacin on indoprol or ibuprofen?

Professor Velo: No. The reason is that it is quite difficult to compare these two experimentally.

16
Responders and non-responders to NSAI drug interactions - a neglected problem?

F Sörgel, R Koob*, M Hemmerlein*, J Braun and E Lang***
IBMP - Institute for Biomedical and Pharmaceutical Research, Harrichstr. 5, 8500 Nürnberg 10, FRG
*Carl Korth Institute, Div. of Clinical Pharmacology, Erlangen, FRG.
**Institute of Nephrology, University of Erlangen-Nürnberg, Nürnberg, FRG

CONTENTS

Side-effects of Anti-inflammatory Drugs. Rainsford, KD and Velo, GP (eds)
Part 1: Clinical and Epidemiological Aspects. (Lancaster: MTP Press)

I. INTRODUCTION

It has been shown that non-steroidal anti-inflammatory drugs (NSAID's) through their inhibition of prostaglandin synthesis, can attenuate the effects of anti-hypertensive and diuretic agents[1-7]. The clinical relevance and therapeutic implications of these findings are not clear at the present time due to the fact that there are large discrepancies between the findings themselves and their interpretation by the respective authors. There is, particularly, very little mention of the fact that there are responders and non-responders to that drug interaction, and very little attention has been given to protocol details that may be necessary to explain the effects observed.

This chapter discusses the discrepancies between different authors, and by the inclusion of our own data[6,7] tends to support the view that subjects or patients may respond quite differently to coadministration of NSAID's to diuretic or anti-hypertensive agents. Particular attention will be given to a critical analysis of protocols, data analysis, statistics and interpretation.

II. INTERACTION OF NSAID's WITH THE ANTI-HYPERTENSIVE ACTION OF BETA-BLOCKERS AND DIURETICS IN PATIENTS WITH HIGH BLOOD PRESSURE

A. Interaction of indomethacin with pindolol and propranolol

The first clinical report of a significant drug interaction between NSAID's and beta-blockers has been described by Durao et al.[1]. In their study they could only analyse the results of seven out of fifteen patients originally in the study. Four patients used pindolol and three received propranolol. All patients were good responders to beta-blocker treatments. Indomethacin was the NSAID studied for potential interaction; it was administered for a period of 10 days. Placebo was included in that single blind study. All but one patient had normal renal function. The blood pressure before beta-blocker treatment was highly abnormal, six of the seven patients had blood pressure of WHO-class 3.

Indomethacin blunted or even abolished the anti-hypertensive effects of either beta-blocker. The authors concluded from their data that, as in previous animal work conducted by them[8], beta-blockers seem to exert their action through prostaglandins, which when blocked can no longer lower blood pressure. The limitations of that study is certainly the small number of patients studied and the heterogeneity of the patients where two out of the seven patients studied had pyelonephritis, with the other five patients being essential hypertensives. The anti-hypertensive equivalence of 15 mg pindolol and 160 mg propranolol was not demonstrated, nor were literature data given to prove this equivalence. The question of circadian variation of blood pressure and the importance of the time of blood pressure measurement during the day, was obviously not addressed, since no information is available on that in the paper. This limits the value of this investigation significantly. It is also the only paper, in which analysis of the individual data does not suggest that there may be responders and non-responders to the effects of indomethacin on the anti-hypertensive action of beta-blockers. The merits of this paper are clearly in the index character and the stimulation of subsequent work by other investigators.

B. Interaction of indomethacin with bendroflumethiazide and propranolol

The Durao paper prompted several other authors to investigate the problem. Watkins et al.[2] studied 15 patients (none with renal or other disease), eight of them on a beta-blocker regime and seven on a thiazide regime. The study was performed in a double-blind randomized cross-over fashion. The doses of the drugs were variable, suggesting that some of the patients may not have adequately responded to a previously suggested dose. That fact limits the comparison with the data by Durao et al.[1] since they used rather unified doses.

Table 1 in this chapter shows the important section of their data taken from their tables. Although indomethacin increased mean

Table 1 Effects of indomethacin treatment on the anti-hypertensive actions of propranolol and thiazide diuretics (data from Watkins et al.[2].) The patients in the propranolol and thiazide group were not identical (supine blood pressure, mmHg)

Patient	Propranolol	Propranolol + indomethacin	Thiazides	Thiazides + indomethacin
I	124/75	134/75	117/84	114/86
II	120/80	139/88	163/101	168/101
III	127/87	152/90	125/85	166/111
IV	123/75	135/87	130/94	155/102
V	114/86	134/95	157/108	159/102
VI	133/82	130/81	146/90	158/106
VII	141/90	164/97	144/82	149/96
VIII	139/96	151/102		
MEAN	128/84	142/89	140/92	153/101
SEM	3/3	4/3	6/4	7/3

blood pressure from 128/84 to 142/89 in the beta-blocker group ($p<0.05$ using a Wilcoxon rank sum and signed tests), it becomes evident, from the individual data of diastolic blood pressure, that their patients can be subdivided into responders and non-responders to indomethacin treatment. The diastolic blood pressure in two of the eight patients studied did not respond to indomethacin. In the group with thiazide regimen, again two patients did not show an increase in diastolic blood pressure. In one case blood pressure even dropped significantly. It should also be emphasized that it is highly questionable whether the small changes in diastolic blood pressure seen in some of their patients are really relevant, if one assumes that blood pressure measurements themselves have their variability. Unfortunately, the authors do not give the blood pressure of patients before they were treated with anti-hypertensives. Therefore it becomes impossible to check the author's claim that the "anti-hypertensive effects of both propranolol and thiazides are almost completely inhibited".

We analysed their data on renal prostaglandin $F_{2\alpha}$ excretion, and could show that there was no correlation between the extent of prostaglandin biosynthesis inhibitions and the increase in diastolic blood pressure (Figure 1). Although that paper again suggests that there seems to be an interaction between indomethacin and anti-hypertensives it does not mention or discuss the fact that in some patients the effects of indomethacin were only marginal, and that in four of the 15 patients studied indomethacin did not affect blood pressure at all.

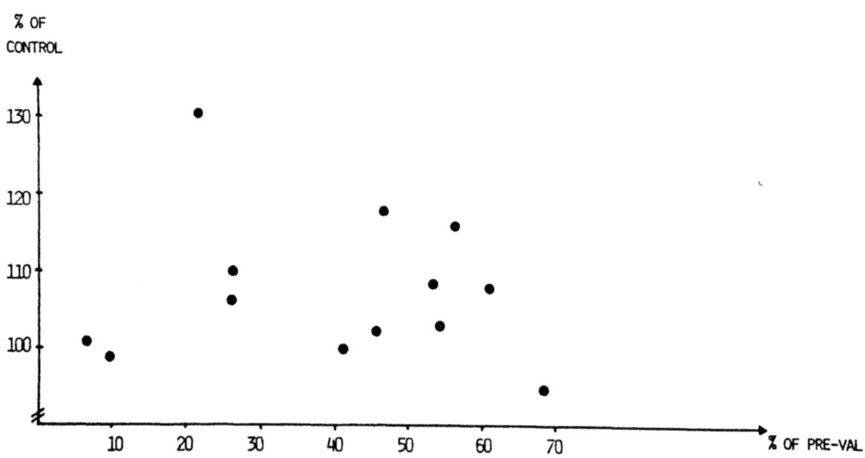

Figure 1 Absence of a correlation between the inhibition of renal prostaglandin $F_{2\alpha}$ excretion and the increase of blood pressure caused by indomethacin treatment (data taken from Watkins et al.[2]).
% of PRE-VAL = Prostaglandin excretion following NSAID dosing (as percentage of the excretion rates before NSAID treatment;
% of CONTROL =Blood pressure increase following NSAID dosing (as percentage of control).

C. Interaction of indomethacin and sulindac with thiazides

A subsequent study by Steiness et al.[4], published two years later, could not confirm their data. Indomethacin given in 100 mg doses did not increase blood pressure. However the individual data show that diastolic blood pressure following indomethacin treatment decreased in four patients and increased in the other four patients. In the case of sulindac they had three patients with no changes or increases in blood pressure, and six patients with decreases in blood pressure. This was enough to reach statistical significance ($p<0.02$) when the Wilcoxon test for paired differences was used. That study at the time of publication was in sharp contrast to what had been thought until then. It also raises the question again, whether prostaglandin synthesis inhibition really increases blood pressure, as suggested by Watkins et al.[2]. The explanation by these authors that the surprising results for sulindac can be explained by the absence of an effect on prostaglandin synthesis in the kidney was not confirmed by subsequent work[9].

D. Interaction of indomethacin, naproxen and sulindac with the anti-hypertensive effects of thiazides

The third paper on that issue, again in the British Medical Journal, appeared recently (Koopmanns et al.[10]). Their data were also in sharp contrast to previous findings. However, unlike other authors they did not leave out that critical point, and tried to explain the discrepancies. They suggested that the drug interaction with indomethacin may be transient, since the increase in blood pressure after 2 weeks vanished after 4 weeks of indomethacin treatment. Our individual analysis of their data once again showed that there seem to be responders and non-responders to that drug interaction.

E. Interaction of indomethacin and pirprofen with oxprenolol

In our study[6] we only included young patients with essential hypertension without any sign of other diseases, such as impaired renal or liver function. For those reasons our group of patients was very homogenous compared to groups studied by other investigators. Only patients with two consecutive blood pressure values above 96 mmHg were included in the study. The type of treatment we used on our patients was very similar to that of Koopmanns et al.[10]. Like them we used the same anti-hypertensive agent and the same dose in all patients, which was oxprenolol in our case. This was done because we did not want to have agents with different pharmacokinetic behaviour or duration or mode of action. Durao et al.[1], for example, used two beta-blockers which differ in their intrinsic activity. Oxprenolol given in a dose of 160 mg as retard formulation, decreased morning blood pressure (supine) from 146/96 to 131/82 mmHg. Standing blood pressure was reduced from 152/103 to 139/91. Heart rate was lowered by five beats/minute (supine) and eights beats/minute (standing). This shows that all patients were good responders to beta-blocker treatment. When pirprofen was added we could not observe any increases in blood pressure, neither during the first few days of treatment nor after 1 or 2 weeks. Most surprisingly we found the blood pressure to decrease even further. This agrees with the findings of Steiness et al.[4], who were able to show that sulindac can have such an effect. Koopmanns et al.[10] could not confirm such findings in a 4-week study. They suggested that the difference between indomethacin and sulindac observed in the first 2 weeks was only transient. Since we treated our patients for 4 weeks with oxprenolol, we can exclude the possibility that the additional decrease in blood pressure was an effect of continuing oxprenolol treatment.

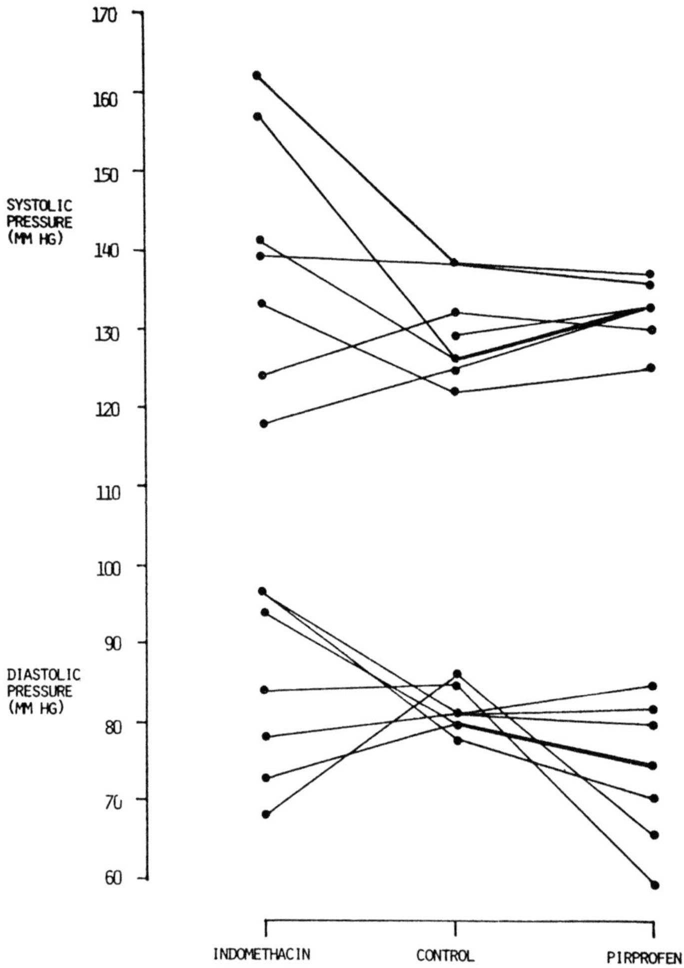

Figure 2 Systolic and diastolic blood pressure for each patient during the control period and during treatment with either indo-methacin or pirprofen.

It is well established that the anti-hypertensive effect of beta-blockers is fully exerted after a 4-week period of treatment, which was confirmed in our study: after three weeks 90% of the 4-week effects were reached. Three of the seven patients participating in the indomethacin study showed an increase in blood pressure, which in three patients could be observed from the first day on (Figure 2). The fourth patient only showed a reaction after two weeks. This finding also shows that late responses to indomethacin can be observed. In the other four patients blood pressure remained unchanged, except in one patient who showed a further decrease in blood pressure. The classification into responders and non-responders was still evident when standing blood pressures were used. A most interesting finding becomes apparent when we include our afternoon blood pressure measurements. Indomethacin, which increased morning blood pressure in the responder group, did not seem to affect the blood pressure of these patients in the afternoon (Figure 3). This suggests that the effects of indomethacin are short-lasting. This would be in agreement with the short half-life and a short duration of action of indomethacin. Unfortunately the other authors do not indicate when they administered indomethacin and the anti-hypertensive agents, and there is no information on how long after drug intake the blood pressure measurements were performed.

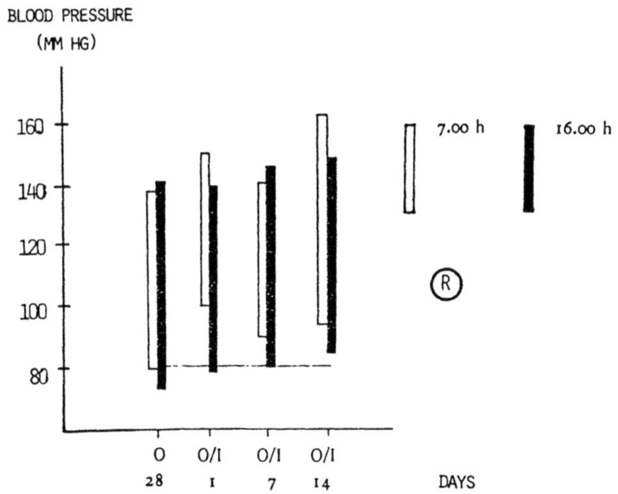

Figure 3 Effect of indomethacin on the systolic and diastolic blood pressure (measured in the morning and in the afternoon) in a representative responder patient: O/I = Oxprenolol + Indomethacin, R = responder.

This limits the value of their data considerably, and may even make interpretation of the clinical significance impossible. Only if the time of drug intake and blood pressure measurement are standardized is one able to discuss the potential interaction. We measured blood pressure each morning between eight and nine o'clock. Indomethacin and oxprenolol were given exactly two hours before the blood pressure measurements. It is, therefore, not surprising that in the afternoon (4-6 pm), there was no effect on blood pressure caused by indomethacin.

III. INTERACTION OF NSAIDS WITH DIURETICS IN HEALTHY VOLUNTEERS AND PATIENTS WITH CONGESTIVE HEART FAILURE (CHF)

No less controversial is the discussion about the effects of NSAID's on the saluretic and diuretic response to diuretics. The major unresolved question still is whether there is a "kidney-sparing" agent. This review includes one drug for which it had often been claimed that it does not affect the kidney, sulindac. We performed two identical studies dealing with the effects of two NSAID's, indomethacin and pirprofen on the diuretic and saluretic activity of furosemide. One study was performed in healthy volunteers and the other was done in patients with congestive heart failure.

A. Effects of pirprofen and indomethacin on the saluretic activity of furosemide in healthy volunteers[6].

Eight healthy volunteers received 100 mg indomethacin or 800 mg pirprofen the night before, and one hour before intravenous administration of 40 mg furosemide. This open randomized cross-over study was performed during a high sodium (300 mEq Na^+/day), and moderate sodium (60-80 mEq Na^+) diet. The means for volume and sodium excretion are given in Table 2. Using analysis of variance there was no statistical significant difference between the two NSAID's and, unlike Chennavasin et al.[11], we did not see an effect of indomethacin on the effects of furosemide. However, individual analysis of the data revealed that our subjects could be divided into responders and non-responders to indomethacin (Figure 4). Due to the lack of such studies on pirprofen by other

Table 2 Effects of indomethacin (I) and piroprofen(P) on the diuretic and natriuretic response to furosemide in healthy volunteers and patients with CHF

	Healthy volunteers						CHF	
	High Na^+			Low Na^+				
	Control	+I	+P	Control	+I	+P	Control	+I
Vol.(1/4 h)	1.92	1.72	1.88	1.81	1.62	1.51	0.859	.402
Na^+(mmol/4 h)	243	226	232	188	155	149	73.0	26.1

authors, critical comparisons are not possible, so we will subsequently only discuss indomethacin where abundant data are available. The interaction with indomethacin was always taken as proof of the involvement of prostaglandins in the saluretic and diuretic activity of diuretics[12]. However, as our study shows, there does not seem to be a signficant interaction when sulindac[13], antrafenin[14], flubiprofen[15]. Many others were also tested for their attenuating effects. Brater et al.[12], who several years ago seemed to have proved that prostaglandins are significant, in their more recent papers take a more careful position[10,16]. The problem of responders and non-responders to the NSAID-drug interaction has only recently been realized by this group. In their 1983 paper in the American Journal of Physiology[16] they used a rather unusual approach to the statistical analysis of the data. They excluded all non-responders from further analysis and collected statistics only on the responder population. These and similar approaches to the NSAID interaction studies do not help elucidate the true nature of that physiologically and pharmacologically important drug interaction.

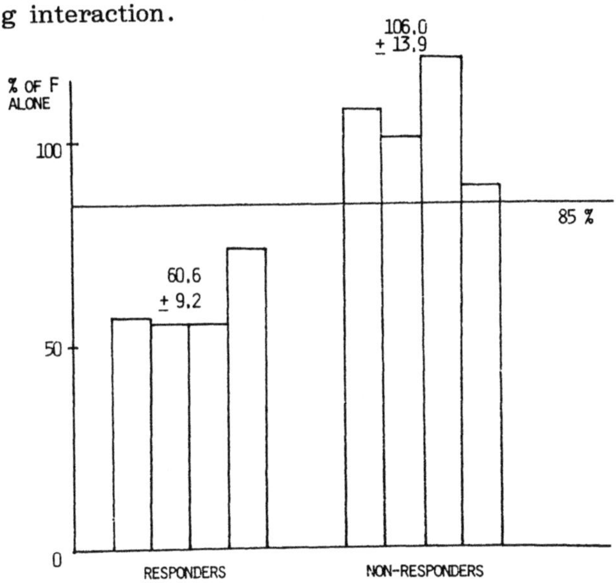

Figure 4 Effect of 100 mg indomethacin on furosemide-induced sodium excretion in eight healthy volunteers during low sodium diet. The 85% line represents the variability of the response to furosemide alone.

B. Effects of indomethacin on the effects of furosemide in patients with congestive heart failure

Seven patients with congestive heart failure (CHF) underwent the same pretreatment with indomethacin as the subjects in the previous study. The patients were on a normal hospital diet of 80-120 mEq Na^+/day. As shown in Figure 5 there is a dramatic blunting of furosemide's effects in this group of patients.

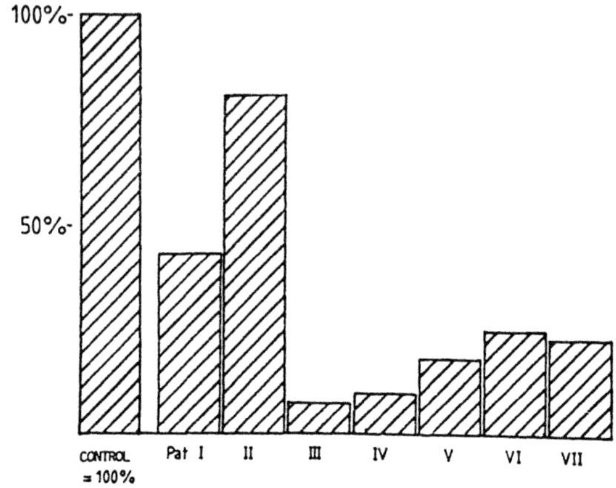

Figure 5 Effect of 100 mg indomethacin on furosemide-induced sodium excretion in seven patients with congestive heart failure. The reduction of sodium excretion caused by indomethacin for each individual patient is shown as a percentage of the control excretion.

It is, however, surprising that even in this group of patients there was one non-responder to the effects of indomethacin (patient II). As Figure 5 also shows, in the rest of the patients there was a variable but significant effect from indomethacin. Pharmacokinetic investigations during this study suggest that the attenuating effects of indomethacin can only be partly attributed to decreases in renal clearance (control: 33.3 ml/min, indomethacin pretreatment: 24.9 ml/min) or impaired tubular delivery of furosemide. Our finding of enhanced effects of indomethacin in CHF patients, but less pronounced effects in healthy volunteers, is in good agreement with animal experiments by Nies et al.[17], who showed that indomethacin has a stronger effect in situations of impaired renal reserve as found in CHF[18].

IV. CONCLUSIONS

A literature review and our own data suggest that the role of prostaglandins in the NSAID-antihypertensive drug interaction is not as established as previously thought. There is no evidence at the present time that the prostaglandins measured in urine are indicators of the effects of NSAID's in the healthy human kidney. Our analysis of the data of Watkins et al.[2] supports that view. Unfortunately, no other data have been published that would allow such analysis. Along with that observation goes our finding of responder and non-responder populations in healthy volunteers. It is highly unlikely, (except for an effect of genetics, which has not been studied), that there are healthy individuals whose proper kidney function needs prostaglandins while that of other individuals does not need it. At least we do not know of such an example in physiology where endogenous compounds play a role in only a part of the healthy human population, but not in the rest. Hypertensives with normal renal function in their response to indomethacin may be very similar to healthy volunteers, as the same percentage of responders to the NSAID-drug interaction was seen in both groups. Our studies in patients show that in CHF the effects of indomethacin -through whatever role they are exerted - are much more pronounced. Since these patients have renal disturbances, many other, possibly unknown, mechanisms of indomethacin may be involved. Most frustrating for the clinical situation at the present time is the fact that the responders cannot be preselected, and that we are still left with a trial-and-error therapy when we have to treat patients with NSAID's.

ACKNOWLEDGEMENT

The secretarial assistance of Mrs. Christine Kraus in preparing this manuscript is greatly appreciated.

REFERENCES

1. Durao, V, Prata, MM, Gonçalves, LMP (1977). Modification of antihypertensive effect of β-adrenoceptor-blocking agents by inhibition of endogenous prostaglandin synthesis. Lancet, 2, 1005
2. Watkins, J, Abbot, EC, Hensby, CN, Webster, J and Dollery, CT (1980). Attenuation of hypotensive effect of propranolol and thiazide diuretics by indomethacin. Br Med J, 281, 702
3. Wing, LMM, Bune, AJC, Chalmers, JP, Graham, JR and West, MJ (1981). The effects of indomethacin on treated hypertensive patients. Clin Exp Pharmacol Physiol, 8, 537
4. Steiness, E and Waldorff, S (1982). Different interactions of indomethacin and sulindac with thiazides in hypertension,Br Med J, 285, 1702
5. Salvetti, A, Arzilli, F, Pedrinelli, R, Beggi, P and Motolese, M (1982). Interaction between oxprenolol and indomethacin on blood pressure in essential hypertensive patients. Eur J Clin Pharmacol, 22, 197
6. Sörgel, F, Hemmerlein, M and Lang, E, (1984). Wirkung von Pirprofen und Indomethacin auf die Effekte von Oxprenolol und Furosemide. Arzneim.-Forsch. Drug Res.34(2), 330
7. Sörgel, F, Koob, R, Gluth, WP, Krüger, B, Lang, E (1985). The interaction of indomethacin and furosemide in patients with congestive heart failure. Clin Pharmacol Ther, 37, 231 (abstr.)
8. Durao, U and Rico, GT (1977). Modification by indomethacin of the blood pressure lowering effect of pindolol and propranolol in conscious rabbits. Eur J Pharmacol, 43, 377
9. Brater, DC, Anderson, S, Baird, B and Cambell, WB(1985). Effects of ibuprofen, naproxen and sulindac on prostaglandins in men, Kidney Int,27, 66
10. Koopmanns, PP, Thien, Th. and Gribnau, Fwj (1984). Influence of nonsteroidal anti-inflammatory drugs on diuretic treatment of mild to moderate essential hypertension. Br Med J, 289, 1492
11. Chennavasin, P, Seiwell, R and Brater, DC (1980). Pharmacokinetic-dynamic analysis of the indomethacin-furosemide interaction in man. J Pharmacol Exp Ther, 215, 77

12. Brater, DC, Beck, JM, Adams, BV and Campbell, WB (1980). Effects on indomethacin on furosemide-stimulated urinary PGE_2 excretion in man. Eur J Pharmacol, 65, 213

13. Roberts, DG, Gerber, JG and Nies, AS (1984). Comparative effects of sulindac and indomethacin in humans. Clin Pharmacol Ther, 35, 269

14. Hassan, SM, Olivesi, A, Fish, A and Turner, PA (1982). A comparison of antrafenin and aspirin on platelet aggregation and furosemide-induced diuresis. Postgrad Med J, 58, 17

15. Symmons, DPM, Kendall, MJ, Rees, JA and Hind ID (1983). The effect of flurbiprofen on the response to furosemide in healthy volunteers. Int J Clin Pharm Therap Tox, 21, 350

16. Kaojarern, S, Chennavasin, P, Anderson, S and Brater, DC (1983). Nephron site of effect of nonsteroidal anti-inflammatory drugs on solute excretion in humans. Am J Physiol, 244, F134

17. Nies, AS, Gas, J, Fadul, S and Gerber, JG (1983). Indomethacin-furosemide interaction: the importance of renal blood flow. J Pharmacol Exp Ther, 226, 27

18. Yeung Laiwah, AC and Mactier, RA (1981). Antagonistic effect of non steroidal anti-inflammatory drugs on furosemide-induced diuresis in cardiac failure. Br Med J, 283, 714

Discussion

Dr Rensing, Switzerland: Did you determine the indomethacin levels?

Dr Sörgel: In plasma you mean?

Dr Rensing: Yes.

Dr Sörgel: No, not in plasma, but we did spot tests in urine to show that our patients really took the drug.

Dr Rensing: So you cannot rule out that the high variation in metabolism of indomethacin is partly due to the different effects?

Dr Sörgel: Yes.

Professor Bennett, UK: I'm a bit worried about your division into "responders" and "non-responders". If you take a scatter about a mean and divide it at the mean, you'll find things above and things below, and you are describing these as "responders" and source of these as "non-responders". I would be convinced if you took the same people who are referred to as "responders" and vice-versa to show that on repeated testing they behaved in the same way. Have you done that?

Dr Sörgel: No, we have not done that yet, but we are doing studies in volunteers in another study. I agree with these limitations, but still when you take the conclusions and those papers are referenced in text books in pharmacology as a significant interaction, you have to show that it is really true for most of your patients, because if you are saying interaction is there and only 50% have that interaction then it may not be quite as insignificant as you think.

Professor Parke, UK: If you get genetic variations in interactions these aren't going to be the same for different kinds of interactions, either between different drugs or between different mechanisms of interactions, so it is quite possible that a patient would be in one category with one type of interaction, but in another category for another, so I'm not worried by your statement.

Professor C Patrono, Italy: I would like to make a few considerations in trying to put your data into perspective with literature data, which as you pointed out is quite confusing in this area. One of the reasons for the confusion is that one basic fact is often entirely ignored and it is that indomethacin can have inherent vasoconstrictor effects which are not due to inhibition of prostaglandin synthesis and are, therefore, not shared by other NSAIDs. This has now been shown quite convincingly in humans both in the cerebral and coronary circulation. The second consideration, which I think comes from your concluding slides is that age may be one variable affecting renal function and this may become an important variable in determining the consequences of the effects of prostaglandin synthesis inhibitors in reducing renal function and their effects on antihypotensive treatment. That is, you may not see anything in a group of young hypotensives whereas you might see some changes in blood pressure in elderly people who have hypotension together with declining renal function.

Dr Sörgel: I agree with that, but when you look at a drug interactions in all age groups you take rather a homogenous patients and that's why we use young hypotensive patients, because when you consider age. As others at this symposium have shown you can discuss nearly everything because you have to go into pharmacokinetics of different prostaglandin synthesis inhibitors and so it becomes very complicated. That is why we selected young patients.

17
Biological implications of the metabolic chiral inversion of 2-arylpropionic acid non-steroidal anti-inflammatory drugs

J Caldwell and AJ Hutt*
Department of Pharmacy, St. Mary's Hospital Medical School, London W2 1PG, UK
*Department of Pharmacy, Brighton Polytechnic, Moulsecoomb, Brighton, West Sussex, UK

CONTENTS

I. INTRODUCTION

Inflammatory disorders of a great many types are widespread in the human population and thus, the non-steroidal anti-inflammatory drugs (NSAIDs) are widely used. Currently, the 2-arylproprionic acids, or "profen" NSAIDs are an important sub-group of this class of drug. Over recent years there has been an increasing interest in the problems of adverse reactions to therapeutic agents of all types, in terms both of their prediction and prevention, and this is particularly so with the NSAIDs. Thus, the toxicity of aspirin has been re-evaluated, and phenylbutazone has been withdrawn in many countries due to the unacceptably high incidence of blood dyscrasias which it causes. Amongst the "profens" attention has focused upon benoxaprofen, zomepirac and indoprofen.

Side-effects of Anti-inflammatory Drugs. Rainsford, KD and Velo, GP (eds)
Part 1: Clinical and Epidemiological Aspects. (Lancaster: MTP Press)

In many areas of toxicology it has been found that a knowledge of the metabolism and pharmacokinetics of compounds is essential in understanding their mechanisms of action, dose-response relationships and adverse reactions. It is, therefore, appropriate to consider how such knowledge of the fate of the "profens" may inform their safety evaluation. Conventional studies in which excreted metabolites are identified, and standard pharmacokinetic parameters of the unchanged drug are defined, have not shed a great deal of light on the problems of the "profens" (see, for example, the paper on Chatfield and Green on benoxaprofen in ref 1). It is the purpose of this chapter to draw attention to the importance of considering stereochemistry in metabolic studies of the "profens", and to the notable biological consequences of the stereochemical aspects of their disposition.

II. CHIRAL PROPERTIES OF 2-ARYLPROPIONIC ACIDS

The 2-arylpropionates, as a class of drug, exhibit optical activity arising from the chiral (asymmetric) centre to which the carboxyl group is attached. They thus exist as pairs of sterioisomers, referred to as (+) and (-) when only their optical activity is known, and R and S when their absolute configuration has been established according to the sequence rule. It is important to note that these two systems of nomenclature are completely unrelated[2]: however, with all the profens so far examined, the two isomers are R(-) and S(+) respectively. Flying wedge diagrams of these are presented in Figure 1.

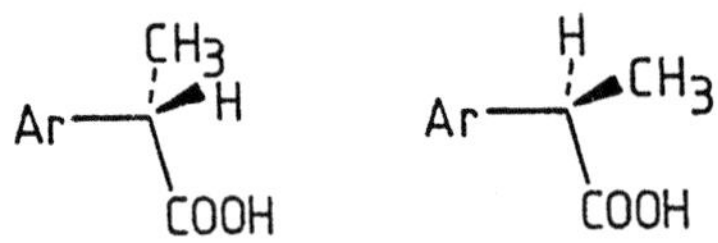

S(+) R(-)

Figure 1 Stereochemical representations of the R(-) and S(+) enantiomers of the 2-arylpropionic acids, shown as flying wedge diagrams.

A. Pharmacological properties

The great majority of compounds exhibiting pharmacological activity possess within their structures a chiral centre, and it is almost always the case that their activity resides partly or wholly in one isomer: the former situation is referred to a stereoselectivity of action, and the latter as stereospecificity[3]. In the case of the "profens" their activity appears to reside in the S(+) enantiomers. The anti-inflammatory action of this group of NSAIDs derives from their ability to block the conversion of arachidonate acid to prostaglandins and other mediators responsible for various features of the inflammatory process[4]. This synthesis of prostaglandins can be studied in vitro in a variety of systems, including microsomes from the seminal vesicles of rams and other mammals, and in blood platelets. Examination of the inhibitory effects of seven therapeutically used or experimental "profen" NSAIDs on prostaglandin synthesis in various systems (see Table 1) shows that the eudysmic ratios[3] [the ratio of the activity of the more active isomer, or eutomer, (here, the S(+) isomer) to that of the less active dystomer (here the R(-) isomer)] are in each case much greater than 1, stereoselectivity of action, and in some cases are so large as to indicate that the action is stereoselective for the S(+) isomer.

Table 1 Stereoselectivity of action of "profen" NSAIDs at putative sites of action

Drug	System examined	Eudysmic (S/R) ratio	Reference
Ibuprofen	PG synthesis inhibition (bovine)	160	5
Flurbiprofen	SRS-A antagonism (guinea pig)	878	6
Indoprofen	PG synthesis inhibition	ca. 100	7
Naproxen	PG synthesis inhibition		
	(sheep)	133	8
	(bovine)	70	9
Pirprofen	PG synthesis inhibition (sheep)	6.4	8
Carprofen	PG synthesis inhibition (sheep)	>16	10
	Platelet aggregation	>23	10
Fenoprofen	PG synthesis inhibition (human platelet)	35	11,12

It is commonly observed that there occur discrepancies between the stereoselectivity of action of pairs of isomers, assessed in vitro on isolated tissue preparations, and in vivo in whole animals. However, such discrepancies are generally small in magnitude, and most often arise from differences between the isomers in their absorption, distribution, metabolism and excretion, factors obviously only operating in vivo, which result in differences between the isomers in their concentrations at their sites of action.

In the case of the "profens", however, a very unusual situation occurs in that the very high degree of stereoselectivity of action which is observed in vitro is greatly obscured, indeed often completely lost, when the activities of the isomers are compared in vivo. This situation is illustrated in Table 2.

Table 2 Differential stereoselectivity of action of "profen" NSAIDs in vitro and in vivo

Drug	Eudysmic S/R ratio[a]		Reference[b]
	In vitro	In vivo	
Ibuprofen	160	1.1- 1.4	5
Flurbiprofen	878	2-16	6
Indoprofen	ca. 100	18.3-31.4	7
Naproxen	133 70	14.7-27.5	14
Carprofen	>16 >23	13.5-16	10
Fenoprofen	>35	ca. 1	11,12

a - see Table 1
b - For in vivo data

B. Metabolic inversion of propionates

The rationalization of the apparently contradictory data quoted in Table 2 is to be found in the study of the stereochemistry of the metabolism of the "profens". The chiral centre of the R(-)-2-arylpropionates undergoes a unique and biologically fortuitous inversion in vivo to give rise to the S(+) enatniomer, without any other change to the drug in question[15]. This reaction is essentially unidirectional, from the R(-) to the S(+) forms: in only two cases, those of ibuprofen[16] and 2-phenylpropionic acid[17], has the reverse reaction of the conversion of the S(+) enantiomer to its R(-) antipode, been reported: in both cases this was far less extensive than the forward reaction.

Since the first observation, in 1967, of the metabolic chiral inversion of ibuprofen[15], at least 10 "profens" have been shown to undergo the reaction, as listed in Table 3, whilst for a number of other such drugs, circumstantial evidence indicates that the inversion reaction may occur.

Most examples of stereoselective drug disposition involve either the preferential enzymic transformation of one isomer, or the preferential formation of one of a pair of isomers from a prochiral drug[13]. These situations obviously cannot apply with respect to the chiral inversion of the "profens", since this latter involves no other change to the drug. Various mechanisms have been proposed to account for the inversion[15], and it seems that this occurs as a consequence of the reversible formation of the acyl-CoA thioester of the "profen" in question.

Table 3 2-Arylpropionic acids known, or suspected, to undergo inversion from their R(-) to S(+) isomers

Conclusively shown (with reference)

Ibuprofen[15]

Cicliprofen[15]

Benoxaprofen[15]

2-[3-(2-Chlorophenoxyphenyl)] propionic acid[19]

2-(2-Isopropylindan-5-yl)propionic acid[15]

Clidanac[15]

Naproxen[15]

Loxoprofen[18]

2-phenylpropionic acid[17]

Suspected to occur with

Carprofen[15]

Ketoprofen[15]

2-(4-Phenylphenoxy)propionic acid[15]

Esterification with coenzyme A is a general reaction of a plethora of carboxylic acids, both xenobiotic and nutrient, and gives rise to acyl CoA's, which in the case of the xenobiotic acids are the obligatory intermediates in amino acid conjugation[20]. Protons alpha to the carboxyl group of acyl-CoA's are highly acidic, and are thus very labile[21]: this is the basis of the reactivity of acetyl and other fatty acyl-CoA's in fatty acid biosynthesis. In the case of the 2-arylpropionyl-CoA's, there occurs exchange of the alpha-methine proton with other protons in the medium, with consequent racemization. The formation of the acyl-CoA shows a high degree of stereoselectivity for the R(-) isomer, leading to the sequence of reactions shown in Scheme 1[22]. In the case of the "profens", the alpha-methyl group militates against the utilization of the acyl-CoA for amino acid conjugation[20,23], and the reactions shown in the Scheme would logically result in the inversion of the R(-) isomer to its S(+) antipode up to 100% if no other process, e.g. metabolism by another route or excretion, operated.

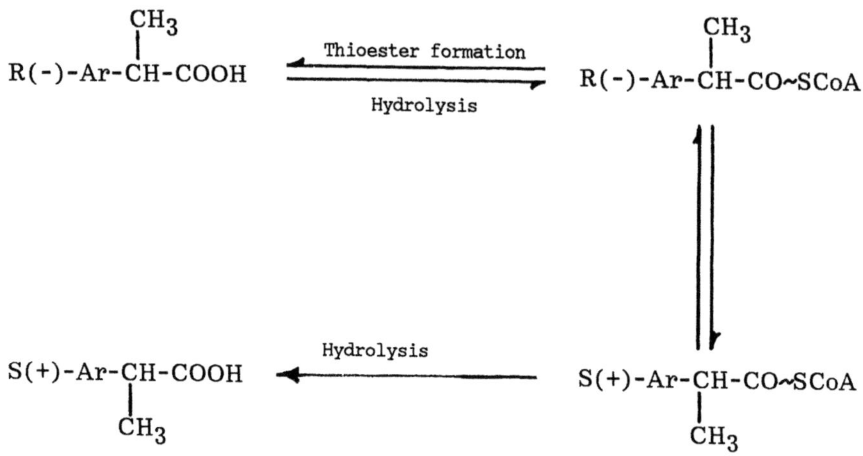

Mechanism involves the exchange of the alpha-methine proton

Scheme 1 Mechanism for the chiral inversion of the 2-arylpropionates.

The species occurrence of the chiral inversion reaction is summarized in Table 4.

Table 4 Species occurrence of the chiral inversion of "profen" NSAIDs

Drug	Species occurrence
Ibuprofen[15]	Man, rat, mouse, guinea pig
Clidanac[15]	Guinea pig, <u>not</u> rat, mouse
Benozaprofen[15]	Man, rat
Cicliprofen[15]	Man, rhesus monkey, rat, dog
Indoprofen[15]	Rat, mouse, <u>not</u> man

Although the reaction is to be regarded as a general feature of the disposition of "profens", there do occur important exceptions to this, which means that the occurrence of the reaction must be established for each "profen" of interest in each species. In addition, there are reported substantial differences between species in the rate and extent of the reaction, e.g. the half-life for the inversion of benoxaprofen in the rat is 2.5 h, but this is extended to 108 h in man[25].

C. Stereoselective disposition

In addition to the fascinating chiral inversion reaction, the isomers of the "profens" also undergo stereoselective disposition, in which the inactive R(-) antipodes are more rapidly eliminated, having shorter plasma elimination half-lives and smaller plasma AUCs. This has been demonstrated with ibuprofen[26], indoprofen[27], carprofen[28,29], and naproxen[30]. These differences may arise variously from stereoselectivity of distribution and/or elimination, or metabolism not involving the chiral centre.

III. POSSIBLE CONSEQUENCES OF CHIRAL INVERSION

What then are the consequences of the chiral inversion of the "profen" NSAIDs which impact upon their therapeutic use? With the sole exception of naproxen, at the time of writing all of the "profen" NSAIDs marketed in the UK and other countries are sold as the racemates, i.e. a 50/50 mixture of the active S(+) and inactive R(-) isomers. The metabolic chiral inversion causes a number of problems in their therapeutic and toxicological evaluation, as follows:

1. The principal biological activity of these agents, inhibition of prostaglandin biosynthesis, which is responsible for their therapeutic actions, resides in the S(+) enantiomers. The progressive inversion of that proportion of the R(-) isomer present in the racemate thus serves to enhance the pharmacological activity of these agents.

2. A number of toxic actions of the "profens" also arise from the inhibition of prostaglandin biosynthesis, e.g. gastrointestinal ulceration. In these cases the inversion of the R(-) enantiomer to the S(+) form will enhance toxicity.

3. It is established that there do occur differences in both rate and extent of the inversion between species (see above). This hinders the interspecies comparison of both pharmacological and toxic effects of "profens" given as the racemates, since the relative proportions of the active S(+) and inactive R(-) isomers will vary between species.

4. Much activity in clinical pharmacology and toxicology is devoted to the elucidation of the relationships between the concentration of a drug in plasma or some other site of interest and the intensity of its effects. However, the majority

of analytical techniques used in such studies are unable to discriminate between enantiomers of chiral compounds. It will be clear from the foregoing discussion that concentration-effect relationships for the "profens" may only be discerned if the enantiomeric composition of the drug is defined, particularly since the R(-)/S(+) (eudysmic) ratio, i.e. the relative amounts of inactive and action isomers, is constantly changing as a consequence of the chiral inversion reaction and of the stereoselective disposition of the isomers. The enantiomeric composition of the "profens" in biological milieux may now be relatively easily determined: the majority of the methods reported involve the formation of diasfereoisomeric derivatives with one isomer of a chiral amine or alcohol, followed by chromatographic resolution of the diastereoisomers: TLC, GLC and HPLC have all been used successfully[15,31].

The use of non-stereoselective assays for such studies cannot be relied upon, unless and until the absence of chiral inversion of any particular "profen" has been established. Assays simply determining the total quantity of active and inactive enantiomers present will be at best of limited value, and may be highly misleading.

5. The occurrence of the chiral inversion of the profens, and the problems which it causes, is suggested to present a strong case for the therapeutic use of only the active S(+) isomers of the "profen" NSAIDs. The R(-) antipodes at best merely function as pro-drugs for the active pharmacophore, which will be liberated in an unpredictable fashion. At worst they may well be an undesirable impurity in the active drug, particularly if there occurs non-stereoselective toxicity, perhaps involving metabolism remote from the carboxyl group and its associated chiral centre. The use of the active S(+) isomers alone would allow dose reduction, and would perhaps avoid problems arising from the R(-) enantiomers. It would also remove variability in the rate and extent of chiral inversion as a source of variability to both desired and adverse responses to "profens". Although the resolution or stereospecific synthesis of the "profen" isomers would add to production costs, in view of the likely significance of the chiral inversion process for the "profen" NSAIDs, a group of drugs with well-documented adverse reactions, the expense of avoiding this particular complication may prove justifiable.

REFERENCES

1. Chatfield, DH and Green, JN (1978). Disposition and metablism of benoxaprofen in laboratory animals and man. Xenobiotice, 8, 133
2. Testa, B (1979). Stereoisomerism arising from a single centre of chirality. In: Principles of Organic Stereochemistry. (New York - Marcel Dekker) ch. 5
3. Ariens, EJ (1983). Stereoselectivity of bioactive agents: general aspects. In: Ariens, EJ, Soudijn, W and Timmermans, PBMWM (eds) Stereochemistry and Biological Activity of Drugs (Oxford: Blackwell) p. 11
4. Flower, RJ, Moncada, S and Vane, JR (1980). Analgesic-antipyretic and

antiinflammatory agents: drugs employed in the treatment of gout. In: Goodman, A, Goodman, LS and Gilman, A (eds), Pharmacological Basis of Therapeutics (New York: Macmillan), ch 29

5. Adams, SS, Bresloff, P and Mason, CG (1976). Pharmacological differences between the optical isomers of ibuprofen: evidence for the metabolic inversion of the (-)- isomer. J Pharm Pharmacol, 28, 256
6. Greig, ME and Griffin, RL (1975). Antagonism of slow reacting substances in anaphylaxis (SRS-Ar) and other spasmogens on the guineq pig tracheal chain by hydratropic acids and their effect on anaphylaxis. J Med Chem, 18, 1127
7. Buttinoni, A, Ferrari, M, Colombo, M and Cesarini, R (1983). Biological activity of indoprofen and its optical isomers. J Pharm Pharmacol, 35, 603
8. Ku, EC and Wasvary, JM (1975). Inhibition of prostaglandin synthetase by pirprofen, studies with sheep seminal vesicle enzyme. Biochem Biophys Acta, 384, 360
9. Tomlindon, RV, Ringold, HJ, Qureshi, MC and Forchielli, E (1972). Relationship between inhibition of prostaglandin synthesis and drug efficacy: support for the current theory on mode of action of aspirin-like drugs. Biochem Biophys Res Commun, 46, 552
10. Gaut, ZN, Baruth, H, Randall, LO, Ashley, C and Paulsrud, JR (1975). Stereoisomeric relationships among anti-inflammatory activity, inhibiton of platelet aggregation and inhibition of prostaglandin synthetase. Prostaglandins, 10, 259
11. Nickander, RC, Kroay, RJ and Marshall, WS (1971). Anti-inflammatory and analgesic effects of fenoprofen. Fed Proc, 30, 563
12. Rubin, A, Knadler, MP, Ho, PPK, Bechtol, LD and Wolen, Rl (1985). Stereoselctive inversion of (R)-fenoprofen to (S)-fenoprofen in humans. J Pharm Sci, 74, 82
13. Trager, WF and Testa, B (1984). Stereochemical considerations. In: Caldwell, J and Paulson, GD (eds) Foreign Compound Metabolsim, (London: Taylor & Francis), p 91
14. Harrison, IT, Lewis, B, Nelson, P, Rooks, W, Roszkowski, A, Tomolouis, A and Fried, JH (1970). Non-steroidal anti-inflammatory agents. I. 6-Substituted 2-naphtylacetic acids. J Med Chem 13, 203
15. Hutt, AJ and Caldwell, J (1983). The metabolic chiral inversion of 2-arylpropionic acids. A novel route with pharmacological consequences. J Pharm Pharmacol, 35, 693
16. Lee, EJD, Williams, K, Day, R, Graham, G and Champion, D (1985). Stereoselective disposition of ibuprofen enantiomers in man. Brit J Clin Pharmacol, 19, 669
17. Hutt, AJ, Fournel, S and Caldwell, J (1986). Application of a Radical Comprehension Column to the HPLC separation of the enantiomers of some 2-arylpropionic acids as diasterioisomeric S(-), 1-Naphthene-1-Y1-ethylamides. in biological samples. J Chromatogr, 378, 409
18. Tamegai, T, Tanaka, T, Kaneko, T, Ozaki, S, Ohmae, M and Kawabe, K (1979). The determination of opticalisomers of 2-[3-(2-chlorophenoxyphenyl)]-propionic acid in rat plasma by high performance liquid chromatography. J Liq Chromatog, 2, 551
19. Nagashima, H, Tanake, Y, Watanabe, H, Hayashi, R and Kawada, K (1984). Optical inversion of (2R)- to (2S)-isomers of 2-[4-(2-oxocyclopentylmethyl)-phenyl]propionic acid (loxoprofen), a new anti-inflammatory agent, and its monohyroxy metabolites in the rat. Chem Pharm Bull, 32, 251
20. Caldwell, J, Idle, JR and Smith, RL (1980). The amino acid conjugations.In: Gram, TE (ed), Extrahepatic Metabolism of Drugs and Other Foreign Compounds. (New York: SP Publications)p. 453

21. Lynen, F (1953). The functional group of Coenzyme A and its metabolic relations, especially in the fatty acid cycle. Fed Proc, 12, 683

22. Nakamura, Y, Yamagucki, T, Takahashi, S, Hashimoto, S, Iwatini, K and Nagagawa, Y (1981). Optical isomerization mechanism of R(-)-hydratropic acid derivatives. J Pharmacobiol Dynam, 4, s1

23. Dixon, PAF, Caldwell, J and Smith, RL (1977). Studies on the metabolism of arylacetic acids. 4. Chemical and biological factors influencing the pattern of metabolic conjugation of arylacetic acids. Xenobiotic, 7, 727

24. Tamassia, V, Jannuzzo, MG, Moro, E, Stegnjach, S, Groppi, W and Nicolis, FB (1984) Pharmacokinetics of the enantiomers of indoprofen in man. Int J Clin Pharm Res, 4, 223

25. Simmonds, RG, Woodage, TJ, Duff, SM and Green, JN (1980). Stereospecific inversion of (R)-(-)-benoxaprofen in rat and man. Eur J Drug Metab Pharmacokin, 5, 169

26. Vangiessen, GJ and Kaiser, DG, (1975). GLC Determination of ibuprofen (d,l-2-(p-isobutylphenyl)propionic acid enantiomers in biological specimens. J Pharm Sci, 64, 798

27. Tosolini, GP, Moro, E, Forgione, A, Ranghieri, M and Mandeli, V (1974). GLC Determination of plasma levels of enantiomers of alpha-[4-(1-oxo-2-isoindolinyl)phenyl]propionic acid. J Pharm Sci, 63, 1072

28. Kemmerer, JM, Rubio, FA, McClain, RM and Koechlin, BA (1979). Stereospecific assay and stereospecific dispostion of racemic carprofen in rats. J Pharm Sci, 68, 1274

29. Stoltenburg, JK, Puglisi, CV, Rubio, F and Vane, FM (1981). High performance liquid chromatographic determination of stereoselective disposition of carprofen in humans. J Pharm Sci, 70, 1207

30. Goto, J, Goto, N and Nambara, T (1982). Separation and determination of naproxen enantiomers in serum by high performance liquid chromatography. J Chromatog, 239, 559

31. Testa, B, (1986). The chromatographic analysis of enantiomers in drug metabolism studies. Xenobiotica, 16, 265

Discussion

Professor Parke, UK: Thank you for that stimulating paper. Putting your paper together with the previous one the obvious question is, do you think the responders and non-responders are people with the ability to transfer the R- to the S- or the inability to transfer the R- to the S-isomer?

Dr Caldwell: Obviously that would depend on the particular situation that was under study. The occurrence of the inversion is established in man with a variety of drugs. The numbers of humans that have been examined is so small that we're really not in a position to do anything other than imagine that inter-individual variation is possible. However, if inter-individual variation did not occur, it would be, I think, the first case that it didn't, and in virtually every other case you can think of, when you have marked differences between animals in any particular metabolic reaction, you usually get wide variations in man. So this is something that is a fascinating thing to do.

Professor Parke: What you're saying is John, that we don't know yet do we? Because going from 800 to 20 a non-responder could have a plasma concentration of a drug some 40 fold different from that of a responder. As far as I know, there's been very little investigation into this and it certainly merits it. I was very surprised to find in another chiral drug, or rather drug with a chiral centre, that the two isomers were oxidatively metabolised at different rates by different populations, in other words we're now looking at polygenetic variations and it gets very complex indeed. This is a drug that's given - well it's not a non-steroidal - but it's given rise to a lot of adverse reations and I think you're onto something very important here. Any further questions?

Dr MW Whitehouse, Australia: This is a very interesting story you've presented but I think you've perhaps overstated it a little inasmuch as there are properties of the inactive isomer. I mean it's only inactive as regards inhibiting the prostaglandin production - and we know that this molecule can certainly penetrate into the mitochondria of certainly, liver cells to undergo this transformation, so presumably other actions as, for example, uncoupling of oxidative phosphorylation which may underlie the slowing down of the leucocyte response of cells on inflammation. That type of pharmacology ought to be independent of the inversion. I'd also like to make the comment that these ratios of activities have been determined in the acute anti-inflammatory assays which depend on prostaglandin production, but how about determining the ratio of activity in chronic arthritic assays, as for example, in treating the adjuvant induced arthritis. What are the ratios there? That may be a little bit more relevant to treatment of rheumatoid disease.

Dr Caldwell: Right! To consider your first point first. I fully agree with you, if there are actions of the wrong isomer that are desirable I'd only really consider situations in which the actions would be undesirable and one would be interested in, if you like, refining prostaglandin synthesis inhibition to the exclusion of, not all else, but to do that, (I mean obviously the point that you make is an appropriate and perfectly valid one), might event represent a case for using the R-isomer only for other purposes. So there are two sides of the coin as you so rightly point out. With reference to your second point, I have to go back to the original literature from which the data that I've presented was drawn. My recollection is that certainly, well, I don't know whether they are what you would call, chronic models, but certainly by no means all of the in vivo data is derived from acute experiments. Certainly talking about up to two weeks administration anyway.

Dr Whitehouse: It's certain that the absolute ratio you gave were derived from in vitro studies weren't they - and you had predicated that the mode of action was in fact to inhibit prostaglandin production?

Dr Caldwell: Oh yes!

18
A medicinal chemist's perspective of side-effects of anti-inflammatory analgesic drugs

TY Shen
Merck Sharp and Dohme Research Laboratories
Rahway, NJ 07065, USA

CONTENTS

I. HISTORICAL DEVELOPMENTS

Following the epoch-making discovery of corticosteroids as antirheumatic drugs and a decade of valiant chemical and biological effort to dissociate their hormonal side-effects from their dramatic anti-inflammatory activity[1], the search for non-steroidal anti-inflammatory drugs, or NSAIDs as they are known today, began in earnest in several laboratories including those at Boots[2], Merck[3] and Parke-Davis[4] in the late 1950s. Pharmacological assays previously developed to measure the anti-inflammatory activity of corticosteroids in the laboratory, such as the cotton pellet granuloma

Side-effects of Anti-inflammatory Drugs. Rainsford, KD and Velo, GP (eds)
Part 1: Clinical and Epidemiological Aspects. (Lancaster: MTP Press)

assay in rats and uv erythema in guinea pigs, were adopted as primary screening assays. Aspirin was not very effective in these models but phenylbutazone became a useful reference standard. The major concern was to achieve adequate anti-arthritic efficacy with a non-steroidal molecule, since the hormonal side-effects of steroids could easily be avoided. Other potential side-effects of anti-inflammatory agents, e.g. gastrointestinal, renal, hepatic, CNS and allergic responses, were not given much attention in the laboratory initially.

In retrospect, this seemingly lesser concern for side-effects in the early days of NSAID research could be attributed to several considerations. First, is the complexity of clinical assessment of side-effects which involves determination of causal relationship, influences of disease conditions, the age and metabolic status of patients (e.g. hepatic and renal dysfunctions) and possible drug interactions. In some cases 1000-2000 patients with 1-2 years drug treatment are needed to generate a fair assessment. Second, the relatively low frequency (<1%, or even <1/10 000) of some severe side-effects after chronic drug administration (e.g. renal and blood dyscrasias), rendered them very difficult to investigate in the laboratory. The situation was further complicated by insufficient biochemical understanding of drug toxicity and the lack of adequate animal models. The CNS side-effect of indomethacin is a good example.

Table 1 Gastrointestinal adverse reactions of major NSAIDs incidence; percentage of total patients on drug therapy

<1%	1-3%	3-9%
Haemorrhage Ulceration	Diarrhoea Constipation Abdominal pain	Nausea Dyspepsia

Medicinal chemists usually excel if molecular information and quantitative structure-activity relationship are available. In the past two decades, potency enhancement of different chemical leads have yielded a large family of clinically effective NSAIDs, but the reduction of side-effects, in the absence of any well-defined structure-toxicity relationship, remains largely empirical and fortuitous. No rational laboratory approach is yet available to tackle the most common gastrointestinal side-effects (Table 1), which are symptoms of gastrointestinal (GI) disturbances, e.g. nausea, epigastric pain and heartburn in 3-9% of patients. Even for the well-publicized acute ulceration or haemorrhage in less than 1% of patients there is still a great deal of uncertainty in extrapolating laboratory findings to long-term clinical expectations.

A. Rational drug developments

Nevertheless, considerable progress towards safer NSAIDs has been made in many laboratories by medicinal chemical approaches based on structure-toxicity assumptions, pharmacodynamic considerations and, more recently, biochemical concepts. Pivotal clinical feedback and encouraging management decisions in some cases were also contributory to the successful outcome. For example, ibuprofen was developed after a sequential clinical testing of four closely related prototypes before the side-effects of skin rash and hepatotoxicity were circumvented[2] (Figure 1).

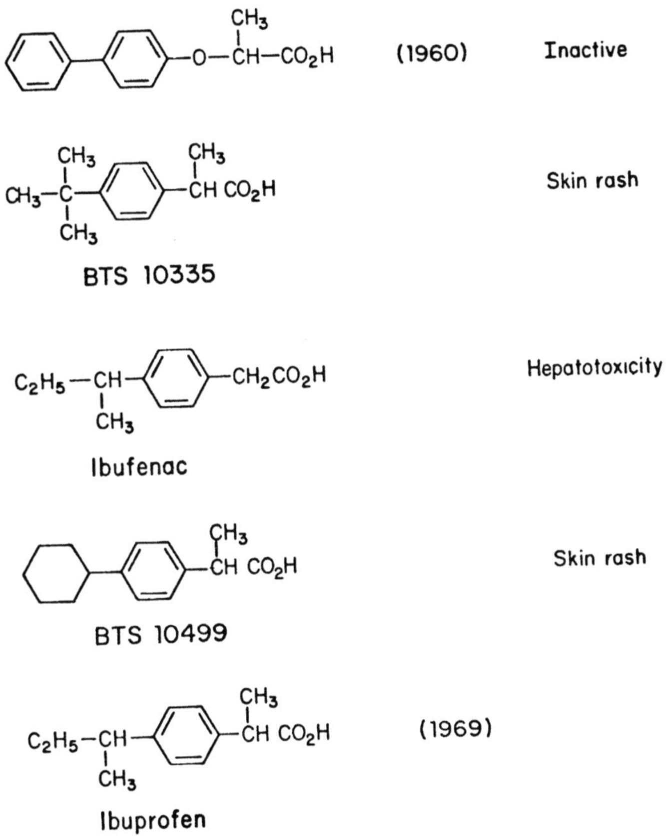

Figure 1 Clinical studies of prototypes of ibuprofen to circumvent side-effects.

The improved safety profile of ibuprofen over its congeners could not be predicted simply on their differences in chemical structure and pharmacological properties. Since then a large family of hydrophobic arylpropionic or acetic acids has been synthesized by many laboratories as potent anti-inflammatory analgesic agents[5]. In these studies various inflammatory models have consistently

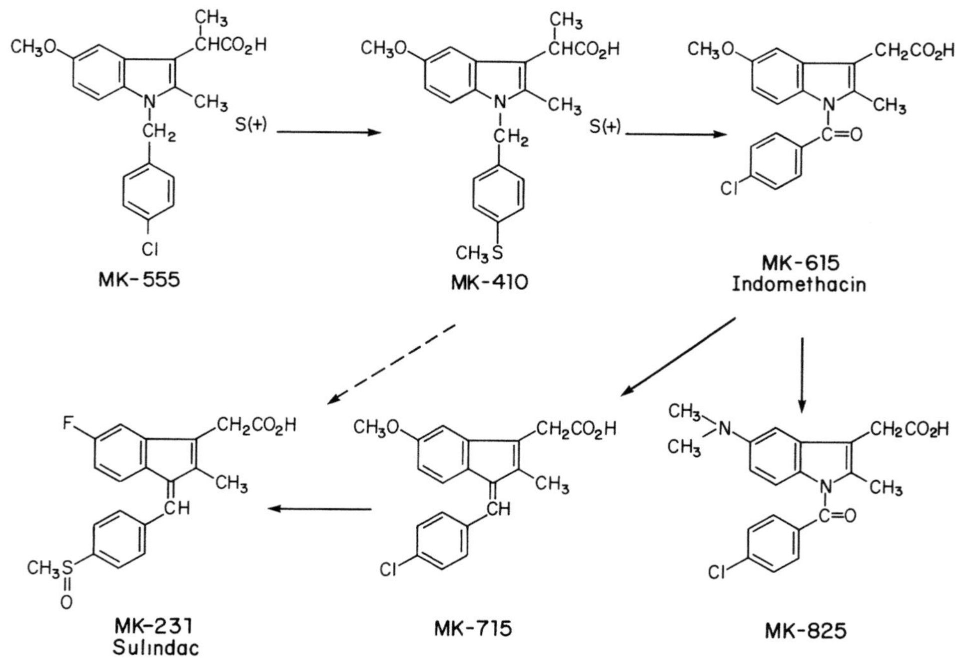

Figure 2 Clinical studies of prototypes of indomethacin and sulindac to improve efficacy and/or tolerance.

guided the selection of clinically efficacious new NSAIDs. Yet, as evidenced by the recent restriction or withdrawal of several agents from clinical trials or marketing (e.g. benoxaprofen, zomepirac, alclofenac, fenclofenac, indoprofen, phenylbutazone and the indomethacin GITS formulation), long-term safety of these compounds remained sadly unpredictable from laboratory experiments or controlled clinical trials.

B. Development of indomethacin and its analogues

In our studies the development of indomethacin also went through two prototypes, MK-555 and MK-410, before a clinical acceptable balance of efficacy and tolerance was achieved[3] (Figure 2). Our observation of GI side-effects of these compounds in man stimulated the development of animal protocols to evaluate the acute ulcerogenicity of newer NSAIDs. However, the complex CNS side-effects of indomethacin were beyond any simple laboratory measurement. Adopting a conceptual pharmacodynamic approach, it was hoped that the introduction of a more basic and more polar dimethylamion substituent as in the analogue MK-825 might alter its tissue distribution pattern and CNS side-effects. In man, MK-825 was comparable to indomethacin in efficacy, but unfortunately in side-effects as well. Luckily, both the central nervous system (CNS) and GI side-effects were reduced significantly with an indene isostere of indomethacin, MK-715. Preliminary clinical results suggested that MK-715 was efficacious and better tolerated than indomethacin. Unexpectedly, the poor solubility of its glucuronide metabolite produced crystalluria in several patients at higher doses. This new side-effect was finally overcome by replacing the chloro substituent with a methylsulphinyl group, which not only increased the aqueous solubility of indene acetic acids more than 100-fold but also provided an active centre for drug metabolism. The anti-inflammatory activity of the sulphide metabolite was anticipated from our previous study of MK-410 and its sulphoxide and sulphone metabolites. Nevertheless, the concept of sulindac being a reversible pro-drug in man was firmly established only after extensive clinical pharmacological experiments[6].

II. RECENT DEVELOPMENTS

A. Pro-drugs

Some common side-effects of NSAIDs are clearly related to their biochemical mechanism(s) of action, notably the inhibition of arachidonic acid cyclo-oxygenase. These side-effects may be modulated to some extent by optimization of the pharmacodynamics of the drug. For instance, with recognizing the association of GI irritation with inhibition of prostaglandin synthesis, pro-drugs of NSAIDs conceivably should minimize the local disturbances of arachidonic acid metabolism in the gastric tissue. Various carboxyl derivatives of NSAIDs have now been investigated as possibly less irritating pro-drugs[5] (Figure 3). Unfortunately, since the metabolic activation process and the pharmacodynamics of the pro-drug and its active metabolite(s) vary in different species, uncertainty remains in the selection of best candidates for clinical trials and in the prediction of clinical efficacy vs. safety (therapeutic index).

Fenbufen was recognized as an irreversible pro-drug only at a late stage of its clinical trial after detailed metabolic studies in man as well as in animals. The correlation of pharmacodynamics with its safety in man was further complicated by the formation of five metabolites in man[7] and up to eleven metabolites in five laboratory species[8] with different pharmacokinetic and pharmacological properties.

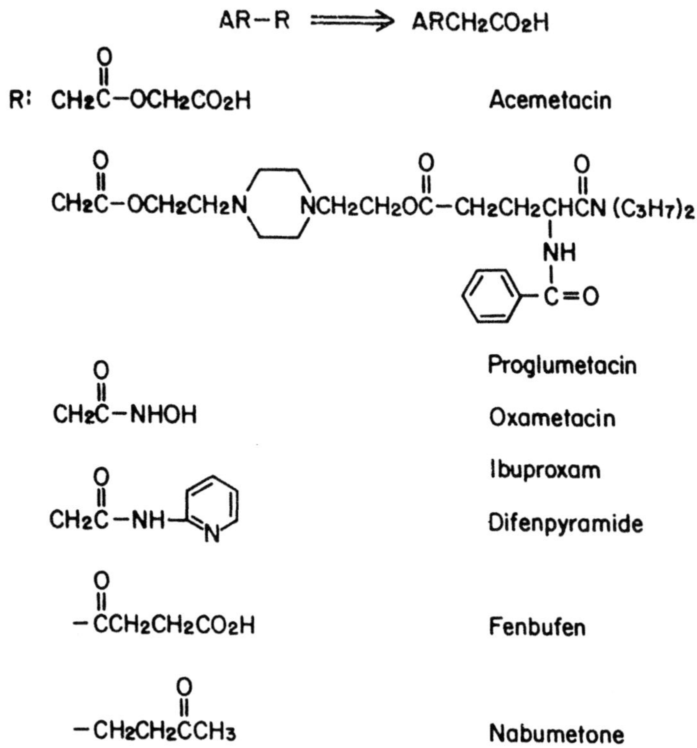

Figure 3 Carboxyl derivatives and metabolic precurcors of aryl acetic acids as irreversible pro-drugs.

With sulindac, the reversible nature of its reduction to the active sulphide metabolite (Figure 4) fortuitously led to the clinical observation that it causes less renal disturbance in patients with impaired renal function[9] and less interference with hypotensive therapy[10]. The local tissue levels of sulindac and its metabolites clearly would be influenced by their different tissue distribution characteristics and by the local oxidative and reductive enzyme capacities[11,12].

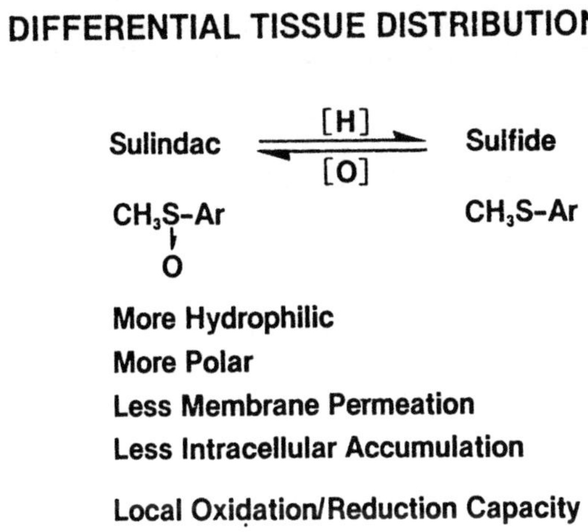

Figure 4 Reversible metabolic reduction and oxidation of sulindac and its active sulphide metabolite.

B. Diflunisal

From the biochemical point of view, knowing the transacetylation potential of aspirin, which irreversibly acetylate cyclo-oxygenase and possibly other macromolecules in vivo, the phenolic diflunisal was selected over other O-acetyl analogues in the series[13]. The addition of a difluorophenyl moiety to salicylic acid not only enhanced its intrinsic potency but also greatly altered its hydrophobicity, protein-binding, tissue distribution characteristics and, consequently, its pharmacodynamics (Figure 5).

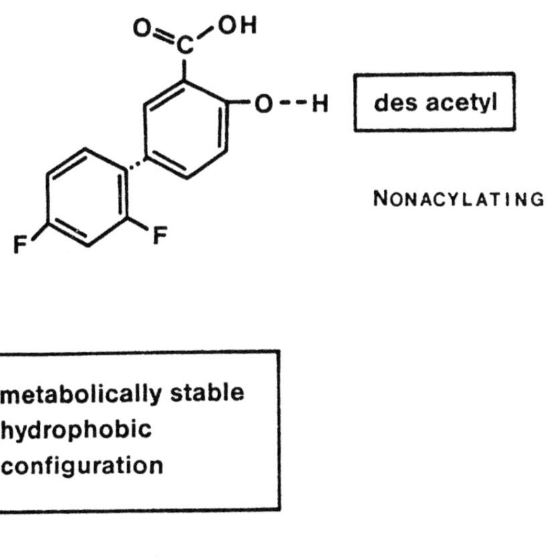

Figure 5 Difunisal as a non-acylating saliicylate.

These changes, presumably, contribute to the improved GI tolerance of diflunisal over aspirin in anti-inflammatory and analgesic therapy.

C. Osmosin (indomethacin GITS formulation)

Using a pharmaceutical approach, the peak and trough pharmacokinetics of indomethacin (t.i.d.) was smoothed to a steady plasma level for 10-12 hours with an innovative zero-order delivery device, the Alza minipump (GITS)[14]. Osmosin gave very encouraging efficacy and safety results in large-scale controlled clinical studies, but its general application was precluded by several unfortunate incidences.

Table 2 Different types of NSAIDs with relatively long duration of action (kinetics/metabolism)

1. Carboxylic pro-drug
Sulindac (reversible)
Fenbufen (degradative)
2. Enolic (slow conjugation)
oxicams: piroxicam, isoxicam, tenoxicam
3. Metabolically stable
Tiflamizole

D. Long half-life drugs

Prolongation of drug action is a desirable feature in anti-arthritic therapy. Naproxen and pro-drugs sulindac and fenbufen require b.i.d. or once-a-day regimen only. Retardation of metabolic inactivation, e.g. glucuronide formation, further prolonged the serum half-life of oxicams[15-17] and several newer NSAIDs (Table 2). The extraordinarily long half-life of tifamizole[18] (approximately 13 days in man) clearly demonstrated the chemical feasibility of achieving very long-acting drugs, if needed. On the other hand, special medical attention should be given to the potential safety and drug interactions of such very long-acting agents, especially in aged patients. The clinical trial of tifamizole was recently suspended because of its intolerance in patients.

E. Locally/topically active drugs

Conversely, with growing interest in developing anti-inflammatory agents for opthalmic, pulmonary and dermatological disorders, chemical structures with facile metabolism may be ideally suited for local and/or topical applications. The rapid metabolic inactivation should minimize their systemic side-effects. A group of 2-aryl oxazolopyridines was previously investigated as non-acidic anti-inflammatory analgesic agents[19]. Later study showed that modification of the phenyl substituents yielded new analogues with comparable topical or local activities, but are totally inactive systemically due to rapid and extensive metabolism (Table 3).

Table 3 Topical oxazolopyridine (OZP)(a total anti-inflammatory agent with minimal side-effects[20]

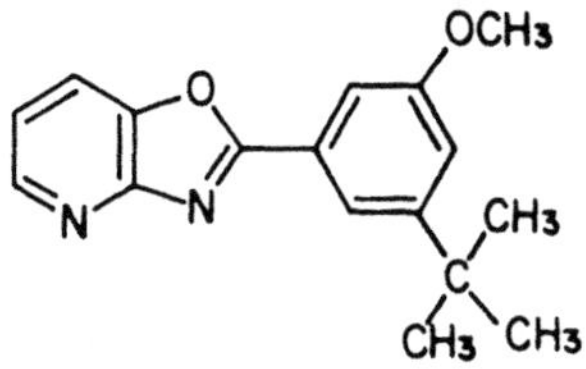

(OZP)

	OZP	IND
In vitro (IC_{50} μM)		
Cyclooxygenase	0.06	0.18
Mφ (PGE_2)	0.09	
Topical (μg/site)		
Rat ear	~220	~ 40
u.v. erythema (2 h)	~ 70	100
Local		
Carrag. oedema/granuloma	+	+
Gastric haemorrhage	>>180 mg/kg	
Extensive metabolism		

For example, the t-butyl methoxy derivative is comparable to indomethacin in the uv erythema assay after topical application but is devoid of GI side-effects[20]. A similar approach has been used successfully to develop other topical enzyme inhibitors or receptor antagonists.

III. EMERGING DEVELOPMENTS

In addition to toxicity-reduction via pharmacodynamics, emerging biochemical concepts have encouraged the development of dual cyclo-oxygenase/5-lipoxygenase inhibitors or the combination of cyclo-oxygenase inhibitors with cytoprotective agents, e.g. stable prostaglandin analogues, H2-receptor antagonists, etc. to reduce their side-effects. The clinical evaluation of these agents or combinations may shed further light on the merit of such biochemical approaches. Alternatively, achieving anti-inflammatory effect through the regulation of inflammatory or immunological mediators (or receptors) other than eicosanoids may also circumvent some common side-effects of current NSAIDs. The profile of a "perfect" NSAID was described by rheumatologist Dr Dudley Hart several years ago[21]:

> The perfect non-steroidal anti-inflammatory agent should be as potent as large doses of corticosteroids, but without their endocrine action. It should be as non-toxic as placebo, leaving the gastrointestinal tract unaffected at both ends and with no toxic effect on the blood, eye, liver or kidney. It should be compatible with other widely used drugs and must not diminish their action . . . . . It should not affect cerebration or mood and should be compatible with alcohol and all desirable food-stuffs. It is doubtful if it has ever been, or ever will be produced, even in Heaven.

Aiming toward that heavenly goal, medical chemists are hopeful that the current investigation of newer anti-inflammatory agents, with novel and specific biochemical and/or immunological mechanisms of action, may provide a new generation of disease-modifying NSAIDs with qualitatively distinct safety characteristics in the not-too-distant future.

REFERENCES

1. Sarett, LH, Patchett, AA and Steelman, S (1963). The effects of structural alteration on the anti-inflammatory properties of hydrocortisone. In: Jucker, E (ed.), Progess in Drug Research, vol. 5. (Basel: Birkhauser Verlag), p. 11
2. Nicholson, JS (1982). In: Bindra, JS and Lednicer, D (eds), Chronicles of Drug Discovery, vol. 1. (New York: Wiley), p. 149
3. Shen, TY and Winter, CA (1977). Chemical and biological studies on indomethacin, sulindac and their analogs. In: Simmonds, AB (ed.), Advances in Drug Research, vol. 12. (New York: Academic Press), p. 89
4. Scherrer, RA (1974). Aryl- and heteroarylcarboxylic acids. In: Scherrer, RA and Whitehouse, MW (eds), Anti-inflammatory Agents, Medicinal Chemical Monographs, vol. 13-1. (New York: Academic Press), p. 45
5. Shen, TY (1984). The proliferation of non-steroidal anti-inflammatory drugs (NSAIDs). In: Parnham, MJ and Bruinvels, J (eds), Discoveries in Pharmacology, vol. 2. (Amsterdam: Elsevier), p. 523
6. Duggan, DE, Hooke, KF, Risley, EA, Shen, TY and Van Arman, CG (1977). Indentification of the biological active form of sulindac. J Pharmacol Exp Ther, 201, 8
7. Chiccarelli, FS, Eisner, HJ and Van Lear, GE (1980). Metabolic and pharmacokinetic studies with fenbufen in man. Arzneim Forsch, 30, 728
8. Chiccarelli, FS, Eisner, HJ and Van Lear, GE (1980). Disposition and metabolism of fenbufen in several laboratory animals. Arzneim Forsch, 30, 707
9. Ciabattoni, G, Cinotti, GA, Pierucci, A, Simonetti, BM, Manzi, M, Pugliese, F, Barsotti, P, Pecci, G, Taggi, F and Patrono, C (1984). Effects of sulindac and ibuprofen in patients with chronic glomerular disease. N Engl J Med, 310 (5), 279
10. Salvetti, A, Pedrinelli, R, Alberici, P, Magagna, A and Abdelhad, B (1984). The influence of indomethacin and sulindac on some pharmacological actions of atenolol in hypertensive patients. Br J Clin Pharmacol,17, 108
11. Ratnayake, JH, Hanna, PE, Anders, MW and Duggan, DE (1981). Sulfoxide reduction - in vitro reduction of sulindac by rat hepatic cytosolic enzymes.

Drug Metab Disposition, 9 (2), 85
12. Light, DR, Waxman, DJ and Walsh, C (1982). Studies on the chirality of sulfoxidation catalyzed by bacterial flavoenzyme cyclohexanone mono-oxygenase and hog liver flavin adenine dinucleotide containing mono-oxygenase. Biochemistry, 21, 2490
13. Shen, TY (1983). Chemical and pharmacological properties of diflunisal. Pharmacotherapy, 3 (2), 3S
14. Roger, JD, Lee, RB, Souder, PR, Ferguson, RK, Davies, RO, Theeuwes, F and Kwan, KC (1983). Pharmacokinetic evaluation of osmotically controlled indomethacin delivery systems in man. Int J Pharmacol, 16, 191
15. Wiseman, EH, Lombardino, JG, Holmes, CL and Perraud, L (1981). Piroxicam. In: Goldberg, ME (ed.), Pharmacological and Biochemical Properties of Drug Substances, vol. 3. (Wasington: Am Pharm Assoc), p. 324
16. Downie, WW, Gluckman, MI, Ziehmer, BA and Boyle, JA (1984). Isoxicam. Clin Rheum Dis, 10, 385
17. Valdes, EF, Barclay, CA and Traballi, CA (1985). Tenoxicam, a novel long-acting anti-inflammatory and analgesic drug of the oxicam class - double-blind comparative study with piroxicam in patients with gona or coxarthrosis. Cur Ther Res Clin Exp, 37, 937
18. Narhi, D, Dromgoole, SH, Rakestraw, DC and Paulus, HE (1984). Tiflamizole elimination from plasma in rheumatoid arthritis. Clin Pharm Ther, 36, 92
19. Clark, RL, Pessolano, AA, Witzel, B, Lanza, T and Shen, TY (1978). 2-(Substituted phenyl)oxazolo [4,5-b]pyridines and 2-(substituted phenyl)-oxazolo [5,4-b]pyridines as nonacidic anti-inflammatory agents. J Med Chem, 21, 1158
20. Bonney, RJ, Olson, BJ, Bach, T, Beveridge, G, Goldenberg, MM, Gitterman, CO, Humes, JL, Lu, AYH, Hucker, H, Dougherty, H and Jensen, N (1985). 2-[3-(1,1-Dimethylethyl)-5-methoxyphenyl]oxazolo [4,5-b]pyridine, a new topical anti-inflammatory and analgesic compound lacking systemic activity and gastric side effects. Arzneim Forsch, 35, 715
21. Hart, FD and Huskisson, EC (1984). Non-steroidal anti-inflammatory drugs: current status and rational therapeutic use. Drugs, 27, 232

Discussion

Dr K Crowshaw, UK: I work for the Ono Pharmaceutical Company and we do have one or two agents which are not specifically free radical scavengers. One of the number is ONO-31/44, and we have another one, ONO-31/22. These agents actually accelerate the conversion of PGG_2, which is an endoperoxide in the pathway of prostaglandin formation to the hydroxy-compound, PGH_2, and the consequence of this is a follow up from the earlier suggestions by Khuel, who said that these free radicals arising from this pathway might well be one of the nasty agents in inflammatory disease. They looked encouraging in animal tests. We are still working on them and I don't have any further information, but they were an interesting extension of some earlier suggestions. I certainly would dearly love to see them prove successful just from the mechanistic point of view, because they are so novel.

Even though they look to be anti-inflammatories if you put them in animal tests, if you measure prostaglandin formation you see large increases of PGE_2 and increases of prostacyclin even though in the animals, they looked to be classical non-steroidal anti-inflammatory agents. Quite interesting!

Professor Parke, UK: Yes. I think you'll find radicals all over the place long before that. I mean, radicals occur in the experimental animal even before you get prostaglandin release or arachidonic release from membranes so it's characteristic of this whole field.

Dr Crowshaw: Well, we've had a few reports that people who've looked at them as typical radical scavengers don't find much activity, which is why I was at pains to say at the beginning they are not general radical scavengers. They do seem to be more specific in that they act within the enzyme pathways that I described.

Dr MW Whitehouse, Australia: You gave us a tantalising glimpse of the oxalapyridines. Do these inhibit cyclo-oxygenase and do you also get the GI toxicity as a consequence?

Dr Shen: As I mentioned that the oxalapyridines the one I showed is a cyclo-oxygenase inhibitor, but it is very quickly metabolised in vivo so therefore it has no GI side effects systemically but still it is effective as an anti-inflammatory agent.

19
Genetic and environmental aspects of drug metabolism relevant to side-effects in arthritic disease

AL Parke* and DV Parke*
*Division of Rheumatic Diseases, University of Connecticut Health Center, Farmington, Connecticut, USA
**Department of Biochemistry, University of Surrey, Guildford, Surrey GU2 5XH, UK

CONTENTS

I. INTRODUCTION

The adverse reactions of a drug are not exclusively due to any inherent toxicity of the drug, but are also the result of the genetic make-up of the patient, the patient's environment and often the patient's disease. In the past, the major cause of adverse drug reactions has been attributed to the intrinsic activity of the drug, or to overdosage, and the contribution of the patient, his environment and his disease state has generally been neglected. In rheumatoid disease the illness is probably a major contributing factor, and some of the major causes of adverse drug reactions in this condition are given in Table 1.

Side-effects of Anti-inflammatory Drugs. Rainsford, KD and Velo, GP (eds)
Part 1: Clinical and Epidemiological Aspects. (Lancaster: MTP Press)

Table 1 Causes of adverse drug reactions in rheumatoid disease

Intrinsic drug toxicity

(a) Non-selective inhibition of eicosanoid biosynthesis results in gastrointestinal, renal and other toxicity.

Patient status

(a) Genetic polymorphism of oxidative drug metabolism may lead to drug accumulation and toxicity

(b) Inflammatory disease destroys the mixed-function oxidase, cytochrome P-450, and may increase cytochrome P-448 and the activation of drugs

(c) Inflammation depletes glutathione, impairing drug conjugation and oxygen radical detoxication[1,2]

(d) Elderly patients are common, and have impaired detoxication and excretion mechanisms

Patient environment

(a) Cytochrome P-448, which is induced by smoking and food pyrolysates, increases the formation of reactive intermediates

(b) Treatment with Fe may exacerbate oxygen radical formation and inflammation.

(c) Nutritional needs (sulphur amino acids, α-tocopherol, eicosapentaenoic acid) for drug detoxication are greater because of the generation of oxygen radicals associated with the disease.

Table 2 Role of cytochrome P-450

1. Generally leads to detoxication of drugs and chemicals
2. In conjuction with superoxide dismutase and catalase, detoxicates tissue oxygen
3. Is involved in biogenesis and deactivation of steroid hormones
4. Is involved in prostaglandin biosynthesis
5. Is induced by drugs and natural chemicals in the diet

Table 3 Differences between cytochromes P-450 and P-448

Cytochromes P-450	Cytochromes P-448
Isoenzymes all have same haem environment	Haem environment different from that of cytochrome P-450 species
Mostly present in liver and gut	Found in all tissues
Oxygenates small globular molecules	Oxygenates large planar molecules
Inserts oxygen into non-hindered positions	Inserts oxygen into hindered (bay-region) and non-hindered positions
Aldrin epoxidation is specific reaction	Ethoxyresorufin de-ethylase is specific reaction
Metyrapone is selective inhibitor	9-Hydroxyellipticine is selective inhibitor
Induced, with the reductase, by drugs	Induced, without reductase, by carcinogenic polycyclic hydrocarbons, smoking and TCDD
Activity increases after birth	Activity decreases after birth
Absent from placenta (not inducible)	Present in placenta (inducible)
Generally leads to detoxication	Activates carcinogens, mutagens and toxic chemicals

II. THE DETOXICATION AND ACTIVATION OF DRUGS AND THE ROLE OF MIXED FUNCTION OXIDASES

A. Oxidases

Drugs are generally deactivated and detoxicated, mostly in the liver, by the processes of biotransformation (oxygenations, oxidations, reductions) and conjugation (with glucuronic acid, sulphate, glutathione). In contrast, drugs, like carcinogens and other chemicals, may undergo metabolic activation to form electrophiles (reactive intermediates), which are not readily conjugated, and therefore react chemically with intracellular nucleophiles, such as proteins, thiol enzymes, glutathione (GSH), and DNA, resulting in toxicity manifested as cell death and necrosis, immunological injury, or mutations and malignancy (se Figure 1). Intracellular GSH is therefore a major defence against the reactive nucleophiles formed in the detoxication of drugs and chemicals, and also protects against the oxygen radicals formed during normal metabolism[1]. Hence, in rheumatoid disease and other conditions of chronic inflammation where the production of reactive oxygen is high, there is great demand for GSH, and the detoxication of drugs and chemicals may consequently be impaired. In this respect it is of interest that D-penicillamine results in an increase in intracellular GSH which correlates with the clinical response seen in rheumatoid arthritis patients[2].

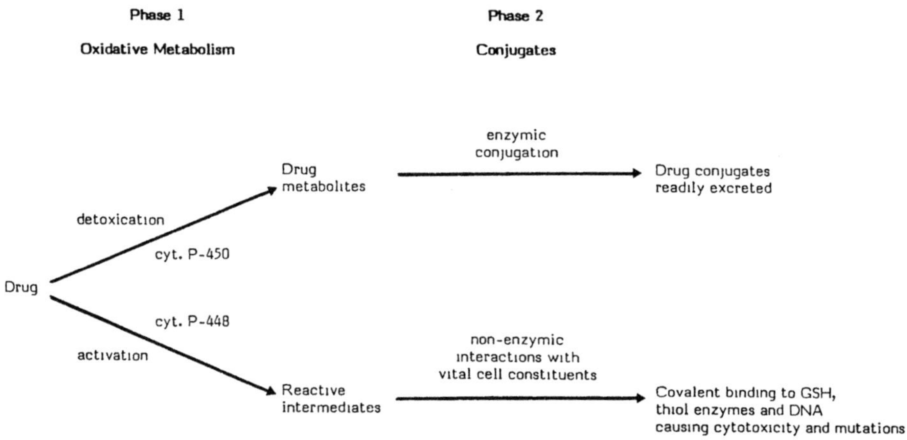

Figure 1 Pathways of detoxication and activation of drugs.

The major mode of biotransformation of drugs and other chemicals is oxygenation by the cytochrome P-450 system of the hepatic endoplasmic reticulum. The cytochromes P-450 comprise a family of isoenzymes with differing substrate specificities, which catalyse oxygenations of exogenous substrates (drugs and other chemicals) and endogenous substrates (fatty acids, sterols, steroids), and are responsible for the biosynthesis of many essential biomolecules, e.g. the steroid hormones and the eicosanoids (prostaglandins, prostacyclin)[3] (see Table 2).

It is now known that there are two distinctly different families of these cytochromes, namely the cytochrome P-450 family of isoenzymes, and the cytochromes P-448 (cytochromes P_1-450). These two families of cytochromes are structurally, functionally, and immunologically quite distinct; they are under different genetic regulation, have different tissue distributions, and exhibit different fetal/neonatal developments[3] (see Table 3).

The significance of the existence of two distinctly different fami-lies of microsomal cytochromes to drug toxicity and chemical carcinogenicity has only recently been recognized. The reason for past confusion between the cytochromes P-450 and P-448 has been due largely to the widespread use of non-specific substrates for the determination of the activities of these cytochromes (e.g. benzo(α)pyrene hydroxylase (AHH) and 7-ethoxycoumarin O-de-ethylase for cytochrome P-448). The development of an enzyme assay specific for cytochrome P-448, namely, the O-de-ethylation of

7-ethoxyresorufin (EROD), has now clarified the basic differences between these two cytochromes[4].

The cytochromes P-448 are distributed mostly in extrahepatic tissue, are exclusive to the placenta, have an affinity for large planar molecules, and insert oxygen in conformationally-hindered positions, resulting in the activation of carcinogens and toxic chemicals (see Table 3). Because of the insertion of oxygen into conformationally-hindered positions, subsequent conjugation is difficult, and the resulting reactive intermediates therefore react non-enzymically with intracellular nucleophiles, which is the basis of chemical toxicity (see Figure 1). In contrast the cytochrome P-450 family of isoenzymes have their highest concentration in the liver and the gastrointestinal tract, they have an affinity for more globular molecules, and catalyse the insertion of oxygen into conformationally non-hindered positions of the substrate molecule, giving products which are readily conjugated, thereby resulting in the eventual detoxication of the drugs and other chemicals[5].

From these recent developments it has been deduced that cytochromes P-448 preferentially activate a certain type of chemical molecule leading to chemical toxicity and carcinogenicity[6]. By computer graphic studies of the X-ray crystallographic data of the structure of specific substrates, inhibitors, and inducing agents of the two families of cytochrome isoenzymes, it has been possible to define the molecular parameters characteristic of the active sites of the cytochromes P-450 and cytochromes P-448, respectively[5]. Furthermore, from these computer graphic measurements, and studies of the potential induction of cytochromes P-448 in vivo from determination of EROD activity in tissue homogenates, it has been possible to identify drugs and other chemicals which have potential toxicity and carcinogenicity.

The inductions of these two different families of cytochromes are also quite distinct, the cytochromes P-450 being induced by the administration of a variety of drugs and chemicals, including the barbiturates, phenytoin and DDT, whereas the cytochromes P-448 are induced by chemical carcinogens, (e.g. benzo(α)pyrene, 3-methylcholanthrene), food pyrolysis products (Tryp-P-1), and by a variety of halogenated chemicals such as Arochlor and TCDD[6]. More recent studies have indicated that cytochromes P-448 are induced by tobacco smoke and by diets high in cooked meat such as charcoal-broiled steaks, whereas the cytochromes P-450 are induced by a variety of substituted indoles and other chemicals mostly found in fresh vegetables[5]. Some of the chemicals known to be activated by the cytochromes P-488, and their molecular dimensions, are shown in

Table 4. Substrates and inducing agents of cytochromes P-488 (e.g. benzo(α)pyrene and ethoxyresorufin) have high area/depth ratios (planar molecules), while subtrates and inducers of cytochromes P-450 have small area/depth ratios (globular molecules).

Table 4 Molecular dimensions of drugs and chemicals activated by cytochrome P-448

Molecule	Function	Length (Å)	Width (Å)	Depth (Å)	Area/depth Ratio
Benzo(α)pyrene	Carcinogen and inducer of P-448	13.6	9.0	3.2	38
Ethoxyresorufin	Specific substrate for P-448	14.6	9.1	3.9	34
Trp-P-1	Food pyrolysis product and P-448 inducer	12.6	9.1	4.2	27
Phenacetin	Analgesic metabolised by P-448	14.1	8.9	5.4	23
Paracetamol	Analgesic metabolically activated by P-448	11.6	7.3	4.2	20
Aldrin	Specific substrate for P-450	10.0	9.0	9.0	10

B. Toxicity of paracetamol

The widely used analgesic paracetamol is generally considered to be a very safe drug, unless given in excessive dosage. The reason for its toxicity is that paracetamol may undergo metabolic activation to form the corresponding quinoneimine[7], which interacts with intracellular glutathione (GSH) per se or may generate oxygen radicals which are then detoxicated by intracellular GSH[8] (see Figure 2). Whichever mechanism is involved, the ultimate event is the oxidation of intracellular GSH to GSSG, thereby removing the ultimate intracellular redox buffer, and the last cellular protection against oxidative damage by free radicals and oxidants. Depletion of cellular glutathione has been associated with an increase in carcinogenicity, either due to removal of the natural protection against DNA damage by free radicals, or by non-genotoxic mechanisms involving lack of protection against the damage of membranes and other vital intracellular macromolecules by free radicals.

The cytochrome P-488-specific activation of paracetamol is shown in Figure 3. As this activation is effected only by cytochrome P-448[7], by free radicals arising from prostaglandin biosynthesis, inflammation, or the specific cytochrome P-450 induced by alcohol, the toxicity of paracetamol is likely to be increased by smoking, the consumption of burnt food, or excessive alcohol, or exposure to TCDD, Arochlor, etc., as well as by chronic inflammatory conditions[9]. Administered repeatedly at high dosage, it may result in chronic depletion of intracellular

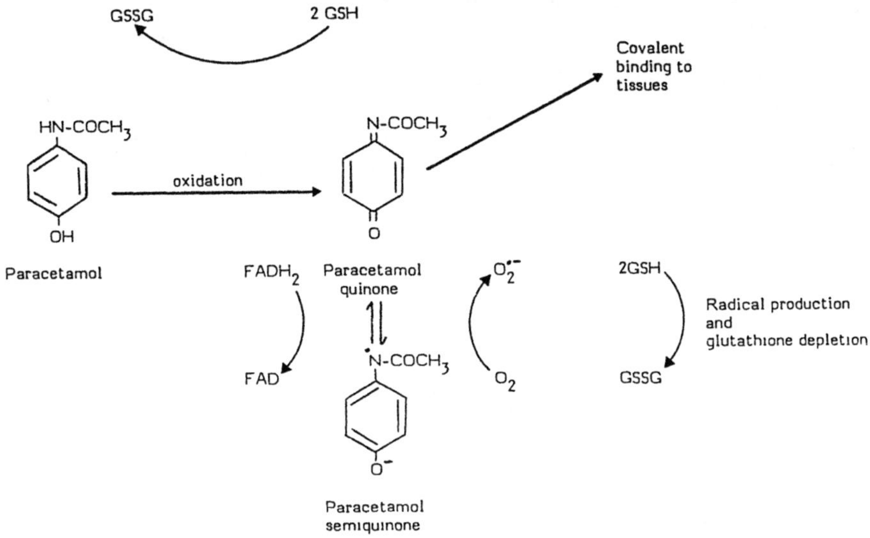

Figure 2 Activation of paracetamol and mechanisms of its toxicity.

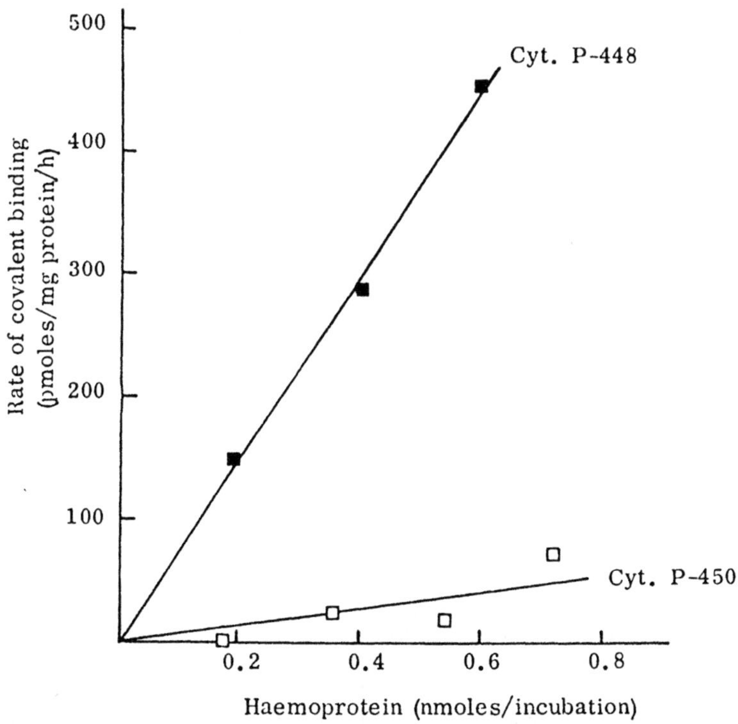

Figure 3 Activation of paracetamol by purified cytochrome P-448 (■---■) and cytochrome P-450 (□---□).

glutathione, which results in chronic toxicity to the hepatocytes and hepatic necrosis, or to malignancy, by its GSH-depleting co-carcinogen action.

Although there have been no equivocal human studies, there are indications that the toxicity of paracetamol may exhibit genetic polymorphism, as other drug oxidative polymorphisms are associated with cytochrome P-488-like activity[10]. Paracetamol is widely used as a non-steroidal anti-inflammatory analgesic by arthritic patients, although its safety has been questioned. In an attempt to avoid critical loss of intracellular hepatic GSH, already considerably depleted by the inflammatory disease, several companies are introducing combination products of paracetamol with methionine and other sources of sulphur amino acids. The combination of paracetamol with dextropropoxyphene, marked as Distalgesic, has also been criticized in terms of its safety, but a recent study conducted by us among rheumatoids and arthritics, who had been taking substantial amounts of Distalgesic for periods up to 5 years, showed that there was no loss of hepatic function, as measured by the highly sensitive and reliable parameter of prealbumin biosynthesis[31].

III. GENETIC POLYMORPHISMS OF DRUG OXIDATIONS

Genetic polymorphisms of drug metabolism in human populations have long been known, and include the "slow" and "fast" acetylators of isoniazid, etc., the "fast" and "slow" deactivators of suxamethonium, etc., and the wide range of activities of glucose-6-phosphate dehydrogenase, an enzyme essential for formation of NADPH, the oxidative metabolism of drugs, the reduction of GSH, and the maintenance of erythrocyte integrity in the presence of oxidants.

The past decade or so has witnessed the recognition of another type of genetic polymorphism, namely, the "extensive" and "poor" metabolizers of debrisoquine (EM_D and PM_D), a drug metabolically deactivated by hydroxylation, a reaction which shows a bimodal distribution in human populations[11]. A number of other drugs, e.g. sparteine, bufuralol, etc., show a similar genetic polymorphism, associated with an aberration of the same mixed-function oxidase enzyme, now known to be an isoenzyme of cytochrome P-450[12,13]. A different type of genetic polymorphism in drug oxidation is shown by propranolol, and this is now considered to be associated with an abnormailty of a different isoenzyme of cytochrome P-450 (see Table 5).

These genetically impaired drug hydroxylations result in the progressive accumulation of the unchanged parent drug, and in some circumstances can give rise to drug toxicity, likely to be associated with idiosyncratic instances of adverse drug reactions. The oxidative metabolism of nortriptyline has recently been correlated closely with the oxidative metabolism of desmethylimipramine, debrisoquine hydroxylation and 7-ethoxyresorufin O-de-ethylase activity, so that all of these activities might be associated with cytochrome P-448[10].

Table 5 Human polymorphisms of drug oxidations

Genetic polymorphism	Oxidative enzyme	Identity with Debrisoquine
Debrisoquine	Debrisoquine 4-hydroxylase	+
Sparteine	Sparteine Δ^5-oxidase	+
Bufuralol	Bufuralol 1-hydroxylase	+
Desmethylimipramine	Desmethylimipramine 2-hydroxylase	+
Nortriptyline	Nortriptyline 10-hydroxylase	±
Encainide	Encainide O-demethylase	±
Propranolol	Propranolol 4-hydroxylase	-
Phenacetin (?)	Phenacetin O-de-ethylase	-

Data from references 10 and 13

Although a genetic polymorphism of cytochrome P-448 is well known in mice, and has been strongly indicated in man, though there is as yet no unequivocal evidence of this. Idle has found some correlation between debrisoquine hydroxylation and the spontaneous incidence of carcinoma of the respiratory tract[14]. Other workers have also claimed correlations between the incidence of cancer and the inducibility of benzo(α)pyrene hydroxylase (AHH) in human leucocytes[15]. As cytochrome P-448 is associated particularly with the activation of carcinogens, and also with an increase in AHH activity, this might be considered as circumstantial evidence of a genetic variation in cytochrome P-448. A genetic polymorphism in cytochrome P-448 activity would not only explain the observed genetic differences in the spontaneous incidence of cancer, but would also account for idiosyncratic instances of drug toxicity, including allergic reactions. For not only does cytochrome P-448 activate drugs and other chemicals to reactive intermediates that may covalently bid to DNA hence causing malignancy, but these may also bind to proteins to form antigens with consequent immunological injury.

IV. CYTOCHROME P-450 ACTIVITIES IN RHEUMATOID PATIENTS

The cytochromes P-450 are rapidly destroyed by free radicals such as hydroxyl radical and singlet oxygen, and this is accelerated by the presence of inorganic iron. Indeed, the role of inorganic iron is so critical that production of active oxygen (hydroxyl radical and singlet oxygen) from superoxy anion and peroxide may not occur in its absence. Conditions of chronic inflammation, such as rheumatoid disease, are associated with a high rate of production of oxygen radicals, the destruction of tissues and the denaturation of cytochrome P-450 to P-420, haem and Fe. In experimental chronic polyarthritis, induced in rat with Freund's complete adjuvant, the resulting biphasic inflammation and foot-pad oedema is preceded by the sequential production of oxygen radicals (peroxide, hydroxyl radical) and is accompanied by increased tissue levels of singlet oxygen malondialdehyde, prostaglandins PGE_2 and 6-oxo $PGF_{1\alpha}$ and thromboxane TBX_2[16,17].

Animals with adjuvant arthritis are characterized by low levels of cytochrome P-450 in their livers and other tissues, and low rates of drug metabolism[18-21] (see Table 6). Iron metabolism is abnormal in rheumatoid patients, with accelerated plasma clearance and excessive tissue deposition of iron. The concentration of iron salts in rheumatoid synovial fluid correlates with lipid peroxidation (measured by the thiobarbituric acid test) and rheumatoid disease activity[22]. Although destruction of cytochrome P-450, or a high rate of turnover of this enzyme, have not been demonstrated explicitly in rheumatoid patients the high rate of production of reactive oxygen species makes this highly probable. This is also the likely cause of the accumulation of Fe in the synovial membrane and fluid, thereby catalysing the further formation of oxygen radicals and lipid peroxidation. Moreover, the iron may also attract inflammatory leucocytes, as these have iron-binding receptors, thus further augmenting the production of reactive oxygen species and the process of inflammation[23].

Table 6 Changes in liver cytochrome P-450 and related parameters in adjuvant arthritic rats

Parameter	Controls	Arthritic	
Cytochrome P-450	0.41±0.04	0.15±0.06	(19)
(nmol/mg protein)	0.45	0.07	(21)
Aminopyrine N-demethylase (μmol HCHO/h per g liver)	9.8±0.6	2.0±0.7	(19)
Propoxyphene N-demethylase (μmol HCHO/h per g liver)	2.2	0.16	(21)
Cyclophosphamide hydroxylation (μmol metabolite/h per mg protein)	21±14	3±0.4 to 7±6	(18)
Haem synthesis (^{14}C glycine dpm/mg protein)	24±3	20±5	(19)

Rats were 14 to 15 days treated.

Data from references 18, 19, and 21, as shown in parenthesis.

Unfortunately, it is often generally assumed that the anaemia of rheumatoid patients is due to a deficiency of iron and an inability to synthesize haem and haemoglobin, so that the condition is frequently treated by the administration of inorganic iron. This could accelerate the production of oxygen radicals, resulting in further denaturation of cytochrome P-450 and increase turnover of haem, haemoglobin and cytochromes, with increasing accumulation of tissue levels of non-haem iron. Treatment of animal models of inflammation with high intraperitoneal doses of the iron chelator, desferrioxamine, results in suppression of inflammation. Further studies in vitro have indicated that desferrioxamine inhibits iron-catalysed lipid peroxidation only when it is poorly saturated with iron, and this effect is lost as the iron saturation of desferrioxamine increases[24]. The administration of iron may further exacerbate this situation and may worsen the clinical condition of the patient. From other studies, where a high turnover of cytochrome P-450 and other haem proteins has been identified, due to the chronic administration of cytochrome P-450-inducing drugs, the associated nutritional deficiency is that of folic acid, not iron.

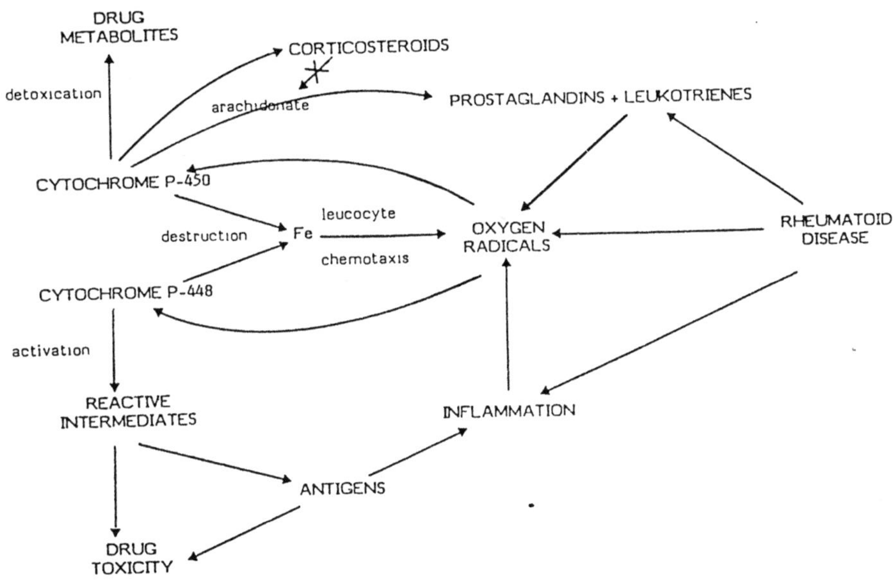

Figure 4 Scheme showing the involvement of cytochromes P-450 and P-448 in drug toxicity in rheumatoid conditions.

Cytochrome P-450 is involved in the biosynthesis of the eicosanoids (prostaglandins and prostacyclin)[25,26], whereas the production of the leukotrienes, involving lipid peroxidation, probably does not require cytochrome P-450. Cytochrome P-450 is also involved in the biosynthesis of the corticosteroid hormones, which is related to the activity of phospholipase A, the release of arachidonate from the phospholipids of the endoplasmic reticulum, and the synthesis of various families of eicosanoids. Deficiency of cytochromes P-450 will therefore result in impaired corticosteroid biosynthesis, increased arachidonate release, enhanced leukotriene formation, lipid peroxidation, inflammatory response, and oxygen radical formation, which in turn would further accelerate the destruction of the cytochromes P-450. These complex interrelationships concerning the many roles of cytochromes P-450 and P-448 are shown in Figure 4. As the total mixed function oxidase cytochromes are destroyed, the cytochromes P-448 tend to predominate, probably because they are more stable to denaturation by oxygen radicals. Hence, in situations of chemical injury such as carbon disulphide poisoning, in chronic inflammation as in rheumatoid disease, and in malignant cell transformation, the intracellular cytochrome P-450/P-448 concentration is progressively depleted with an increasing predominance of the cytochromes P-448. Inflammatory conditions therefore tend to increase the tissue activities of cytochrome P-448, with a simultaneous increase in the activation of drugs and toxic chemicals, possibly to decrease still further the intracellular glutathione, and to increase the formation of reactive intermediates that bind to tissue proteins forming antigens or to DNA resulting in mutations with the possibility of malignancy.

Penicillamine toxicity is greater in rheumatoid arthritis than in Wilson's disease or cystinuria[27]. This toxicity is associated with impaired sulphoxidation of the penicillamine in rheumatoid patients, as is the presence of HLA-DR3, but these appear to be independent risk factors[28] (see Table 7). Sulphoxidation is catalysed by cytochrome P-450 or flavoprotein oxidoreductases, and the impaired sulphoxidation seen in rheumatoid disease may well be associated with decreased cytochrome P-450 activity.

Table 7 Drug and chemical toxicity in rheumatic disease

HLA Antigens	(i)	DR3 - gold and penicillamine toxicity
	(ii)	DR4 - hydralazine-induced lupus
	(iii)	DR5 - vinyl chloride disease
Acetylator status	Drug-induced lupus	
Sulphoxidation status	Pencillamine toxicity	
Disease state	Pencillamine toxicity more common in rheumatoid arthritis than in Wilson's disease	
Age	Benoxaprofen toxicity-impaired clearance	

Penicillamine may also induce autoimmune disease in susceptible individuals, and is capable of inducing autoantibodies to acetylcholine receptors, intra-epithelial cement substance, and basement membranes, with the consequent occurrence of myasthenia gravis, pemphigus, and Goodpasture's syndrome[29]. Penicillamine is also one of the few drugs capable of inducing autoantibodies to native double-stranded DNA. It is possible that increased tissue activity of cytochrome P-448 with consequent production of reactive intermediates, neo-antigen formation and DNA mutation may account for drug-induced antoimmune disease seen with drugs such as penicillamine, and for the increased drug toxicity seen in rheumatoid disease.

V. FUTURE PROSPECTS

Perhaps one way forward would be to use free radical scavengers and antioxidants as anti-rheumatoid drugs, or at least to attempt to break the vicious spiral of autoxidative cellular injury by inhibiting the biosynthesis of leukotrienes and other chemotactic agents which enhance the cellular response. If nutritional supplements are to be given for rheumatoid disease, folate and sulphur amino acids (methionine) might be considered to offset the high turnover of haem protein synthesis, α-tocopherol and ascorbate might be valuable as antioxidants, and eicosapentaenoic and docosahexaenoic acid would be valuable in limiting the production of leukotrienes and other eicosanoids from arachidonate[30].

REFERENCES

1. Hodgkiss, RJ, Jones, NR, Watts, ME and Woodcock, M (1984). Glutathione depletion enhances the lifetime of oxygen-reactive radicals in mammalian cells. Int J Radiat Biol, 46, 673
2. Munthe, E, Käss, E and Jellum, E (1981). D-Penicillamine-induced increase in intracellular glutathione correlating to clinical response in rheumatoid arthritis. J Rheumatol, 8, Suppl 7, 14
3. Parke, DV (1983). Survey of drug-metabolizing enzymes. Biochem Soc Trans, 11, 457
4. Phillipson, CE, Godden, PMM, Ioannides, C and Parke, DV (1984). Determination of cytochrome P-448 activity in biological tissues. Biochem J, 221, 81
5. Parke, DV, Ioannides, C, Iwasake, K and Lewis, DF (1985). Microsomal enzymes and toxicity-conclusions. In: Boobis AR et al. (eds), Microsomes and Drug Oxidations (London: Taylor & Francis), p 402
6. Ioannides, C, Lum, PY and Parke, DV (1984). Cytochrome P-448 and the activation of toxic chemicals and carcinogens. Xenobiotica, 14, 119
7. Steele, CM, Masson, HA, Battershill, JM, Gibson, GG and Ioannides, C (1983). Metabolic activation of paracetamol by highly purified forms of cytochrome P-450. Res Commun Chem Path Pharmacol, 40, 109
8. Mitchell JR, Jollow, DJ, Potter, WZ, Gillette, JR and Brodie, BB (1973). Acetaminophen-induced hepatic necrosis. IV. Protective role of glutathione. J Pharmacol, Exp Ther, 187, 211
9. Parke DV and Ioannides, C (1984). Reactive intermediates and oxygen toxicity in liver injury. In: Keppler D et al. (eds), Mechanisms of Hepatocyte Injury and Death, Falk Symposium No 38 (Lancaster: MTP Press), p 37
10. von Bahr, C, Birgersson, C, Morgan, ET, Eriksson, Ö, Göransson, Spina, E and Woodhouse K (1986). Oxidation of tricyclic antidepressant drugs, debrisoquine and 7-ethoxyresorufin in human livers in vitro, Xenobiotica, 16, 391
11. Smith, RL (1985). Genetic polymorphisms of drug oxidation in man. In: Boobis AR et al. (eds), Microsomes and Drug Oxidations, (London: Taylor & Francis),

p 349

12. Boobis, AR, Murray, S, Hampden, CE, Harries, GC, Huggett, AC, Thorgeirsson, SS, McManus, ME and Davies, DS (1985). Enzymic basis for polymorphisms of drug oxidation in man. In: Boobis AR et al. (eds) Microsomes and Drug Oxidations (London: Taylor & Francis), p 361
13. Guengerich, FP, Distlerath, LM, Reilly, PEB, Wolff, T, Shimada, T, Umbenhauer, DR and Martin MV (1986). Human liver cytochromes P-450 involved in polymorphisms of drug oxidation. Xenobiotica, 16, 367
14. Ayesh, R and Idle, FR (1985). Evaluation of drug oxidation phenotypes in the biochemical epidemiology of lung cancer risk. In: Boobis AR et al. (eds) Microsomes and Drug Oxidations. (London: Taylor and Francis), p 340
15. Kouri, RE, McKinney, CE, Levine, AS, Edwards, BK, Vesell, ES, Nebert, DW and McLemore, TL (1984). Variations in aryl hydrocarbon hydroxylase activities in nitrogen-activated human and non-human primate lymphocytes. Toxicol Pathol, 12, 44
16. Dowling, EJ, Jasani, MK, Parke, DV, Peters, RF and Symons, AM (1985). Free radicals, lipid peroxidation and prostaglandins during the development and maintenance of foot-pad oedema in the Koch model. Br J Pharmacol, 84 35P
17. Dowling, EJ, Jasani, MK, Parke, DV, Peters, RF, and Symons, AM (1985). Characterisation of ex-vivo luminol-amplified chemiluminescence accompanying the initiation of foot-pad oedema in the Koch model. Br J Pharmacol, 84, 79P
18. Beck FJ and Whitehouse, MW (1973). Effect of adjuvant disease in rats on cyclophosphamide and isophosphamide metabolism. Biochem Pharmacol, 22, 2453
19. Cawthorne, MA, Palmer, DE and Green, J (1976). Adjuvant-induced arthritis and drug-metabolizing enzymes. Biochem Pharmacol, 25, 2683
20. Mathur, PP, Smyth, RD, Witmer, CM and Carr, GS (1978). Effects of a non-steroidal anti-inflammatory agent and phenobarbital on hepatic microsomal mono-oxygenases in adjuvant disease in the rat. Boichem Pharmacol, 27, 1771
21. Morton, DM and Chatfield, DH (1970). The effects of adjuvant-induced arthritis on the liver metabolism of drugs in rats. Biochem Pharmacol, 19, 473
22. Rowley, D, Gutteridge, JMC, Blake, D, Farr, M and Halliwell, B (1984) Lipid peroxidation in rheumatoid arthritis: thiobarbituric acid-reactive material and catalytic iron salts in synovial fluid from rheumatoid patients. Clin Sci, 66, 691
23. Blake, DR, Hall, ND, Bacon, PA, Dieppe, PA, Halliwell, B and Gutteridge, JMC (1981). The importance of iron in rheumatoid disease. Lancet 2, 1142
24. Blake, DR, Hall, ND, Bacon, PA, Dieppe, PA, Halliwell, B and Gutteridge, JMR (1983). Effect of a specific iron chelating agent on animal models of inflammation. Ann Rheum Dis, 42, 89,
25. Williams, DE, Hale, SE, Okita, RT and Masters, BSS (1984). A prostaglandin α-hydroxylase cytochrome P-450(P-450_{PG-}) purified from lungs of pregnant rabbits. J Biol Chem, 259, 14600
26. Capdevilla, J, Marnett, LJ, Chacos, N, Prough, RA and Estabrook, RW (1982). Cytochrome P-450-dependent oxygenation of arachidonate to hydroxyicosatetraenoic acids. Proc Natl Acad Sci USA, 79, 767
27. Lancet, (1975). D-penicillamine in rheumatoid arthritis. Leading article, Lancet, 1, 1123,
28. Emery, P, Panayi, GS, Huston, G, Welsh, KI, Mitchell, SC, Shah, RR, Idle, JR, Smith, RL and Waring, RH (1984). D-Penicillamine induced toxicity in rheumatoid arthritis: the role of sulphoxidation status and HLA-DR3, J Rheumatol, 11, 626
29. Lyle, WH (1979). Penicillamine. In: Clinics in Rheumatic Diseases, No. 5. (London: Saunders)

30. Lee, TH, Hoover, RL, Williams, JD, Sperling, RI, Ravalese, J, Spur, BW, Robinson, DR, Corey, EJ, Lewis, RA and Austen, KF (1985). Effect of dietary enrichment with eicosapentaenoic and docosahexaenoic acids on in vitro neutrophil and monocyte leukotriene generaton and neutrophil function. N Engl J Med, 312, 1217

31. Hutchinson, DR, Childs, AKS, and Parke, DV (1986). Liver function in patients on long-term paracetamol (co-proxamol) analgesia. J Pharm Pharmacol, 38, 242

Discussion

Professor J Dequeker, Belgium: This is not really a question, just a little comment about the associated between the HLA-typing DR3 and gold and D-penicillamine toxicity. I think the association is not so strong as it has been suggested. There have been may other duplications coming later on with larger studies, systematic studies which could not show this association or showed it in a very low proportion, but I will elaborate on this this afternoon in my paper on immuno-genetics.

Professor Parke: I certainly agree that there's controversy in the literature.

Dr G Wormsley, UK: NSAIDs frequently give rise to gastro-intestinal troubles and we often use drugs like cimetidine to treat the ulcer disease that results. How does cimetidine affect the two cytochrome P's.

Professor Parke: Cimetidine is a much more specific inhibitor of P-448 than P-450. In other words it's probably the best drug to use.

Dr K Crowshaw, UK: Just a small point please. On the last slide, under dietary supplements you have I think eicosapentaenoic acid. I just wonder if you could explain why you have that there?

Professor Parke: There has been quite a lot of work recently, looking at the role of diet in the inflammatory arthritides, and you may or may not be familiar with some of this evidence. There has been quite a lot of work to show that, in animals, if you supplement their diets with eicosapentaenoic acid there are changes in their rates of prostaglandin synthesis.

Dr Crowshaw: Yes, I am familiar with that, but I think that further up the slide, you suggest that some of the biosynthetic pathways for prostaglandins are impaired in rheumatoid arthritis, so the same enzymes which you want to use to convert the eicosapentaenoic acid products, may be impaired.

Professor Parke: No. There are two control mechanisms on arachidonic oxygenation. One is the corticosteroids and the other is the eicosapentaenoic and docosahexaenoic acids. Even if their metabolism is impaired, if these are present, they will make the corresponding eicosanoid analogues, which are much less toxic than the leukotrienes. Analogues from those two polyunsaturates are much less toxic than arachidonic acid. As we attempted to show, arthritis and the drug-toxicity associated with it, is a very complex series of events and I think the eicosa-acids would restore part of the balance.

Dr J Lunec, UK: I think you mentioned that cytochrome P-450 was more reactive with hydroxyl radical. Is that correct?

Professor Parke: Not more reactive, but is more easily destroyed. If you expose animals (and I think this work has only been done in animals), if you expose animals to radical generating mechanisms such as iron nitrilotriacetate acid, or peroxide, or xanthine-oxidase, you will find that the cytochrome P-450 is very rapidly destroyed in a matter of minutes - and the P-450 activity and drug metabolizing activity drops very rapidly over some 20 minutes. If you expose the animals chronically to radical generators you will find that the P-450/P-448 ratio in the liver changes with the P-448 increasing and you can reach a situation where you only have P-448 there. The explanation that has been given for this is that P-448 is much more stable to free radical damage than P-450 and there is a massive increase as the body attempts to correct this disruption by increasing the rate of synthesis. In fact people have suggested that it is the free oxygen radical which is responsible for the induction of cytochrome P-450 and P-448, but you reach a situation where there is very little if any P-450 left and it's pretty well all P-448. This situation may - we don't know in humans - may pertain in some severe cases of inflammatory disease in humans.

Dr Lunec: Why should that be? With cytochrome P-450 - is there something inherently different about the structure compared to the others which makes it capable of acting on these radicals?

Professor Parke Yes, oh yes! That's the important thing, you see these two cytochromes have - they're both cytochromes but they have very different structures and functions. One doesn't have to have a 90% difference in structure to make a 100% difference in stability. The normal turnover of these two enzymes are very similar. It appears only in the presence of large concentrations of reactive oxygen free radicals that the P-450 is more easily destroyed. One sees this in a number of industrial disease states - carbon disulphide exposure causes loss of cytochrome P-450. This is associated with hypertension as you probably know, so P-450 is involved in the etiology of a whole series of human disease.

Dr Lunec: But proteins tend to have high reactivity with hydroxyl radicals often because they contain metals. The two cytochromes have iron but is it because the iron is on different sites than each of the cytochromes?

Professor Parke Yes. You may be getting near it, but they both contain iron as haem and the haem is in the active site pocket and the active sites of these two enzymes are the main differences. The rest of the molecule is very much the same. So you may have a very important point there and I think its the way the haem is liganded to the rest of the molecule. We could discuss this in more detail later if you like.

Professor JC Roujeau, France: Is it known if infectious disease, for example viral disease, alters cytochrome pathways?

Professor Parke No, it isn't. Another very interesting thing about cytochrome P-450 is that it is the binding site of the ribosomes for the synthesis of protein in the liver and the gastro-intestinal tract particularly, and these proteins are glyco-proteins. The first thing a virus does when it takes over a cell is to take over the glyco-protein synthesising equipment, so there may be some possible inter-relationship there but it hasn't been identified yet.

Dr A Callin, UK: Could I ask you to clarify the situation with the adjuvant rat model. You said that P-450 is reduced before the arthritic phase. Is this strain-dependent or is it after the adjuvant is given?

Dr A Parke, USA: It's after the adjuvant. It's as soon as the animals start to show evidence of inflammation so it seems to be related to the association with the oxygen radicals rather than the strain. I mean the mouse doesn't actually have to have arthritis, they even found it when they injected a microplasma intra-peritoneally in those animals. They did not actually have arthritis but they also had impairment of P-450.

Professor Parke: We've been making various kinds of adjuvant arthritis in animals and examining their paws by chemiluminescence and it's interesting that we see two bursts. The initial burst is of singlet oxygen formation which precedes any swelling. That's followed by stimulation of prostaglandin and leukotriene formation, and also peroxide formation, followed then by a second burst of hydroxyl radicals which is probably associated with the leucotactic effects of the first aspect of inflammation. P-450 is destroyed by the singlet oxygen in that first burst. It goes very, very quickly indeed. That's probably why you get it before the first manifestation of inflammation.

20
Disease-drug interactions: utility of the conditional concept for experimental pharmacology and toxicology in the context of inflammation

MW Whitehouse
Adelaide Rheumatology Research Group
c/o Department of Pathology
University of Adelaide
Adelaide, South Australia 5001

CONTENTS

> The most powerful antigen known to man is a new idea. **Wilfred Trotter**
>
> There is nothing new under the sun.
> **Jesus ben-Sirach**

I. THE "CONDITIONAL" CONCEPT

The discipline of physical chemistry has long recognized the non-ideality of the phenomena it describes, the behaviour and interactions of ions and molecules. Thus even the simplest mathematical

Side-effects of Anti-inflammatory Drugs. Rainsford, KD and Velo, GP (eds)
Part 1: Clinical and Epidemiological Aspects. (Lancaster: MTP Press)

description of the properties of gaseous molecules (P=RT/V) has to be modified by the Van der Waal's corrections, which allow for the intermolecular associations and other departures from ideal behaviour. This leads naturally to the concept of molecular "activity" for describing the effective quantity of a reagent and to allow for the various factors which cause the activity to be less than the concentration (except in the most dilute solutions). A third example of the chemist's critical recognition of a departure from ideal behaviour is provided by the use of a conditional association/ dissociation constant, K', to describe for example the binding of a metal ion (M^+) by a metal ligand (L^-). Since the experimental studies to measure $M^+:L^-$ interactions have of necessity to be conducted in non-ideal media, rarely at a standard temperature (0 °C), probably not at standard pressure, almost certainly with extraneous solutes (counterions to solubilize M^+ and L^- respectively and other additives to control pH); it is only realistic to accept the value of K' derived from such experiments as not an absolute constant and only invariable if the experimental conditions are adequately defined (by pH, ionic strength, temperature, solvent composition, etc.). Nevertheless such conditional constants are of immense practical value. Together with other chemical constants obtained under defined conditions (particularly pH), such as equilibrium constants for enzyme reactions or redox potentials for electron transfer reactions, they are invaluable for both interpreting and for making predictions about the chemistry of biological systems.

The idea I wish to stress here - and carry over to experimental toxicology from these simple physicochemical concepts - is that fruitful analyses of quite complex biosystems can be made that may not be absolute but are still immensely useful. Their value is, however, conditional, i.e. strictly determined by the experimental conditions, which must therefore be clearly defined. We are all aware that there is little hope of exactly reproducing any experimental observations, no matter how simple the test system, if the conditions of the experiment and the manner of recording the observations have been poorly defined. The "picture" that emerges from any enquiry into the natural universe is in fact "framed" by these conditions of experiment/observation. However, as we step back from the bench and try to integrate our mental picture(s) of a phenomenon with those made by others, the various conditional descriptors ("frames"), that ought to rightly surround these pictures, risk being lost - being thought cumbersome, inelegant or, worse still, irrelevant. This is strange because real pictures are rarely displayed or sold without a frame and the quality of the frame may enormously affect the visual impact of what it surrounds. A conditional constant is useless to a chemist if there is no allusion to the conditions for deriving it or implied sensitivity to some variable (pH, ionic strength, irradiation, altitude or whatever). Yet even the simplest of toxicological data, the LD_{50}, can be proffered with little or no reference to the many known factors influencing its numerical value such as sex, strain, diet, age, ambient temperature(s), light exposure, microbial and other infestation, physical stresses (noise, draughts, etc.), density of housing, environmental factors (feed additives, insecticides, deodorants, bedding used, etc.). Where these are so difficult to enumerate, or even identify, and rarely likely to be reproduced in toto, it seems more than expedient to procure a practical frame of reference - as for example, including the LD_{50} for a standard drug simultaneously derived under the same conditions. This would in essence calibrate the conditions, without having to define them in detail. The LD_{50} for the new/reported drug could then be seen as relative to the LD_{50} for the standard, the value of which could be quickly scrutinized for acceptability.

II. SOME APPLICATIONS OF THIS CONCEPT: PHARMACOLOGY OF INFLAMMATION (TABLE 1)

Table 1 Pharmaco-activity of some arthritic drugs (these illustrative examples are discussed briefly in the text)

1.	Antipyretics are only effective in fever <u>but</u> not hypothermic in normals
2.	Antimalarials inhibit leucocyte activation (with certain stimuli) <u>but</u> have no effect on leukocyte activation by other stimuli
3.	Sulphinpyrazone inhibits metabolism of some drugs <u>but</u> induces metabolism of others
4.	Aspirin increases bleeding time in most people <u>but</u> decreases bleeding time in Eskimos
5.	Aurothiomalate shows anti-arthritic, no, or pro-arthritic, activity in different rat strains

Five examples will be given to illustrate the concept that a frame of reference is often essential to give a complete "picture", i.e. convey a clear understanding, of a drug's behaviour. Failure to define the particular conditions that may determine the drugs properties will inevitably underrate, even falsify, the perception of a drug's potential for causing good or harm.

1. Antipyretic drugs are accepted as beneficial because they reduce only an elevated body temperature, not that of a normal subject/animal. Compounds which are hypothermic, i.e. indiscriminately reduce a fever and normal body temperature, are rightly regarded as toxins. Indiscriminate temperature reduction is not the quality required of an antipyretic but normalization of a fever is. These conditions of acceptability can be readily assessed in (a) sick, i.e. fevered, and (b) normal animals. By such differential screening tests the antipyretic is disclosed by only being effective in sick animals. (This same generalization would apply to a great many drugs of practical value.)

2. The antimalarial/antiarthritic quinoline/acridine drugs such as chloroqine and mepacrine show very selective effects in vitro on activated leucocytes. When cells such as peripheral blood monocytes are stimulated by opsonized zymosan or the chemotactic peptide, fMLP, membrane phospholipid methylation is induced and this is inhibited by these antimalarials in vitro. Unstimulated cells are not affected by these drugs. Other leucocyte stimulants, e.g. phorbol diesters, bypass this lipid-methylation step in inducing superoxide formation, arachidonate oxygenation, etc., and their effects are not counteracted by the antimalarials.

   This leucocyte-regulant property of these antimalarial is clearly determined by the nature of the leukocyte stimulant. The drug action is therefore selective, conditioned by whether phospholipid methylation is involved or not. Some of the anti-arthritic gold drugs show rather similar selectivity, acting at other stages involved in leukocyte activation but with their effects also depending upon the nature of the leukocyte activator. It is almost impossible to describe this type of leukocyte pharmacology without having to refer to how the leukocytes are stimulated.

3. This third example does not involve the pre-history of the test system determining a drug's response (as in examples 1 and 2) but presents a problem that comes "ready-made" in the clinic. Metabolic interactions between two or more drugs can be quite devastating and unfortunately are still not entirely predictable. They are due to induction or inhibition of drug-metabolizing enzymes, increasing or reducing drug clearance respectively. The problems arise because of the multitude of cytochrome P-450 oxygenases. Each has its own substrate selectivity, inhibitor sensitivity and induction pattern. So for example the uricosuric and antiplatelet durg, sulphinpyrazone, is a potent inhibitor of the oxidative metabolism of tolbutamide, warfarin and phenytoin but it is also a good inducer of the metabolism of theophylline, antipyrine and verapamil. This seemingly ambivalent property of the one drug, affecting the metabolism of other drugs in two contradistinct ways, can only be fully comprehended by referring to (a) which of the P-450 enzymes are involved, and (b) how their particular drug substrates might be affected.

4. In normal subjects, aspirin usually prolongs the bleeding time by inhibiting platelet aggregation. It does so by preferentially acetylating platelet cyclo-oxygenase, thereby reducing the production of pro-aggregatory thromboxanes from arachidonate (20:4). The natural counterbalancing mechanism, namely arachidonate cyclo-oxygenation to form the anti-aggregatory prostacyclin (PGI_2) within endotheliol cells, is rather less sensitive to aspirin. However in Eskimos, who normally consume a diet rich in eicosapentaenoic acid (20:5/EPA) and are relatively impoverished in arachidonate precursors, the effect of aspirin can be quite different. Instead of extending bleeding times (what we ex-

pect of this drug), aspirin may actually shorten them for the Eskimo. The explanation for this exceptional effect of the aspirin appears to lie partly in the fact that EPA is metabolized to a prostacyclin, PGI_3, that is anti-aggregatory and whose effect is lost with aspirin. Since EPA is only a poor precursor of pro-aggregatory thromboxanes, the levels of PGI_3 normally ensure tardy platelet aggregation until it is accelerated by aspirin (sic). In this context the effects of aspirin upon eicosanoid-regulated phenomena can only be understood after defining the ambient dietary levels of the eicosanoid precursors (20:3, 20:4, 20:5). I suspect that this example, of how a drug effect is conditioned by the diet, may not be as rare as it might seem at first sight.

5. This last example is cited to illustrate again the vital role of the genetic constitution in determining drug action. It has been difficult to establish the anti-arthritic activity of goldthiocomplexes in rat models of polyarthritis: some laboratories were successful but others were not. A recent analysis of this problem indicated several variable factors had to be controlled, including the nature of the arthritogen, the time of administering the reference gold drugs and the rat strain. Depending on which strain was used, aurothiomalate either inhibited the arthritis, had no effect on its development or <u>even</u> provoked the arthritis in a low-responder strain[1].

These five examples have indicated how a drug effect may be related to disease state, concurrent therapy, diet or genetic factors; conditions that must be considered in describing the biological effects of many xenobiotics

III. FURTHER APPLICATIONS OF THIS CONCEPT: TOXICOLOGY OF ANTI-ARTHRITIC DRUGS

This section discusses some of our own experimental observations, which are summarized in Tables 2 and 3. These data essentially compare the properties of a few drugs in normal rats, with their effects in diseased or physiologically distinct littermates. This section will focus on drug interaction with three organs only: the kidney, the stomach and the chief drug-metabolizing organ, the liver.

A. Effects on the kidney

It has previously been noted how the nephrotoxicity of some heavy metals is reduced by concurrent inflammation[2]. This is of more than academic interest because it is only the most refractory patients with arthritis or cancer who are treated with metal complexes such as aurothiomalate and cisplatin. These, the most diseased, patients (who have made insufficient responses to less potent drugs) may in fact be the most tolerant - if the experimental animal studies can be considered a guide to human drug tolerance.

Table 2 Lesser nephrotoxicity of some heavy metal drugs in female hooded rats

		% Increase in kidney body weight	
Drug, i.p.	Dose (mg/kg)	Male	Female
Mercuric chloride	1 x 3	35	3
Cisplatin	4 x 3	38	2
Aurothiomalate	10 x 3	75	16

Toxicity was measured by kidney oedema 24 hours after the last of three daily doses. Males were approximately the same body weight as females to equalize volumes of distribution.
Relative to ratio for control animals injected with saline only. Data compiled from groups of six rats (weighing 200-240 g)

In the course of trying to quantify this nephroprotective effect of extra-renal inflammation we rediscovered the well-known fact that males are not the same as females! As Table 2 shows, non-inflamed females will tolerate doses of several metal complexes that are quite nephro-irritant to males of the same body weight. This sex difference in renal susceptibility is also known for other drugs, e.g. gentamycin, and may be more a property of the organ than a peculiarity of metal toxicity. The interesting question is of course to what degree can this nephro-protectant/metal-detoxicant property of the female be transferred to the more susceptible male, without resorting to drastic sex-change procedures? One common feature of both inflamed males and normal females, is the higher circulating level of caeruloplasmin. Inflamed animals also contain higher levels of metal-binding polypeptides, the metallothioneins, which are partly induced (in the rat) by one of the pro-inflammatory monokines, interleukin-1. This brief survey indicates how the sex and inflammatory status of a rat will condition its survival and response to potentially intoxicating metal complexes.

Table 3 Gastroxicity of some NSAIDs in rats with inflammatory disease (conditions given below)

	Gastric lesion indices[a] with			Relative values of		
	ASA	MFA	PBZ	PST[d]	Serum SH[e]	Alb[f]
Normal, not-inflamed	24	08	04	(1.0)	(1.0)	(1.0)
17-day polyarthritis	92	94	56	4.7	0.4	0.6
-treated with PBZ			26	0.9[g]	0.6	0.6
-treated with IX			19	2.7	0.6	0.7
-treated with PX			17	2.9	0.7	0.7
31-day polyarthritis	64	28	48	3.1	0.7	0.9
99-day polyarthritis	51	21	36	1.3	0.9	1.1
4-day inflammation	71	50	36	3.7	0.6	0.8
-treated with 6-MP			0	1.9	0.7	0.8
17-day inflammation	19	16	0	1.1	0.9	1.0

Footnotes

(a) All groups of three to six male hooded rats were fasted overnight; challenged with drugs = gastrotolerance probes, administered orally in 0.02% Tween-20; stressed by brief cold exposure (25 min, -20 °C) and sacrificed after 2 h. Gastric lesion indices were compiled (3). Blood samples were taken wherever possible from undrugged animals, otherwise when determining GLI. Drugs used as probes: ASA = 30 mg/kg aspirin; MFA = 50 mg/kg mefenamic acid; PBZ = 50 mg/kg phenylbutazone

(b) Polyarthritis was induced by injecting 50 μl adjuvant (= 1% Mycobacterium tuberculosis dispersed in squalane) into tailbase and treated on days 12-16 only with phenylbutazone (40 mg/kg) isoxicam (IX) (3 mg/kg) or piroxicam (PX) (0.8 mg/kg) given once daily orally

(c) Inflammation was induced by injecting 0.1 ml oleyl alcohol into tailbase and treated on days 0-3 with 50 mg/kg 6-mercaptopurine

(d) PST = mean sleep time after 25 mg/kg pentobarbital i.p., an an index of drug metabolism, compared to controls

(e) Serum thiol level, determined with Ellman reagent, relative to controls

(f) Albumen level, determined with bromcresol green relative to controls. (Controls for (d)-(f) were non-inflamed, co-aged littermates

(g) Insignificant, since PBZ reduces PST in normal rats too.

B. Effect on gastric mucosa

An accompanying report illustrates how the degree/severity of mucosal haemorrhage caused by a single dose of an anti-inflammatory drug is conditioned by:

1. The nature of the drug, its formulation and route of administration;
2. physical/physiological stresses, including prior starvation;
3. concurrent inflammation (and other pathogenic stresses) suffered by the test animal.

The data in Table 3 provide further evidence that the pathological condition of the animal may determine very largely how toxic the drug may be. Even rats with long-standing adjuvant-induced polyarthritis (at least 3 months duration), that have apparently recovered from the florid inflammation manifested in the first month of this disease, can be still hypersensitive to doses of drugs that are not gastro-irritant in normal rats. These drugs include diplosal (salsalicylate), phenylbutazone and mefenamic acid at marginal anti-inflammatory doses given orally, which have proved quite useful as probes for diagnosing the severity of systemic inflammation by the gastric bleeding they elicit. Other suitable probes, which are not anti-inflammatory agents, include clofibric acid and the 2,3- or 2,5-diacet-oxybenzoates that only cause significant gastric damage in highly stressed/rather inflamed rats. Some of these drugs are not readily available but even a low dose of aspirin can be used for this type of probing exercise - the only disadvantage being that the lesion index in normal animals is nearly always finite, not usually zero (as with the above-mentioned drugs).

As Table 3 shows, rats were still very sensitive to oral phenylbutazone, low-dose aspirin or mefenamic acid in the late/permanent phase of the polyarthritis (at day 99), even though they had (a) almost normal levels of albumen or serum thiols (which are depressed during the earlier, rather inflammatory, phases of this disease) and (b) minimally impaired capacity to metabolize xenobiotics, as indicated by near-normal pentobarbital sleep times. Treatment of the aggressive inflammatory phase of this polyarthritis (days 12-16) considerably ameliorated the gastrotoxicity of phenyl-butazone when monitored on day 17.

The lower half of Table 3 shows how useful this gastroxic probing can be. Animals inflamed by an injection of 0.1 ml oleyl alcohol (octadec-9-en-1-ol) in the tailbase suffer minimal local injury, temporary loss of weight gain but a considerable impairment of their capacity to metabolize xenobiotics. This latter dysfunction is largely normalized by giving the anti-proliferative drug, 6-mercaptopurine (6-MP). That this effect of 6-MP is upon the grosser inflammation, rather than an inductive effect on drug metabolism, is amply demonstrated by the fact that the MP-treated inflamed rats showed almost no gastric bleeding with oral phenylbutazone. This may seem a devious type of analysis for recognizing the contra-inflammatory effect of 6-MP but this drug shows very little anti-inflammatory activity in orthodox animal assays. The justification lies in the fact that 6-MP has proved beneficial in the clinic, and it is only through experiments of this type that we might hope to substantiate its beneficial effects in animals with a view to understanding the molecular mechanisms involved.

There are serious doubts that experimentation with painful and aggressive tissue-damaging diseases, such as the adjuvant-induced polyarthritis, can be ethically justified. By employing alternate inflammagens such as oleyl alcohol, which initiate much the same spectrum of biochemical changes that follow the injection of an adjuvant (consequent to mononuclear phagocyte activation) including compromised drug-resistance, it may be possible to largely reduce our dependence on the polyarthritis model for investigating drug efficacy and toxicity. Many experiments can be completed within one working week when oleyl alcohol is the inflammagen and the inflammation is normally self-remitting (see Table 3, 16-day gastrotoxicity data). There is probably no need to use an adjuvant-inflamed rat to disclose the cryptotoxicity of a drug to the gastric mucosa, when the same test can now be carried out in rats pre-inflamed with oleyl alcohol or some other less aggressive but self-limiting inflammagen.

A number of other physical/physiological/pathogenic stressors will compromise the resistance of the gastric mucosa to an otherwise well-tolerated dose of phenylbutazone (50 mg/kg) or other probes for gastro-tolerance. In this list we would include noise (both intermittent and continuous), physical injury (tail or foot damage), the social stress of isolating individual rats and diseases with minimal overt inflammation such as allergic encephalomyelitis (EAE) or rats made tolerant to an arthritogenic adjuvant by prior treatment with a dummy adjuvant. Whilst many of these conditioning events undoubtedly include monocyte activation, a few may not (e.g. starvation, noise, isolation) - suggesting the more classical aspects of stress are involved, e.g. adrenal activation.

C. Effect on drug metabolism/detoxication

It is now well known that inoculation of adjuvant or other "heavy" inflammagens such as oleyl alcohol will alter the levels of many drug-metabolizing enzymes in rats. At least two mechanisms may be involved: (1) the production of interleukin (IL-1) by mononuclear phagocytes activated by the foreign irritant; and (2) the production of reactive oxygen metabolites (ROM) by these same, and other, phagocytes. IL-1 signals hepatocytes to produce more fibrinogen and several plasma glycoproteins (the so-called "acute phase reactants"). It may concurrently switch off albumen synthesis and the replacement of hepatic xenobiotic-metabolizing enzymes. The state of "oxidant stress", due to ROM production accompanying inflammation, reduces the level of both serum thiols and liver glutathione, a co-factor required for normal drug metabolism and to protect the hepatocyte from many toxins. The outcome of these and other sequelae of inflammation is that the liver, the primary drug-detoxifying organ, is compromised in this essential function.

What may not be so well known is the rapidity of this metabolic impairment. We have found that 12 hours after inoculating rats with sufficient brewers yeast to set up a fairly enduring fever (=39 °C after 18 hours), the metabolism of many drugs is quite seriously compromised. This is indicated after 12 hours by doubling/trebling of sleep times in response to a standard dose of a barbiturate or trichloroethanol. What this means in practical terms is that both the toxicity and the effective half-lives of antipyretics disclosed in such yeast-fevered rats are likely to be over-estimated. This could be the pharmacological illustration of both Heisenberg's uncertainty principle and the Ying-yang enigma.

Attempts over several years to find pyrogens other than brewer's yeast which might not unduly compromise hepatic drug metabolism were consistently unsuccessful. Nor is this surprising now in the light of recent discoveries that IL-1-like molecules are both pyrogens and modulators of liver function.

This fever-metabolism-toxicity interrelationship is not always as easily unravelled as we might wish it to be. Some drugs that are well tolerated in normal rats certainly become rather lethal in rats with pre-established fever, e.g. phenylbutazone, presumably due to (pyrogen-related) insufficient detoxication. Other drugs which will actually suppress the onset of fever, e.g. aurothiomalate (20 mg/kg), are poorly tolerated at doses that are quite acceptable to normal rats. However, the converse is true for certain other fever-suppressants, particularly experimental drugs containing Pt(II) or Cu(I), that are comparatively well tolerated by inflamed animals but seem far more toxic in normal rats. Undoubtedly the non-metabolizing, detoxicant, role of the RES is involved in some of these phenomena; particularly where the metal drugs are concerned. Yet another property of IL-1, that of reducing plasma zinc levels by inducing extra metallothionein synthesis in the liver, may also protect inflamed animals from those metal drugs that are thionein-bound. This raises an interesting paradox: the same inflammatory mediator (IL-1) acting on the same organ (the liver) might well induce intoxication by one drug (reducing its metabolism or detoxication of another drug (enhancing its sequestration).

Overloading phenomena may then become decisive as any one of at least three levels:

1. too much inflammagen for the RES to remove efficiently;
2. too much drug to be accommodated by the RES (perhaps already sated with other foreign material);
3. too much drug to be rapidly detoxified by an IL-1/ROM-compromised liver.

IV. DRUGS IN AN INFLAMMATORY MILIEU

The theme has now become a refrain: inflammation, wherever it originates, may have systemic effects that alter the pharmacoactivity and toxicity of the drugs applied to suppress it. This bidirectional interaction can be conveniently represented as:

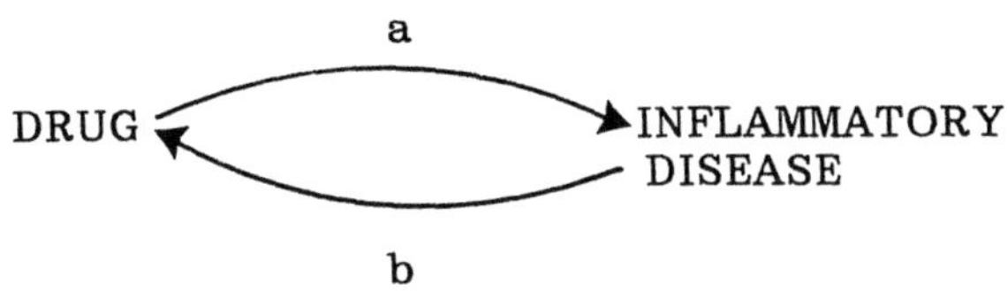

but even such a simple picture still needs a frame of reference to include the relative "pressures" of (a) the drug action on the inflammation, and (b) the effect of the inflammatory disease on drug handling or performance. These pressures will inevitably change, as each exerts its effect on the other. Even in the absence of an exogenous modulator, inflammation is an ever-changing process until it is totally superseded by complete healing.

Table 4 Some reasons for discriminant effects of a drug/toxin

A. Presence/lack of:
1. Delivery system
2. Receptors/concentrating mechanisms
3. Metabolic activation of pro-drug
4. Co-agonists/receptor activators

B. Lack/presence of:
5. Systemic removal systems
6. Local inactivation mechanisms
7. Antagonists

The constitution of a drug is easily defined; other aspects of its nature can only be described in the context of certain conditions that will determine its principal biological effects (Table 4). However, there are yet other conditions that cannot so conveniently be summarized while we know so little of (or indeed want to know about) the pathogenic milieu within which an inflammation-regulant must act - and in turn, be acted upon. Table 5 is included here (1) as an attempt to partly supplement Table 4, and (2) to list a few of the many factors that might cause drugs to change in efficacy with increasing inflammation. Many in fact increase in potency, as seen by comparing their ED_{50} values to inhibit a carrageenan paw oedema with their ED_{50} to repress the established/developing inflammation of a polyarthritis model. Some drugs, e.g. Clozic, Cu(I) complexes or azapropazone, are almost impotent in the oedema assay while very active in the arthritis assay (without being immunosuppressant). There are yet other explanations too; for example, the greater drug sensitivity of a monocyte population (recruited to an "aged" inflammation) compared to a granulocyte population (that is likely to dominate a "new" inflammation) as demonstrated for diclofenac in vitro[4]. Another example might be the production of cyanide by stimulated phagocytes interacting with circulating macromolecular aurothiocomplexes to locally generate the cytotoxic aurocyanide anion, as a basis for the selective and localized anti-arthritic effect of the clinical gold(I) drugs[5].

Table 5 Some further conditions determining activity of "anti-inflammatory" drugs

A.	Local	
	1.	Decreased pH of inflamed site*
	2.	Protease action on albumin-drug complexes*
	3.	Accumulation of drug in phagocytes (± albumin)
	4.	Non-enzymic metabolism, e.g. salicylate + ROM $\longrightarrow$ antoxidant 2,3-/2,5-dihydroxybenzoates[4]
	5.	Monocyte as target cell for drug effect[4,5]
B.	Systemic	
	Severe inflammation may cause:	
	6.	Slower drug inactivation
	7.	less albumin-binding of drug (less albumin, more fatty acids)*
	8.	? less efficient renal/biliary clearance
	9.	increase in circulating antoxidants (e.g. caeruloplasmin), corticoids and other endogenous modulators of inflammation

* These effects would facilitate transfer of drug from circulating albumin-drug complexes

V. FINAL COMMENTS

Until we attempt to understand rather more about the inflammatory milieu which conditions a drug's effects it will be very difficult to define and then discover the drugs that are so badly needed to improve the current treatment of chronic inflammatory disorders.

Ridding ourselves of the rather unhelpful notions that drugs have effects in isolation (absolutism) and replacing them with a concept of conditional action, i.e. efficacy or toxicity within a specific context, will allow us to accommodate many pragmatic observations of quite variable drug potency/toxicity in different contexts, e.g. with/without stress, diurnal rhythms, altered diets, different strains of test animal, or with different inflammatory stimuli/"age" of inflammation, etc. Drugs will then no longer be unwisely or loosely labelled with blanket but almost meaningless terms such as "anti-inflammatory", but more appropriately described, for example, as "anti-oedemic" or "IL-1-regulating" or "tissue-conserving", etc.; that is, with terms that clearly state the conditions under which a drug's performance was assessed experimentally.

These terms or descriptors might then be carried over to monitor the performance of these same drugs in the ultimate clinical context.

REFERENCES

1. Garrett, IR, Whitehouse, MW and Vernon-Roberts, B (1986) Ambivalent properties of gold drugs in adjuvant-induced polyarthritis in rats. J Rheumatol (accepted for publication)
2. Whitehouse, MW and Garrett, IR (1984) Heavy metal nephropathy: studies in normal and inflamed rats. In: Rainsford, KD and Velo, GP (eds), Side Effects of Anti-inflammatory Analgesic Drugs. (New York: Raven Press), pp291-294
3. Betts, WH, Whitehouse, MW, Cleland, LG and Vernon-Roberts, B (1986) Antoxidant properties of some salicylates and 4-aminophenazone. J Free Radical Biochem Toxicol (accepted for publication)
4. Ku, E, Kothari, H, Lee, W, Kimble, W, Tjan, J and Lian, H (1985) Regulatory role of diclofenac on arachidonic acid release and metablism in cellular and animal models. Abstr F-20, XVI Int. Congr. Rheumatol., Sydney
5. Graham, GG (1985) The cellular uptake of gold: relevance to the action of gold compounds. Abstr R-195, XVI Int. Congr. Rheumatol., Sydney

Discussion

Dr J Caldwell, UK: A comment and a question. Firstly, I want to extend what you said, Dr Whitehouse, about the effective modulation of host defence mechanism on drug metabolism. We've been very interested in the effects of such modulations on aspirin metabolism in relation to the pathogenesis in Reys' Syndrome and we've looked at the effect of various perturbations of host mechanism akin to the brewer's yeast experiments that you've described and these in fact have succeeded in doing one remarkable thing, that is abolishing the formation of gentisic acid from aspirin. It's quite a remarkable effect and apparently we have no other effect on the metabolism of aspirin at all, which in the context of our setting out on the experiments, is a disappointment, but it does lead me to enquire what evidence you have for the formation of oxidised products from salicylate other than gentisic acid, particularly since some time ago we made a very rigorous examination of human urine for other hydroxy benzoates and could only find gentisic acid. I was just wondering if this was in vitro data only that you were quoting?

Dr Whitehouse: Yes, the evidence is patchy. First of all of course, we know that all these three agents are very good anti-oxidants, for example in preventing chemiluminescence by activated polymophononuclear leucocytes. Secondly we know that 2,3-dihydroxy-benzoate is very and catechol of both and very rapidly destroyed under these circumstances, you therefore still get a deletion of the active molecule which implies consumption and reaction.

Dr KD Rainsford, UK: A couple of points. One follows on actually, to what Dr Caldwell was saying and that is concerning 2,3-dihydroxy-benzoate to which you ascribe an anti-oxidant activity. Of course this drug was shown, many years ago by Tony Cerami of the Rockefeller University in New York, to be a very efficient iron chelator and since the iron is a central part of the pathogenesis of some of the injury that we're seeing in liver and other manifestations of rheumatic disease, then I think it's a key factor there relating to the action of this. The second point I wanted to make was concerning your desire to have explicit descriptive terms relating to the reactions of drugs particularly the anti-inflammatory group of drugs. I agree with this in the sense of describing a particular action where you're looking at that particular action. Unfortunately, these drugs are polyvalent, they're acting on very many systems and we see this with chloroquine which has got at least three primary actions, i.e., on interleukin-1, oxyradical and phospholipase. So I think it would be very difficult to describe that in your context because you'll end up with a mouthful of descriptive terms.

Dr Whitehouse: Yes, but as you are well aware there are drugs like clozic, and in our experience copper [1] drugs or even azapropazone which are totally inactive in some assays and yet we know probably very good in the clinic.

Dr Rainsford: May I ask you a very general question? We all know how conventional animal toxicology testing is performed today with regard to the development of new drugs. Do you believe that a lot of the general conventional toxicology testing can be substituted for studies in diseased animals?

Dr Whitehouse: No, not at all. I think as long as we had some reference drugs put through the same tests at the same time that would calibrate the conditions.

Dr AJ Lewis, USA: Both to Dr Whitehouse's and Dr Parke's comment. You concentrated very much on adjuvant arthritis and demonstrated very clearly that this model is that the drug metabolism is dramatically altered. We have done similar studies in collagen arthritic rats and there is no such similar drug metabolic defect which is just, as I say, of interest. It's obviously not related to the inflammation again.

Dr Whitehouse: Yes, but I don't think you've got anything like the activation of phagocytic cells producing interleukins amongst other things, in the collagen-induced arthritis.

Dr Lewis: I don't think you've got any evidence that interleukin-1 plays a role in adjuvant arthritis either. To my knowledge there's been no evidence of that.

Anonymous: Do you get free radical generation in collagen-arthritis?

Dr Lewis: I presume so. I don't think anybody has measured it.

Anonymous: It would be interesting to measure it.

21
Pharmacokinetic profile of ketoprofen in elderly subjects*

WF Kean, H Howard-Lock, G Caille, J Bourgouin, J Gauthier, JA Rischke, CJL Lock, R Tocchio, E McNiven and A Buchanan
McMaster University, Canada and University of Montreal, Canada

CONTENTS

I. STUDY OUTLINE

In order to investigate the pharmacokinetic profile of ketoprofen in elderly patients, the pharmacokinetic parameters of ketoprofen were measured in nine elderly non-smoking patients (69±0.8 years), six with rheumatoid arthritis and three with osteoarthritis. Each subject was asked to discontinue all non-steroidal anti-inflammatory drugs 72 hours prior to the study (piroxicam and phenylbutazone were stopped 2 weeks prior to the study) and to refrain from fatty foods and alcohol during the study period. All subjects fasted for 8 hours prior to the start of the study. History and physical and routine blood work were taken prior to the commencement of the study (day 1) and at the end (day 8). Single dose (ketoprofen 50 mg capsule on day 1) and multiple dose (29 ketoprofen 50 mg

*This is a summary of a poster presentation.

Side-effects of Anti-inflammatory Drugs. Rainsford, KD and Velo, GP (eds)
Part 1: Clinical and Epidemiological Aspects. (Lancaster: MTP Press)

capsules day 1-8) pharmacokinetic studies were undertaken. On days 1 and 8 the first 50 mg capsule of ketoprofen was taken with 200 ml of water only, and light lunch was permitted after 3 hours. Blood samples on day 1 and day 8 were taken at time 0.00, 0.25, 0.50, 0.75, 1.00, 1.50, 2.00, 4.00 and 6.00 hours. Trough samples were taken at 6 hours on day 3 and day 5.

Urine samples on day 1 and day 8 were collected at 0-2, 2-6, 6-12, 12-18 and 18-24 hours.

All plasma and urine samples for the study were measured by a standard HPLC technique in the laboratory of GC.

II. RESULTS

There was no significant difference for the elderly patients studied when kinetic values for day 1 were compared to day 8 (day 1 x ± S.E.M. vs day 8 x ± S.E.M.): Cmax 6.15 ± 0.75 vs 6.67 ± 0.71 mcg/ml not significant (N>S>); Cmin 0.58 ± 0.10 vs 0.55 ± 0.09 mcg/ml N>S>; Tmax 1.25 ± 0.38 vs 0.92 ± 0.20 h N>S>; $t_{\frac{1}{2}}$ 1.80 ± 0.23 vs 1.48 ± 0.10 h N>S>; and AUC 12.42 ± 1.32 vs 13.38 ± 1.58 mcg h/ml N>S. Drug urinary values indicated that 74% of the excreted drug appeared as a glucuronide.

III. CONCLUSIONS

Ketoprofen has a short half-life and did not demonstrate any change in kinetic values, nor evidence of accumulation in the elderly patients we studied.

22
The effects of frusemide and Dorbanex on the pharmacokinetic profile of benoxaprofen in elderly subjects*

RC Hamdy and B Murnane
Department of Clinical Gerontology, St. John's Hospital, London, SW11, UK

CONTENTS

I. STUDY OUTLINE

The pharmacokinetic profile of benoxaprofen following a single oral administration of 600 mg was studied in twelve elderly subjects. Six received concomitantly 40 mg of frusemide and six received 10 ml of Dorbanex. These findings are compared to the previously determined pharmacokinetic profile of benoxaprofen in elderly subjects at St John's Hospital, London SW11.

II. RESULTS

The main findings are shown in Table 1. Statistical comparison, using Student's t-test, shows a significant difference ($p<0.01$) in the mean plasma levels at 1 h and in the half-lives. The half-life

*This is a summary of a poster presentation.

Side-effects of Anti-inflammatory Drugs. Rainsford, KD and Velo, GP (eds)
Part 1: Clinical and Epidemiological Aspects. (Lancaster: MTP Press)

in those taking the diuretic (mean = 154 h) was significantly higher ($p<0.01$) than in those taking the laxative (mean = 58 h) and this was significantly shorter than the previously determined half-life in elderly subjects[1].

Table 1

No.	Sex	Age (years)	Weight (kg)	Urea mmol/l	Creat. µmol/l	$t\frac{1}{2}$ (hours)
Initial kinetic study: duration of follow-up 120 hours						
1	F	87	39.1	9.0	110	137
2	F	84	65.5	5.8	96	59
3	F	80	58	11.3	163	136
4	F	83	61.8	4.6	87	138
5	F	76	42.1	9.9	129	90
6	F	81	63.5	4.4	92	104
Mean		81.8	62.9	7.5	112.8	111
Second kinetic study: duration of follow-up 504 hours						
7	F	81	48	8.2	116	132.2
8	F	71	53.6	2.9	48	127.3
9	F	86	43	4.0	86	158.8
10	F	80	42	4.9	128	173.1
Mean		79.5	46.7	5.0	94.5	147.9
Mean		80.9	51.7	6.7	105.5	125.5
Benoxaprofen + Dorbanex						
11	M	68	76.5	4.3	99	37.2
12	M	83	50.0	7.1	128	
13	M	85	59.0	6.2	87	52.0
14	M	80	43.0	4.0	103	68.2
15	M	70	63.0	5.3	74	61.1
16	M	80	60.0	9.1	144	71.0
Mean		78	58.6	6.0	106	57.9
Benoxaprofen and frusemide						
17	F	88	40.7	4.7	78	139.0
18	F	87	47.8	17.8	143	194.0
19	F	84	44.5	5.7	87	142.2
20	M	91	50.8	6.7	122	67.9
21	F	85	50.5	14.0	120	154.1
22	M	82	49.0	19.0	174	225.6
Mean		86	47.2	11.3	121	153.8

III. CONCLUSIONS

These findings may have relevant clinical implications as both diuretics and laxatives are frequently administered to elderly patients and might significantly interfere with the pharmacokinetic profile of anti-inflammatory preparations.

ACKNOWLEDGEMENT

We wish to acknowledge the help of Lilly Research Centre Ltd for assaying the plasma benoxaprofen levels.

REFERENCE

1. Hamdy, RC et al (1982). Eur J Rheum & Inflam, 5 (2), 69

Discussion

Dr R Jones, UK: I'm just a bit worried about the data presented because Dr Hamdy is using retrospective data from work done on benoxaprofen several years ago, to work done, I presume more recently. The subjects are quite different in that, in his original work, it was all female subjects and I think it's all males in the present one of the studies. I'm therefore just a bit worried on the interpretation of his data. Would he like to comment on that, particularly on weight differences and that sort of thing?

Dr Hamdy: Thank you. The three studies were done very shortly after each other. The time gap is not years, it is in fact months. For reasons that I won't elaborate on we had not published the data at that time. The differences in weight are not really all that remarkable if you look at the first study, 600 mg on six female patients. Their average weight was 62.9 kg. If you looked at the group that was getting Dorbenox, their mean weight is 58.6 kg. The patients who were on diuretics tended to have a lighter weight and their creatinine was slightly elevated but then these are patients and they had other concomitant diseases. If you look at the number of elderly people who are on diuretics, it will be well over a third. At the same time they would be on non-steroidal anti-inflammatories and we were interested to see how these diuretics would interfere with the kinetic profile, whether you should increase or decrease the dose or the frequency they're receiving.

23
Enantioselective disposition of a model non-steroidal anti-inflammatory drug 2-phenylpropionic acid*

PJ Meffin*, BC Sallustio*, YJ Purdie* and ME Jones**
Department of Clinical Pharmacology and **Human Morphology, Flinders University of South Australia, Adelaide, Australia

CONTENTS

I. INTRODUCTION

Non-steroidal anti-inflammatory drugs such as ketoprofen and fenoprofen are racemic mixtures of substituted 2-phenylpropionic acids. 2-phenylpropionic acid (2PPA) has been used as a model compound in order to study the enantioselective disposition of such drugs. Several 2PPA derivatives have been shown to undergo inversion from the pharmacologically inactive R to the active S enantiomer in vivo[1], but there are no reports of a model which allows the prediction of the relative concentrations of the enantiomers in plasma upon administration of racemic drug.

II. METHODS

Six NZW rabbits received an i.v. bolus (40 mg/kg) of S-2PPA, and

*This is a summary of a poster presentation.

Side-effects of Anti-inflammatory Drugs. Rainsford, KD and Velo, GP (eds)
Part 1: Clinical and Epidemiological Aspects. (Lancaster: MTP Press)

an hourly infusion of R-2PPA to steady state (10 mg/kg) in order to estimate the model parameters, the clearances of R-2PPA (CLr) and S-2PPA (CLs), the clearance of R-2PPA to S-2PPA (CLrs) and the fraction of the dose of R-2PPA converted to S-2PPA (Fr-s). The model was evaluated using the estimated parameters for each animal to predict the fraction of S enantiomer in plasma at steady state resulting from a racemic infusion (Fs pred.) and the value was compared with that observed during such an infusion (Fs obs.) Because the plasma protein binding of 2PPA was found to be enantioselective, binding data from three additional rabbits were fitted to a binding model which incorporates both non-specific binding sites and specific sites at which there is competition between the R and S enantiomers. The binding model was used in conjunction with that of 2PPA disposition to calculate the above model parameters for unbound R- and S-2PPA and to predict the unbound Fs pred.

III. RESULTS (Table 1)

Table 1 Model parameters for total and unbound 2PPA

Parameter	CLs (l/h/kg)	CLr (l/h/kg)	CLr-s (l/h/kg)	Fr-s	Fs pred	Fs obs
Total 2PPA						
mean	0.136	0.132	0.034	0.268	0.549	0.535
S.E.M.	0.008	0.013	0.001	0.022	0.020	0.013
Unbound 2PPA						
mean	0.311	0.480	0.138	0.313	0.657	0.689
S.E.M.	0.022	0.074	0.008	0.037	0.027	0.009

IV. CONCLUSIONS

The model is able to predict the fraction of S enantiomer in plasma upon infusion of racemic drug to steady state for both total and unbound 2PPA. The mean ratio of the plasma concentrations of the S to the R enantiomer at steady state upon racemic infusion is 1.14 for total 2PPA but 2.22 for unbound 2PPA.

ACKNOWLEDGEMENTS

The work is supported by the National Health and Medical Research Council of Australia.

REFERENCE

1. Hutt, AJ and Caldwell, J (1983). J Pharm Pharmacol, 35, 693

SECTION III

GASTROINTESTINAL TRACT (CLINICAL ASPECTS)

24
Anti-inflammatory drugs and upper gastrointestinal perforation

D St J Collier and JA Pain
Department of Surgery,
Addenbrooke's Hospital,
Cambridge, UK

CONTENTS

I. INTRODUCTION

> If you are an aspirin salesman you can say that taking aspirin is safe because so few aspirin users get ulcers or bleeding, but if you are an ulcer doctor you will say that these drugs are important causes of ulcers and bleeding because up to 30% of persons with these diseases are regular users of aspirin. (A quotation from the late Morton Grossman)[1].

As surgeons we frequently encounter patients presenting with perforated peptic ulceration (PPU). Often these patients are currently receiving medication with non-steroidal anti-inflammatory drugs (NSAIDs), and in view of previous reports of an association between NSAIDs and PPU[2-4] we undertook a retrospective study of all patients (n=269) admitted with PPU over a 10-year period (1973-82).

Side-effects of Anti-inflammatory Drugs. Rainsford, KD and Velo, GP (eds)
Part 1: Clinical and Epidemiological Aspects. (Lancaster: MTP Press)

II. SUSCEPTIBILITY OF THE ELDERLY FEMALE

This study has led us to the conclusion that there are important factors that determine susceptibility to NSAID-associated PPU, and these include being aged over 65 years, especially for females.

The annual incidence of PPU remained unchanged at 8.9 per 100,000 population in the first and second halves of the study period. Thirty-four per cent of patients were taking NSAIDs on admission compared to 7% of controls matched for age, sex and time of admission. The two groups were subdivided into those aged over and under 65 years, and compared by chi-square analysis Table 1. There was a highly significant difference ($p<0.001$)

Table 1 NSAID ingestion in patients and controls in specified age groups

	Under 65		Over 65	
	Taking NSAID	No NSAID	Taking NSAID	No NSAID
Controls	6	95	12	156
Patients	13	88	79	89

Patients under 65: $chi^2 = 2.09$; $p<0.5$, with Yate's correction
Patients over 65: $chi^2 = 67.65$; $p<0.001$

in NSAID ingestion between patients and controls in those aged over 65, but no difference in those aged under 65. Furthermore when the number of patients each year taking NSAIDs were correlated with the annual number of prescriptions for NSAIDs issued in this population region by Spearman's rho (Table 2) there was a highly significant correlation in those aged over 65 ($p<0.0001$) but no correlation in those aged under 65[5]. In specified age/sex groups there were marked differences in the prevalence of patients with perforated peptic ulcers taking NSAIDs (Figure 1). These differences cannot be explained by the precribing patterns of NSAIDs in the UK to these age/sex groups (Figure 2). The largest number of prescriptions in the UK were issued to females aged under 65, yet perforation was rare in this group. Although there was an increase in NSAID prescribing to all groups the percentage of patients with perforations taking NSAIDs only increased in those aged over 65, and this was especially so in females.

An increase in the incidence of perforated peptic ulcers in women has been reported by others[6-9], and the susceptibility of the elderly, especially females, to NSAID-related PPU reported by others[10,11] is confirmed by this study. Such a finding raises interesting questions about the pathophysiology of NSAID-related PPU, and furthermore has important implications for the prescribing of NSAIDs.

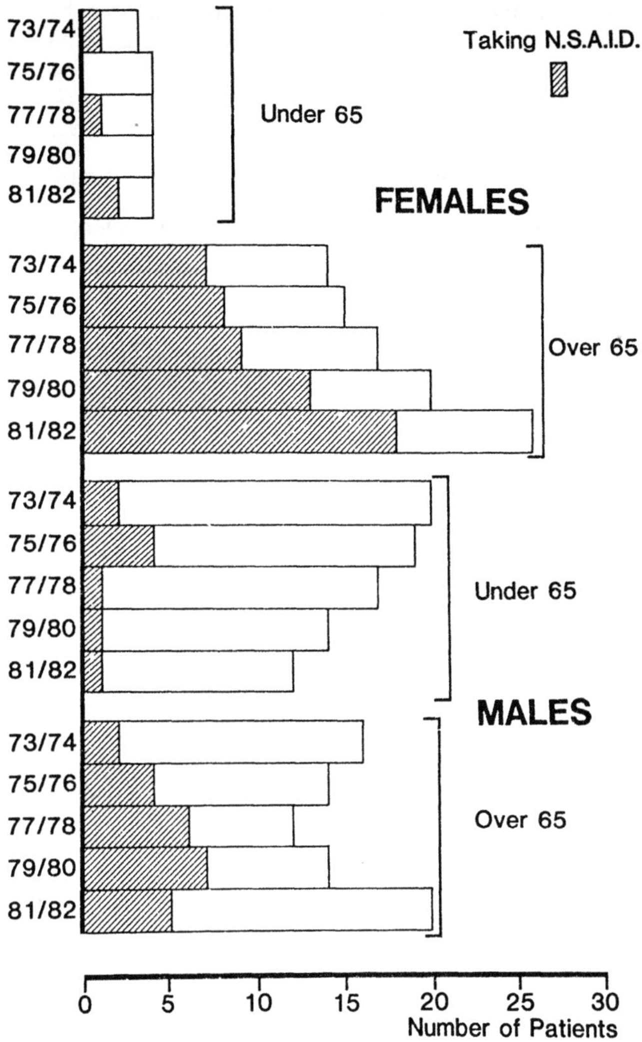

Figure 1 Number of perforated peptic ulcers in specified age and sex groups.

Why should the elderly be susceptible? Local ischaemia caused by atherosclerosis may predispose to ulcer formation[12], and this may be compounded by NSAIDs inhibiting prostaglandin synthesis, so leading to reduced gastric mucosal blood flow[13,14]. Altered pharmacokinetics occur in the elderly[15], and may influence the action of NSAIDs; however no sex difference in the rate of phenylbutazone metabolism has been found[16]. Dietary factors that have been implicated in the aetiology of PPU include low fibre intake[17,18], low vitamin C[19] and coffee[20]. The elderly are recognized as having a poor dietary intake of fibre and vitamin C.

Table 2 Number of perforated peptic ulcers in patients taking NSAIDs in specified age groups and number of prescriptions for NSAIDs in the region annually

Year	Patients taking NSAIDs		Prescriptions
	Aged < 65	Aged > 65	NSAID ('000)
1973	0	5	262
1974	3	4	307
1975	2	5	322
1976	2	7	359
1977	1	9	429
1978	1	6	405
1979	0	6	409
1980	1	14	471
1981	0	13	471
1982	3	10	515

Spearman's rho
Patients aged under 65: rho = -0.19; p N.S.
Patients aged over 65: rho = 0.93; p <0.0001

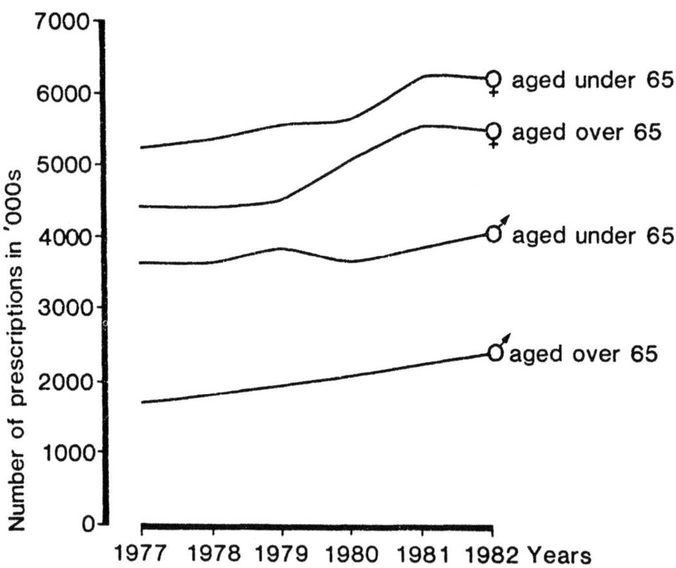

Figure 2 Annual number of prescriptions for NSAID issued to specified age and sex groups in the United Kingdom between 1977-1982. (Source: IMS)

Why should elderly females be especially susceptible? Postmenopausal hormonal changes may be important. Oestrogens and progestogens increase the production of mucus in the stomach[21], postmenopausal women may have a lowered mucus production, and this could be further reduced by the effect of NSAIDs on the gastric mucosa[22] leading to loss of mucus cytoprotection. As oestrogens have been used successfully in the treatment of peptic ulceration[23] the low incidence of perforations in premenopausal women may suggest a hormonal protective effect. Smoking has been implicated in the pathogenesis of PPU[24] and during the 10-year period of this study smoking in elderly females remained constant but decreased in all other groups (Ash, personal communication).

Further factors that should be investigated include the type, dose and duration of NSAID treatment. Table 3 shows the frequency of ingestion of specified NSAIDs in our study; however it is difficult to draw conclusions since overall prescribing figures for these individual drugs remain commercial secrets.

> "The gun must be loaded in order for an explosion to occur when salicylates pull the trigger" (Morton Grossman[25]).

We suggest that being elderly, and especially female, makes it more probable that the gun is loaded, and it remains to be seen which NSAIDs are more likely to pull the trigger.

Table 3 NSAID ingestion in patients with perforated peptic ulcers according to specified drugs

NSAID	Perforated duodenal ulcers	Perforated gastric ulcers
Indomethacin	31	10
Phenylbutazone	10	1
Aspirin	8	1
Piroxicam	5	4
Ketoprofen	5	1
Indomethacin suppositories	3	3
Ibuprofen	4	1
Benorylate	3	1
Diflunisal	2	1
Mefenamic acid	2	0
Others	9	4

Some patients were taking more than one NSAID

REFERENCES

1. Kurata, JH, Elashoff, JD and Grossman, MI (1982). Inadequacy of the literature on the relationship between drugs, ulcers, and gastrointestinal bleeding. Gastroenterology, 82, 373

2. Thompson, MR (1980). Indomethacin and perforated duodenal ulcer. Br Med J, 280, 448
3. Glarborg Jorgenson, T (1977). Drug consumption before perforation of a peptic ulcer. Br J Surg, 64, 247
4. Duggan, JM (1972). Aspirin ingestion and perforated peptic ulcer. Gut, 13,631
5. Collier, DStJ and Pain, JA (1985). Non-steroidal anti-inflammatory drugs and peptic ulcer perforation. Gut, 26, 359
6. Coggon, D, Lambert, P and Langman, MJS (1981). 20 years of hospital admissions for peptic ulcer in England and Wales. Lancet, 1, 1302
7. Barker, DJP, Power, C, Lambert, PM and Smith, CL (1981). Perforated duodenal ulcer in England and Wales time trends, and regional and urban-rural differences. Health Trends, 13,13
8. Dark, JM and MacArthur, K (1983). Perforated peptic ulcer in south-west Scotland 1966-1980. J R Coll Surg Edinb, 28, 19
9. Brown, RC, Langman, MJS and Lambert, PM (1976). Hospital admissions for peptic ulcer during 1958-72. Br Med J, 1, 35
10. Gleeson, MH (1982). A survey of peptic ulcers associated with NSAIDs. Eur J Rheumatol Inflamm, 5, 41
11. Cooke, P and Thompson, MR (1981). Old ladies, drugs and gastric ulceration. Gut, 22, A430F
12. Avery Jones, F (1979). Pathogenesis of gastric ulcer. In: Truelove, SC and Willoughby, CP (eds), Topics in Gastroenterology, vol. 7. (Oxford: Blackwell Scientific Publications), p. 35
13. Kauffman, GL, Aures, D and Grossman, MI (1980). Intravenous indomethacin and aspirin reduce basal gastric mucosal blood flow in dogs. Am J Physiol, 238, G131
14. Main, IHM and Whittle, BJR (1975). Investigation of the vasodilator and antisecretory role of prostaglandins in the rat gastric mucosa by use of nonsteroidal anti-inflammatory drugs. Br J Pharmacol, 53, 217
15. O'Malley, K, Crooks, J, Duke, E and Stevenson, IH (1971). Effect of age and sex on human drug metabolism. Br Med J, 111, 607
16. Whittaker, JA and Price Evans, DA (1970). Genetic control of phenylbutazone metabolism in man. Br Med J, 4 323
17. Tovey, FI (1975). Duodenal ulcer and diet. In: Burkitt, DP, and Trowell, HC (eds), Refined Carbohydrate Foods and Disease: some implications of dietary fibre. (London: Academic Press), p. 279
18. Rydning, A, Berstad, A, Aadland, E and Odegard, B (1982). Prophylactic effect of dietary fibre in duodenal ulcer disease. Lancet, 2, 736
19. Russell, RI, Williamson, JM, Goldberg, A and Wares, E (1968). Ascorbic-acid levels in leucocytes of patients with gastrointestinal haemorrhage. Lancet, 2, 603
20. Paffenbarger, RS, Wing, AL and Hyde, RT (1974). Coffee, cigarettes and peptic ulcer. N Engl J Med, 290, 1091
21. Parbhoo, SP and Johnston, IDA (1966). Effects of oestrogens and progestogens on gastric secretion in patients with duodenal ulcer. Gut, 7, 612
22. Menguy, R and Desbaillets, L (1967). Influence of phenylbutazone on gastric secretion of mucus. Proc Soc Exp Med Biol, 125, 1108
23. Truelove, SC (1960). Stilboestrol, phenobarbitone and diet in chronic duodenal ulcer. Br Med J, 2, 559
24. Solomon, TE and Jacobson, ED (1972). Cigarette smoking and duodenal ulcer disease. N Engl J Med, 286, 1212
25. Grossman, MI, Matsumoto, KK and Lichter, BS (1961). Fecal blood loss produced by oral and intravenous administration of various salicylates. Gastroenterology, 40, 383

Discussion

Professor J Dequeker, Belgium: I would like to ask about the different diseases these patients had, also the condition for which the NSAIDs have been prescribed? Is there more for osteoarthritis, for rheumatoid arthritis, for backache, for periarthritis, because I think it is very important to know the most dominant of the disease which is associated with perforated ulcer?

Dr St John-Collier: Right, amongst patients with a perforated peptic ulcer, there were twenty three with rheumatoid arthritis, nineteen of which were taking NSAIDs. Amongst these patients there were seventy eight with osteoarthritis of which seventy three were taking NSAIDs. In the control group, two of three patients had rheumatoid arthritis and were taking NSAIDs and sixteen of twenty five had osteoarthritis and were taking NSAIDs in the controls.

Dr TJ Daymond, UK: Can you tell us whether any of these patients were on steroids at all and whether you had patients on steroids who had perforated ulcers?

Dr St John-Collier: Yes. Amongst the patients with the perforated peptic ulcers, sixteen with duodenal ulcers, i.e. 7% were taking steroids and ten (19%), with a gastric ulcer. However, of these twenty six, fifteen were also taking NSAIDs. Amongst the controls, nine were taking steroids out of the two hundred and sixty nine.

Dr A Calin, UK: To what extent do the non-steroidal agents mask early symptoms thereby preventing the patient reaching the physician?

Dr St John-Collier: Well, as far as indigestion is concerned, (and I presume that's the question that you're asking), of the patients with perforated peptic ulcer 50% of those taking NSAIDs had a history of indigestion, and by a history of indigestion we meant a history of longer than three months. In those who were not taking NSAIDs, had a history of indigestion lasting longer than three months. Interestingly enough also, as far as previous medical history is concerned we looked at those who had a definite history of peptic ulceration and this we defined that they'd either had an operation for an ulcer or they'd had an ulcer shown either endoscopically or by barium meal. Amongst those with a perforated peptic ulcer who were taking NSAIDs, 13% had this history as opposed to those who were not taking NSAIDs where 26% had a history, a positive history, of previous peptic ulcer, but it's rather surprising that 13% who had a positive history were prescribed NSAIDs by their doctor.

Anonymous: One of the things that surprises me is that this very obvious conclusion that you've come to wasn't reached by others.

Dr St John-Collier: Well it has been reached by others.

Anonymous: Has it?

Dr St John-Collier: Yes.

Anonymous: So that's my ignorance - but you hadn't alluded to it. I would have thought that you would have alluded to it.

Dr St John-Collier: Well Gleason and others have shown this. As I said at the beginning, in view of the previous reports of the association between NSAID intake and peptic ulcer, Gleason showed that there was an association between indomethacin consumption in elderly females, which was written up in BMJ. Gleason also showed (I think it was in the European Journal of Rheumatology), and Thompson gave a presentation at the Gastroenterology Society showed the same thing.

Anonymous: When was that?

Dr St John-Collier: That was about three years ago - it was in the journal Gut about three years ago, I think the abstract was called, "Old Ladies, NSAIDs and Peptic Ulceration". In fact he found one thing we haven't found, that amongst the people with a perforated peptic ulcer, they were much more liable to be taking diuretics. We didn't find that, we found equal numbers of both the controls and the patients with perforated peptic ulcers.

Dr H Guess, USA: What about anti-coagulants? Did you find any usage of anti-coagulants in these patients?

Dr St John-Collier: There were none in the gastric ulcer and three in the duodenal ulcer group.

Anonymous: Were any of the patients taking a buffer product like butazole and anachole when it was available or were they regularly taking antacids or an H_2-receptor blocker for their dyspepsia?

Dr St John-Collier: Of those with a duodenal ulcer, fifty were taking antacid. Amongst the gastric ulcer patients, six people were taking antacids. As far as cimetidine goes, five patients were admitted who were taking full dose cimetidine at the time of their perforation but none of those were taking NSAIDs. However, they all smoked and were smoking while taking a full course of cimetidine.

Professor SJ Konturek, Poland: Do you have any information about the histology of the mucosa or gastroduodenal mucosa in these subjects or any data on secretory rates?

Dr St John-Collier: As far as histology is concerned, they were all considered to be benign peptic ulcers, and as you know, the treatment of this condition is variable. With gastric ulcer - some people oversew it, some people biopsy to oversew it, some people excise the ulcer, some people perform a partial gastroectomy. As far as duodenal ulcers, the usual treatment was oversewing, not usually with biopsy, but they all have been followed up and either the ulcer has been shown to have healed or they've had further treatment for continuing ulcer symptoms. We have excluded any with a gastric malignancy.

Professor Dequeker: Would the lesson from your paper not be that too many osteoarthritics are getting NSAIDs at a much too high dose and should preferably have another drug which is a more pure analgesic rather than an anti-inflammatory drug?

Dr St John-Collier: Sorry?

Professor Dequeker: Would not the lesson from your paper be that too many NSAIDs are prescribed for conditions where they are not necessary, for example, the osteoarthritis or backache not due to inflammation? Should we not be more inclined to push the use of more analgesic drugs with less drastic effects on the gastric mucosa for these conditions in the elderly?

Dr St John-Collier: Yes.

25
Piroxicam and gastrointestinal ulceration

FR Vicary, PJM George and KH Fok
Department of Gastroenterology
Whittington Hospital
Highgate Hill
London N19, UK

CONTENTS

I. INTRODUCTION

Piroxicam (Feldene) is now established among the favourites of the non-steroidal anti-inflammatory drugs, and the most widely used worldwide[1]. Its advantages include high efficacy, long plasma half-life (a mean of 38 hours) enabling it to be taken as a single daily dose, and its supposedly relatively low incidence of gastrointestinal (GI) side-effects. However, we have recently seen six cases of piroxicam-related peptic ulcers (four gastric and two duodenal) over a period of 11 months. All patients were taking piroxicam for minor arthritic problems. None had dyspeptic symptoms in the past and all developed GI symptoms only after taking piroxicam. None were concurrently taking any known ulcerogenic drugs other than piroxicam.

Side-effects of Anti-inflammatory Drugs. Rainsford, KD and Velo, GP (eds)
Part 1: Clinical and Epidemiological Aspects. (Lancaster: MTP Press)

II. CASE REPORTS

Case 1

A 79-year-old housewife with a 40 year history of arthritis was treated with phenylbutazone for 5 years before being changed over to piroxicam 20 mg a day by her doctor. Three months later she developed symptoms of anaemia and epigastric discomfort responding to antacids. Investigations showed she had an iron deficiency anaemia with a haemoglobin of 5.9 g/dl (MCV = 30.6). She was not taking any medication other than piroxicam at that time. Endoscopy showed a pre-pyloric ulcer. Piroxicam was stopped and she was given a 6-week course of cimetidine. Repeat endoscopy showed complete healing of the ulcer.

Case 2

A 50-year-old Nursing Officer had symptomatic multiple joint pain for 3 years. She was given aspirin 2 years ago but later changed to piroxicam 20 mg daily, with good relief. She developed typical ulcer pain soon after taking piroxicam and was given antacids by her doctor. She was taking piroxicam, was on no other medication and was a non-smoker. Investigations showed she had normal haematological indices and biochemistry, but endoscopy showed three benign gastric ulcers. Piroxicam was stopped and after a course of ranitidine repeat endoscopy showed a complete healing of the ulcers.

Case 3

An 87-year-old female taking piroxicam for arthritis, was admitted with a 5-day history of melaena and a massive haematemesis immediately prior to admission. She was shocked, with a blood pressure of 90/70 mmHg and a pulse of 110/min. Her haemoglobin was 6 g/dl. A total of 4 units of blood were transfused and she remained stable afterwards. Endoscopy showed a duodenal ulcer with blood clot in the ulcer crater. She recovered on conservative treatment, and cimetidine. Repeat endoscopy was not performed.

Case 4

An 81-year-old high-graded educationally subnormal man was admitted because of massive haematemesis and melaena. He was taking piroxicam 10 mg b.d. for arthritis. In addition to piroxicam, he was also on frusemide 40 mg and amiloride 10 mg b.d. for his minimal heart failure. He was shocked when admitted, with a blood pressure of 60/0 mmHg and a thready pulse of 110/min. His haemoglobin was 8.2 g/dl. A total of 5 units of blood were given in the first 24 hours before his blood pressure became stable. However, 36 hours after admission he re-bled with a massive melaena, and collapsed with the blood pressure dropping from 140/80 to 90/60 mmHg. Three more units of blood were transfused and emergency endoscopy showed a deep posterior duodenal ulcer with stigmata of active haemorrhage. A polyagastrectomy was performed as an emergency, and he made a good recovery.

Two further patients, both taking piroxicam 20 mg and no other medication, were seen during the period. Both presented with gastrointestinal bleeding, and both had endoscopically proven gastric ulceration.

III. RETROSPECTIVE STUDIES

We have looked retrospectively at endoscopy records over this period. 203 patients had benign gastric or duodenal ulcers (see Table 1). Thirty-two per cent of patients were taking an NSAID either alone or in combination with another drug. More patients were taking piroxicam than any other medication.

Table 1 Upper gastrointestinal system: anti-inflammatory drugs and ulceration

Patients taking an NSAID	41	32% (first three rows)
Patients taking an NSAID and another drug not known as ulcerogenic	17	
Patients taking an NSAID and another drug which is recognized as ulcerogen	7	
Patients taking other drugs	37	
Patients in whom drug history not clear from notes	23	
Patients not taking any medication	66	
Records not traceable	12	
Total	203	

IV. DISCUSSION

We are concerned by this high incidence of piroxicam-related ulceration occurring within such a short period. The current comparative clinical trials conducted with piroxicam showed a very low incidence of serious GI side-effects. Ando and Lombardino in their analyses did not find a single case of ulcer/GI bleeding in 537 patients[2]. Various large-scale multicentre surveillance studies involving over 73,000 patients reported an incidence of ulcer of between 0.1 to 0.7%[3-5]. Pitts[6] had shown that at 20 mg daily dose the prevalence of ulcer with piroxicam was 0.9%. Criticisms that these studies have underestimated the real incidence of ulceration were borne out by the fact that recent gastroscopic studies in arthritic patients with ulcers showed that many have no overt symptoms[7].

Furthermore there is a big discrepancy between the data based on clinical studies and the large number of cases of ulcers due to piroxicam reported to the UK Committee of Safety of Medicines.

We suspect that piroxicam may be associated with considerable upper gastrointestinal ulceration. The only way to prove or disprove this hypothesis would be to endoscope patients before, and some weeks after, a course of this drug.

In the absence of this proof we need to look at all our information on this whole area of NSAIDs and gastrointestinal bleeding and ulceration. On the one hand we have strong evidence from the three drug safety committees from the UK, USA and Sweden. On the other hand we have evidence from prescription-event monitoring[8] (see Chapter 7 in this volume) that there is no increase in events noted for piroxicam.

It is in the interest of all concerned - physicians, patients, and drug companies - that we must evaluate the risk and efficacy of drugs and come to a rational scientific conclusion. I suggest that we introduce a formula to combine our conflicting data. We must consider the "risks" as embodied by:

1. Clinical reports, whether they be case reports, post-marketing surveillance or clinical trials.
2. Committees of Safety of Medicines - undoubtedly the Swedish Committee is of great importance in view of the care of their documentation, but the UK and USA Committees make valuable contributions.
3. Prescription-event monitoring.

From these three sets of data we need to come up with an estimate of "risk".

Against this we need to set "efficacy". If a drug cures cancer, patients will not mind taking a few "risks". If the drug is of dubious efficacy, even a minor risk will be unacceptable. Thus efficiency will need to be judged by (a) clinical trials, and (b) patient acceptability. I suggest we weigh piroxicam or any other NSAID by this formula:

<u>The risk</u>		<u>The efficacy</u>
1. Clinical reports 2. CSMs 3. Prescription-event monitoring	versus	1. Clinical trials 2. Patient acceptability

If we fail to find some acceptable formula we run the continuing danger of arbitrary decision-making to ban useful drugs, influenced by misleading reporting in popular newspapers.

REFERENCES

1. Nuki, G (1983). Non-steroidal analgesics and anti-inflammatory agents. Br Med J, 287, 39
2. Ando, GA and Lombardino, JG (1983). Piroxicam, a literature review of new results from laboratory and clinical studies. Eur J Rheum Inflamm, 6, 3
3. Langloh, N (1981). Experience with Feldene in general practice. Therapiewoche, 31, 5501
4. Alvart, R (1981). Etude Multicentrique du Proxicam en Rheumatologie Ambulatoire. Gazette Medicale, 11 December, p. 3
5. Huskission, EC et al (1983). UK Hospital and General Practitioner Group - Treatment of Oesteoarthritis with Piroxicam. Eur J Rheum Inflamm, 6, 73
6. Pitts, NE (1980). Piroxicam, a new non-steroidal anti-inflammatory agent. Proceedings of the Ninth European Congress of Rheumatology, p. 48
7. Caruso, I and Porro, GB (1980). Gastroscopic evaluation of anti-inflammatory agents. Br Med J, 1, 75

Discussion

Dr G Cox, UK: You have shown that you have had six out of two hundred and twenty three patients that bled on piroxicam and by comparison not more than three on any other drug. Did all these patients come from your health district?

Dr Vicary: No they did not all come from the same region.

Dr Cox: So some were migrants?

Dr Vicary: I beg your pardon?

Dr Cox: Some were immigrants - to your district?

Dr Vicary: That's a very nice way of putting it - yes!

Dr Cox: What I want to know is how does this compare with the total prescribing habits in the district?

Dr Vicary: We've tried to look at it, it's incredibly difficult.

Dr Cox: I mean, is piroxicam the most frequently prescribed non-steroidal?

Dr Vicary: I cannot answer that because we've been unable to get the information for this. We've made enormous efforts to get the information for this. We've had terrible difficulty and I heard yesterday how one does it. So I can't answer it but perhaps I could go on from that and make the point about retrospective studies that I wanted to make earlier and that is that you know there's only a limited amount of information that you can get from a retrospective study. I'm comparatively new to all of this business of taking drug histories even though I qualified and was a medical student and was taught how to do it. If you actually sit down with a patient and you take a history, as I'm sure you know, a very careful detailed history and you bully them and push them and are very careful about it, you actually get a completely different answer to the answer that the houseman got in the middle of the night when the patient was admitted as an emergency. I think, therefore, that one has to be very careful, and I've learned this recently, about what information you can actually get out of studies such as ours which are retrospective. So what we're going to try and do in future is, (in fact what we've just started doing), is a prospective view of this which I hope, will give us a better perception when all the medical staff are sensitised to really being careful with drug histories. I don't know whether you go along with that or what?

Dr KE Giersky, Norway: Being a surgeon I certainly share your concern about non-steroids and GI tract problems and a similar story. In a prospective series of GI bleeding following piroxicam appeared in Norway three years ago and I was asked to give general practitioners some general advice on this problem and we did not want to use others' retrospective data. We, therefore, made a prospective study over the following fourteen months. We found that 50% of all GI drug related bleeding was related to aspirin alone, but we also found that 50% of patients developing GI bleeding following non-steroids had previously been treated for severe dyspeptic symptoms or ulcers. To our surprise, when the number of drug related bleedings were related to drug consumption using the method Professor Wiholm told you about yesterday, we found that indomethacin gave some more GI bleedings than the other, but there was no significant difference between piroxicam, naproxyn and ibuprofen. We tried the only four drugs that are used in Norway.

Dr Vicary: Was that because the numbers are very small?

Dr Giersky: For ibuprofen the number is very small for that drug is used very seldom in Norway, but the numbers were not small for the other drugs. So I wonder if you are now going to do a prospective study where you can involve the consumption of the different drugs, because this is a very serious problem?

Dr Vicary: Yes. I absolutely agree and I think without that information. Part of our difficulty relates to what I think Dr Cox referred to as our immigrant population. The overlap in the district is much more difficult in the United Kingdom and people move around. I, for instance, get a lot of patients referred up from Luton and Dunstable, which complicates things enormously.

Dr RD Montgomery, UK: I would like to endorse everything that Dr Vicary has said and I very much like the plan he's got on the board at the moment, the problem of course, is to implement it. You hear a lot of talk about the value of anecdotal reports and they have their place, and we have a lot of talk about the CSM reports. I would like to emphasise once more how totally unreliable these voluntary reporting figures must be. In our real world in Birmingham, in my hospital, we see about one hundred and twenty cases of haemorrhage every year and we have upper GI haemorrhage of whom about one third have chronic ulcers and about 15% overall are on these drugs. The principal drug that we see every year is still indomethacin. Piroxicam comes somewhere way down quite a long list. It is important, of course, that piroxicam has only been in use for a few years, but we have seen no change in fact, in the past three years. To my knowledge, none of these cases is ever reported on a yellow card because physicians know that this sort of thing is happening and they have no incentive in a case like indomethacin where as with new drugs of course, they may do. Particularly, the more unusual the drug effect, the more they're going to be reported, but that does not apply to haemorrhage.

Dr Vicary: Yes. Thank you very much. I think we have to do something about improving reporting to the CSM and I would think that the fact that there is no follow-up from the CSM back to us when we send in the yellow card means that we have no reward for sending in those cards. So I would have thought that if we had some feedback and somebody came along and looked at our notes or whatever, we'd be much more interested and we'd have a bit of a reward. I was horrified to discover that of these six patients, four of whom I'd actually written in a case report and the BMJ as you may know, two of them still haven't had a yellow card put into the CSM.

Professor K Brune, FGR: May I take advantage of your selective view on the GI tract? Can you discriminate between gastric ulcers and duodenal-jejunal ulcers which I think you can and, if so, can you make an estimate if you see more ulcers with aspirin in the stomach and maybe more with more modern non-steroidals in the deeper GI tract, or is there no way of answering this question?

Dr Vicary: Our numbers are not big enough to give you definite statistical answers to that and I cannot answer the point about ulcers in the region beyond the second part of the duodenum because we deliberately excluded that. However, you will, I believe, be hearing about that from Professor Langman.

Professor A Bennett, UK: There are some gaps in your information. For example, you didn't tell us the ages of the two other people, (two of your females were seventy nine and eighty seven), and you are making a comparison of numbers where you don't know the relative rates of prescribing. You haven't told us the ages or the sexes of these people. Do they fall into the same age range as all the others that you've equated them with?

Dr Vicary: If I could answer the first five questions first. The prescribing we've already alluded to and the extreme difficulties of cross district flow relating to that. I'd like to hear an answer to that, let alone the difficulty of getting the information from our district. The two patients to whom I've not alluded were both elderly females. One was sixty nine and the other was seventy four. We actually stopped looking at this because I was so worried about the information that we were getting in our retrospective study I wasn't really convinced of its value. I hope, if we have this meeting again next year, to come up with a prospective study, of which I'll give you all of that information.

26
Anti-inflammatory drugs and gastrointestinal disease

Reasons for the failure of adverse reaction reporting and surveillance systems to detect a significant association

MJS Langman
University Department of Therapeutics
Queens Medical Centre
Nottingham NG7 2UH, UK

CONTENTS

I. INTRODUCTION

Amongst clinicians there is a clear perception that non-steroidal anti-inflammatory drugs (NSAIDs) commonly cause acute upper gastrointestinal (GI) bleeding, whereas those responsible for surveillance programmes have difficulty in detecting serious GI problems. By contrast adverse reaction reporting bureaux have quantities of reports associating GI disease with the use of individual NSAIDs but have difficulties in deciding whether the voluntary reporting of events has any general significance. Thus the increased reporting of events in takers of, say, piroxicam but not indomethacin, might reflect real differences in toxicity profiles. On the other hand the prescribing of the newer drug piroxicam deliberately by clinicians for patients with known GI problems, because the new drug is believed from its pharmacokinetic or animal toxicological profiles to be safer, could in fact lead to an increased number of reports of events post hoc, but not necessarily propter hoc. Thirdly spontaneous reports must reflect physician prejudice about what seems appropriate for reporting.

Side-effects of Anti-inflammatory Drugs. Rainsford, KD and Velo, GP (eds)
Part 1: Clinical and Epidemiological Aspects. (Lancaster: MTP Press)

The problem of perception is illustrated by United Kingdom experience with the controlled-release indomethacin preparation Osmosin, which was banned after two cases of intestinal perforation were reported and were perceived to be unique events demonstrating undoubted drug toxicity. No attempt seems to have been made prior to the prohibition of prescribing of Osmosin to determine if the event of intestinal perforation was unique.

II. LOWER INTESTINAL DAMAGE

That the event of lower intestinal perforation was not unique was demonstrated by a retrospective study in Nottingham[1]. In this study antecedent drug histories were examined in 268 patients aged 40 and over admitted between 1977 and 1982 with lower intestinal perforation or bleeding believed not to be due to ulcerative colitis, Crohn's disease or cancer, and where an upper GI cause was not suspected. The drugs taken by the 268 patients were then compared with the drugs taken by an age- and sex-matched group of patients admitted with uncomplicated lower bowel disease.

Table 1 Drug histories given by patients admitted with and without complicated bowel disease

	Total no.	Drug-takers	Non-takers	Uncertain
Haemorrhage	161	71	23	6
Perforation	107	65	21	14
Total	268	69	22	9
All others	472	68	23	9

Table 1 shows that patients with perforation or bleeding were in general about as likely to be takers of drugs of any type as controls, with approximately two-thirds being recorded as definite takers, about a quarter to a fifth as definite non-takers, and a tenth having no drug history recorded. However, when data recorded about all anti-inflammatory drug intake were examined separately clear differences between patients and controls were present. About a quarter of those with haemorrhage or perforation were noted to be takers compared with half as many of the controls. None were taking Osmosin (Table 2), and most of the difference was accounted for by NSAIDs.

The data obtained did not seem explainable by greater intensity of questioning of patients compared with controls about general drug intake, for no trend was found for potassium intake which has been associated with intestinal ulceration in the past, nor for overall numbers of items recorded in test and control groups. The rate of anti-inflammatory drug intake in the controls was also of the same order as has since been found in a random population sample of patients over 60 years of age, a comparison which is appropriate because almost all the colonic disease patients we studied were over the age of 60 rather than near the lower limit of 40 initially set for the study.

We therefore concluded that controlled-release indomethacin (Osmosin) was not uniquely likely to cause intestinal complications.

Table 2 Percentage takers of anti-inflammatory drugs

	Total no.	Percentage takers of NSAIDs alone	Percentage takers of Cortico-steroids alone	Both	Percentage overall takers
Haemorrhage	168	18.0	2.5	1.9	22.4
Control	168	6.2	3.7	0	10.0
Perforation	107	15.9	3.7	6.5	26.2
Control	107	9.3	1.9	0.9	12.1

III. UPPER GI BLEEDING

The difficulty which clinicians have in accepting that NSAIDs are not an important cause of peptic ulcer and its complications is illustrated by more recent studies of ours[2]. In these we have taken drug histories from consecutive patients admitted with acute upper GI bleeding, and have matched all patients with confidently diagnosed gastric and duodenal ulcers who were over 60 years of age with a hospital inpatient control and a community control. The community control was obtained by contacting the general practitioners responsible for the patients admitted with bleeding, and taking off their registration list an age- and sex matched individual, who would not necessarily be an attender, but would simply be registered for care. Histories of NSAID intake, excluding aspirin and paracetamol and other simple analgesics, were obtained in one-third of the patients with bleeding compared with just over a tenth of those admitted with other medical complaints or in the community controls.

IV. "PERCEPTION" OF GI TOLERANCE

At first sight it is difficult to reconcile this large difference with the apparent non-toxicity to the GI tract of NSAID as perceived by surveillance groups. However this difficulty is resolvable. About 20 million prescriptions for NSAIDs are dispensed each year in England and Wales. There is no reason to believe that the Nottingham population are atypically low or high consumers, although the type of NSAID will probably vary from place to place. We also know that the 700,000 population is served by only two hospitals, and we collected data from both of these.

In Nottingham in general we can thus expect the total number of NSAID scripts each year to be 20,000,000 x 700,000/50,000,000, using 50 million as the denominator for the total population of England and Wales. This gives 280,000 scripts for NSAIDs in Nottingham each year. We also know that 230 patients over 60 years of age were admitted with acute upper GI bleeding due to gastric and duodenal ulcer in 2 years, of whom 80 were NSAID takers. Now the control groups contained about 30 takers each, so that the 2-year excess is 50 and the 1-year excess to relate to the total 280,000 prescriptions is 25, or about 1 in 10,000. Whether this is deemed significant is a matter of individual judgment, but grossed up to the population at large this gives a national event rate of 2000 episodes annually, and if ordinary mortality rates of 10% were to apply would indicate 200 deaths attributable to treatment.

REFERENCES

1. Langman, MJS, Morgan, L and Worrall, A (1985). Use of anti-inflammatory drugs by patients admitted with small or large bowel perforations and haemorrhage. Br Med J, 290, 347
2. Somerville, KW, Faulkner, G and Langman, MJS (1986). Non-steroidal anti-inflammatory drugs and bleeding peptic ulcer. Lancet, 1, 462

Discussion

Dr A Herxheimer, UK: I think that's a very convincing demonstration that we actually need to do something rather than go on collecting lots more data first, which is the point which I was getting at yesterday. I would like to hear discussions from many people here concerning realistic things that we can do with the information that we now have to improve the situation. One obvious possibility is to ask ourselves if all the people who were taking these NSAIDs and suffered serious ill effects, actually needed the NSAIDs? Did they benefit from them? Then we can discuss what we can do to discourage those people from being given the drug. There may be other things we can do too.

Professor Langman: I suppose the answer to that is yes. There are things to say about that data first and that is that the controls are not complete but I'm pretty sure what the answer will be. However, I've not got all the drug data together for every other variety of drug, so there may be inbuilt biases that people are generally drug takers, so my "attributable risk" may be too great. I suspect it's not and there is something odd, otherwise why is this happening to elderly women because I suspect the same amount of drug taking is actually happening in elderly men - they're different, but I agree that something needs doing and I suspect it means things like reducing dosage for relatively trivial conditions and perhaps a two tier drug list.

Professor K Brune, FGR: I think I like your data but I disagree with your calculations and I think you contradict yourself a little bit in making the point concerning your group of patients at risk. Now you cannot simply calculate from the number of prescriptions a risk and I think what you more clearly defined was, that there is a group of patients which may be at risk. We therefore should not calculate an effective number which may be suffering but we should elucidate or evaluate the risk, why it comes and which drugs are involved. I'm sure not all non-steroidals are equally ulcerogenic in your old female group. Then we should reach for solutions, otherwise I think this calculation is leading up to a couple of deaths per year and it is too simple, too trivial and could be misused in public.

Professor Langman: Thank you. I was not prepared to talk about the individual drugs because the data are not complete and they won't be for another month. I think I disagree about the calculation. I think it is a reasonable enough calculation and I think it's helpful, because it explains where people who are doing "conveyance" studies where they collect twenty-thousand scripts are failing to find something. You have got to collect a hell of a lot more scripts and you've actually got to look at a group of people who've got the problem. That was the only point I wanted to make.

Dr RD Montgomery, UK: I would like to congratulate you on putting the situation so clearly for us once more. I would just like to make the point that your findings agree with a study which we made retrospectively on cases of haemorrhage. I'm glad to say that we also found a 90% positive record in our notes about drug taking showing that there was an increase of haemorrhage due to these drugs in elderly women but not in any other group. I would like to emphasise that we are talking about haemorrhage and not about the incidence of ulcers and I would still say that we have no evidence that any of these drugs actually cause a chronic ulcer. I don't know whether you would agree with that?

Professor Langman: Yes. I take your point about the previous studies. I'm sure that the answers they produced were correct. What they needed, I think, was some validation to show that if one collected data in a planned manner with a good control, and I think we have got a good control, everything we said was true. It does appear to be true.

Professor Parke: Coming back to Andrew Herxheimer's question, what's your view about using anti-ulcer drugs prophylactically? I mean this was started twenty years ago with carbenoxolone and we've run through the range of different anti-ulcer drugs right up to cimetidine. Many GPs do it quite routinely.

Professor Langman: Broadly speaking, there's a shortage of evidence as to what is the best policy and what is the best drug to use and you can produce theoretical arguments for saying that you should deliberately use prostaglandins. You can produce other arguments for saying you should use H_2-antagonists but by and large they would seem to be reasonably safe in elderly people. Whether they're effective is not so sure. I don't know the right answer. I don't think anybody else does either yet.

27
An evaluation of the frequency of anti-inflammatory and analgesic drug intake among patients with acute gastrointestinal bleeding

U Haglund, L Frost and BE Wiholm
Department of Surgery, University of Lund, Malmö General Hospital, Malmö, and Department of Clinical Pharmacology, Karolinska Institute, Huddinge University Hospital, Huddinge, Sweden

CONTENTS

I. INTRODUCTION

Many anti-inflammatory and analgesic drugs are cyclo-oxygenase inhibitors, and thus inhibit prostaglandin synthesis[1]. This is true for acetylsalicylic acid and other NSAIDs except paracetamol. All these drugs are known to induce gastric mucosal damage, gastric bleeding and ulceration[2-6]. The damaging effects on the gastric mucosa are prevented if patients are provided with exogenous prostaglandin E_2 or a synthetic analogue with prostaglandin E_2 effects, in addition to NSAID[7-10]. Cyclo-oxygenase inhibition in the gastric mucosa suppresses several components of the mucosal defence mechanism. However, such inhibition only produces gastric ulceration in the presence of acid. The depressant effect on the mucosal defence mechanisms includes compromising the mucus-bicarbonate barrier[11], but other factors, such as mucosal blood flow and the ability of rapid mucosal cell reconstitution, may also be involved, as discussed elsewhere[12,13].

Side-effects of Anti-inflammatory Drugs. Rainsford, KD and Velo, GP (eds)
Part 1: Clinical and Epidemiological Aspects. (Lancaster: MTP Press)

It has thus been natural to associate acute upper gastrointestinal bleeding and intake of anti-inflammatory and analgesic drugs. Several studies have indicated a high frequency of intake of such drugs among patients with acute upper gastrointestinal bleeding[3,14,15],. However, because of difficulties in obtaining adequate objective reliable measurements on the intake of analgesic and anti-inflammatory drugs, it remains an open question whether patients with acute upper gastrointestinal bleeding as a group have an overconsumption of such drugs. Furthermore, whether some NSAIDs are more associated with upper gastrointestinal bleeding than others also remains an open question.

The present study was performed to evaluate different techniques to study the frequency of anti-inflammatory and analgesic drug intake and the type of drugs taken among patients with acute gastrointestinal bleedings. Healthy men born in 1931, participating in a health study, served as controls.

II. MATERIALS AND METHODS

The study was performed at the Department of Surgery, Malmö General Hospital, which serves a population of approximately 235,000 as the only available hospital. Approximately 350 patients are admitted each year with more or less pronounced acute bleeding from the upper gastrointestinal tract.

1. A retrospective analysis of patient records for 1981 was performed with the aim of studying the intake of anti-inflammatory and analgesic drugs among patients with acute gastrointestinal bleeding.
2. A prospective study was performed from June 1983 to May 1984. During this period all patients with acute upper gastrointestinal bleeding (except bleeding from oesophageal varices), that were admitted to one surgical ward, were included. This ward specialized in upper gastrointestinal diseases, and treated the majority of the patients with severe gastrointestinal bleeding during that period. For reasons not related to this study patients admitted in December and January were not included. In total 49 patients were included. The mean age for the 36 men was 56 years (range 29-79), and for the 13 women 63 years (range 54-86). All patients were studied in the following way:
   - (a) A retrospective analysis of the patient records regarding intake of anti-inflammatory and analgesic drugs was performed.
   - (b) A few days after admission, but while the patients were still on the ward, they were interviewed by a specially trained nurse regarding intake of anti-inflammatory and analgesic drugs. This interview included questions on different conditions, such as headache, back pain, common cold, etc., which were likely to constitute a rationale for anti-inflammatory and analgesic drug intake.
   - (c) One or two days later the patients were interviewed by

means of a special form with the aim of finding conditions related to intake of anti-inflammatory and analgesic drugs, as above. In addition, a list of the anti-inflammatory and analgesic drugs sold in the region was presented to the patients, and they were asked whether they had taken any of these drugs in the days prior to their bleeding.

3. Fifty-nine consecutive men who, during November 1984-February 1985, participated in a population health study in Malmö of men born in 1931, served as controls. They were subjected to an interview by a specially trained nurse and by the specially designed form as described above (2a and 2b).

III. RESULTS

The retrospective analysis of the patient records for 1981 revealed that 22% had an intake of anti-inflammatory or analgesic drugs. The retrospective analysis of the records for the 49 patients admitted during June 1983-May 1984 revealed that 38% of the patients had such drug intake. The nurse interview revealed anti-inflammatory and analgesic drug intake in 42% of the patients. The investigation by the drug list, however, revealed that 76% of the patients had taken anti-inflammatory or analgesic drugs; 71% had an intake of drugs with an inhibiting effect of cyclo-oxygenase while 5% had taken drugs with other mechanisms of action (paracetamol). Among the healthy men born in 1931, 47% had taken analgesic or anti-inflammatory drugs within the week preceding the health study (Table 1).

Table 1 The frequency of anti-inflammatory and analgesic drug intake among patients admitted to a surgical ward for acute upper gastrointestinal bleeding, and among men born in 1931 participating in a health control study.

	Patients 1983-84 (%) (n=49)	Health study 1985 (%) (n=59)
Patient records	38	-
Nurse interview	42	<5
Drug list	76	47

The most frequent drugs used by the patients were pure acetylsalicylic (ASA) drugs (20 of 37 patients - 54% - had taken pure ASA drugs). In addition, 14% had an intake of drugs in which ASA are combined with other analgesics. Thus in total, 68% had an ASA intake before admission. NSAIDs, except ASA, were taken by 24% and paracetamol-containing drugs by 8%. Among healthy men born in 1931 ASA intake constituted 80% of the total anti-inflammatory and analgesic drug intake. An analysis of the amount and type of these drugs sold within the region (expressed in defined daily doses) revealed that pure ASA-containing drugs constituted 17% of the total, paracetamol 12% and NSAID 36%. Various combinations of analgesics constituted 35% of the total amount sold (Figure 1).

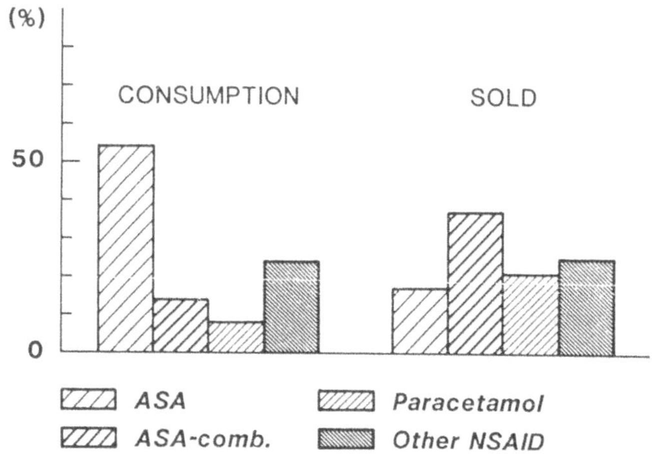

Figure 1 Distribution of consumed and sold anti-inflammatory and analgesic drugs among pure acetylsalicylic acid, combinations of acetylsalicylic acid and other compounds, paracetamol and other non-steroidal anti-inflammatory drugs. Consumption is expressed as a percentage of the total number of patients, and the selling figure as a percentage of total defined daily doses.

IV. DISCUSSION

In the present study it was demonstrated that if investigated with special emphasis the intake of anti-inflammatory and analgesic drugs is high among patients with upper gastrointestinal bleeding but also in a control group. The increase in the routine patient records from 1981 to 1983-84 is probably due to interest in the subject evoked among residents at the department. Whether there is a difference in the frequency between bleeders and non-bleeders cannot be evaluated from the present study. However, the present study clearly shows that the frequency of drug consumption found is very much influenced by the investigative method used. A retrospective analysis is clearly inadequate with a large number of false negative answers. It is our impression that many patients deny intake of acetylsalicylic acid-containing drugs of this type because they do not consider them as medical drugs. The indications for drug intake are in many of these cases not related to the pharmacological effects of the drugs, but instead may be due to habit only, or a vague feeling that the drug induces well-being in general. In our study the list of drug trade names increased the number of consumers significantly (Figure 1). We believe that similar difficulties may exist when other types of drug intake are investigated. In addition, other difficulties are likely to prevent true figures on consumption among patients of agents not fully accepted by society, e.g. alcohol.

It was demonstrated that the drugs most frequently used among patients and healthy controls are acetylsalicylic acid-containing drugs, which in Sweden are freely available without prescription. It should be noted that in Figure 1 the sold quantities are expressed as defined daily doses. For ASA this is 3 g daily, or six tablets of the most often used brands. Most patients in our study had a daily intake of less than 3 g. If this reflects the intake habits of the population of Malmö, which is very likely to be the case, it means that the quantities of ASA sold are distributed to a proportionally larger fraction of the population than is the case with other drugs requiring a doctor's prescription. For other NSAIDs except paracetamol, the defined daily doses are probably closer to the daily intake. However, with this reservation in mind we feel that, at least during the study period, there was an overconsumption of pure ASA as compared to other NSAIDs among patients with upper gastrointestinal bleeding. The consumption of non-ASA drugs was found to be about equal to the frequency expected from the quantities sold. In other words, we found no over-representation of NSAID intake among the patients with acute gastrointestinal bleeding. This is probably due to the fact that these drugs are available only after prescription, and the result thus reflects a restrictive and careful attitude among the prescribing physicians. The fact that the gastrointestinal side-effects of anti-inflammatory and analgesic drugs were being debated in the medical community at the time of the present study might have influenced the results obtained.

REFERENCES

1. Vane, JR (1971). Inhibition of prostaglandin synthesis of a mechanism of action for aspirin-like drugs. Nature New Biol, 231, 232
2. Lövgren, O and Allander, E (1964). Side-effects of indomethacin. Br Med J, 1, 118
3. Langman, MJS (1970). Epidemiological evidence for the association of aspirin and acute gastrointestinal bleeding. Gut, 11, 627
4. Kivilaakso, E and Silen, W (1979). Pathogenesis of experimental gastric-mucosal injury. N Engl J Med, 301, 364
5. Lanza, FL, Royer, GL and Nelson, RS (1980). Endoscopic evaluation of the effects of aspirin, buffered aspirin, and enteric-coated aspirin on gastric and duodenal mucosa. N Engl J Med, 303, 136
6. Caruso, I and Bianchi Porro, G (1980). Gastroscopic evaluation of anti-inflammatory agents. Br Med J, 280, 75
7. Colton, DG, Callison, DA and Dajani, EZ (1979). Effects of a prostaglandin E_1 derivative, SC-29333, and aspirin on gastric ionic fluxes and potential difference in dogs. J Pharmacol Exp Ther, 210, 283
8. Bolton, JP and Cohen, M (1979). Effect of 16, 16-dimethyl prostaglandin E_2

on the gastric mucosal barrier. Gut, 20, 513

9. Johansson, C, Kollberg, B, Nordemar, R, Samuelson, K and Bergström, S (1980). Protective effect of prostaglandin E_2 in the gastrointestinal tract during indomethacin treatment of rheumatic diseases. Gastroenterology, 78, 479

10. Cohe, MM, McCready, DR, Clark, L and Sevelius, H. Protection against aspirin-induced antral and duodenal damage with enprostil. A double-blind endoscopic study. Gastroenterology, 88, 382

11. Ross, IN and Turnberg, LA (1983). Studies of the "mucus-bicarbonate" barrier on rat fundic mucosa: the effects of luminal pH and a stable prostaglandin analogue. Gut, 24, 1030

12. Miller, TA (1983). Protective effects of prostaglandins against gastric mucosal damage: current knowledge and proposed mechanisms. Am J Physiol, 245, G601

13. Johansson, C, Aly, A, Befrits, R, Smedfors, B and Uribe, A (1985). Protection of the gastroduodenal mucosa by prostaglandins. In: Johansson, C et al (eds), Frontiers in Gastroduodenal Disease, vol. 20, suppl. 110. Scand J Gastroenterol, 41

14. Levy, M (1974). Aspirin use in patients with major upper gastrointestinal bleeding and peptic-ulcer disease. N Engl J Med, 290, 1158

15. Coggon, D, Langman, MJS and Spiegelhalter, D (1982). Aspirin, paracetamol, and haematemesis and melaena. Gut, 23, 340

Abbreviations used: AR(s), adverse reaction(s); ADR(s), adverse drug reaction(s); NSAID(s), non-steroid anti-inflammatory drug(s)

INDEX

INDEX

INDEX

GPSR Compliance

The European Union's (EU) General Product Safety Regulation (GPSR) is a set of rules that requires consumer products to be safe and our obligations to ensure this.

If you have any concerns about our products, you can contact us on ProductSafety@springernature.com

In case Publisher is established outside the EU, the EU authorized representative is:

Springer Nature Customer Service Center GmbH
Europaplatz 3
69115 Heidelberg, Germany

Batch number: 10607220

Printed by Printforce, the Netherlands